# Essential Urology

Melanie D'Souza

1993

# Essential Urology

**Nigel Bullock** MD, FRCS
Consultant Urologist, Addenbrooke's Hospital,
Cambridge and Associate Lecturer,
University of Cambridge

**Gary Sibley** DM, MCh, FRCS
Clinical Lecturer in Urology,
University of Cambridge

PAEDIATRIC UROLOGY BY
**Robert Whitaker** MD, MChir, FRCS
Consultant Urologist, Addenbrooke's Hospital,
Cambridge and Associate Lecturer,
University of Cambridge

*Illustrations by Peter Cox* MMAA

CHURCHILL LIVINGSTONE
EDINBURGH LONDON MELBOURNE AND NEW YORK 1989

CHURCHILL LIVINGSTONE
Medical Division of Longman Group UK Limited

Distributed in the United States of America by
Churchill Livingstone Inc., 1560 Broadway, New
York, N.Y. 10036, and by associated companies,
branches and representatives throughout the world.

First published 1989
Reprinted 1991

ISBN 0-443-03841-4

British Library Cataloguing in Publication Data
Bullock, Nigel
  Essential urology.
  1. Man. Urinary tract. Diagnosis & therapy
  I. Sibley, Gary II, Whitaker, Robert H.
  616.6

Library of Congress Cataloging in Publication Data
Bullock, Nigel.
     Essential urology/Nigel Bullock, Gary Sibley, with a
contribution by Robert Whitaker: illustrations by
Peter Cox.
     p.    cm.
  Bibliography: p.
  Includes index.
  ISBN 0-443-03841-4
  1. Genitourinary organs—Diseases.  2. Urology.
I. Sibley, Gary.
II. Whitaker, R. H. (Robert H.)  III. Title.
  [DNLM: 1. Urologic Diseases.
WJ 100 B938e]
RC871.B85 1989
616.6—dc19
DNLM/DLC                                        88–30225

Produced by Longman Singapore Publishers (Pte) Ltd.
Printed in Singapore

# Preface

Urology is a rapidly expanding specialty. New diagnostic and therapeutic techniques are constantly being added to the surgeon's armamentarium and many fundamental changes have occurred over the last 10 years. These new techniques have allowed us to diagnose and treat diseases which were hitherto poorly understood and to introduce new, safer methods of investigation and treatment for common urological problems.

It is all too easy, however, for clinicians and students to be left behind by this rapid progress. This book, therefore, is intended primarily for medical students, to aid them in grasping the fundamental concepts behind current urological practice. It is hoped that nurses and surgical trainees will also find useful practical hints. At the same time, we have endeavoured to give a flavour of some of the new and exciting developments in urology that have taken place in recent years.

This book makes no attempt to produce a comprehensive catalogue of all known urological diseases. Instead, we have endeavoured as far as possible to concentrate on a practical approach to patient management, rather than listing urological diseases by anatomical regions.

Whilst there can be no substitute for medical students talking to and examining patients, we believe that it is important to obtain a grasp of how to approach the patient with urological symptoms. This is particularly important now that a bewildering array of new and sophisticated investigative measures are available. Our aim is to encourage students, when faced with a patient with urological symptoms, to develop a sensible, balanced approach to patient management by concentrating on the basics of clinical medicine — the history, examination, investigations and appropriate treatment options. By concentrating on these factors, we hope to encourage the development of that indefinable quality possessed by the best surgeons, *clinical sense*.

The authors are indebted to their many clinical colleagues who have advised, encouraged and criticised sections of this book. We also acknowledge our debt to medical artist Mr Peter Cox who constructed meaningful drawings from our rough scribbles and whose contribution to the overall pattern of the book is invaluable. Finally, we must thank our wives and families for their forbearance whilst we spent endless hours sitting in front of our word processors.

Cambridge, 1989                                                          K.N.B.
                                                                         G.N.A.S.
                                                                         R.H.W.

# Contents

# Contents

# 1

# Structure and function of the upper urinary tract

## EMBRYOLOGY

The primitive kidney in lower vertebrates is known as the pronephros. Although this structure exists in the human embryo, it cannot be identified as a separate organ. The mesonephros, however, arises after 4–5 weeks' gestation from the intermediate cell mass of mesoderm in the upper thoracic region (Fig. 1.1). Vesicular spaces appear within the mesonephros and elongate transversely; the medial end of each space expands to resemble a Bowman's capsule (*internal glomerulus*) whilst the lateral end fuses with the rudimentary pronephric duct to form the mesonephric duct. This entire structure bulges into the abdominal cavity to form the *urogenital fold*.

After 6 weeks, the more cranial tubules of the mesonephros begin to degenerate and this process proceeds in a caudal direction so that only the most cranial and caudal tubules persist. In the fully-formed fetus these form the paradidymis/paraoophoron and the vasa efferentia of the testis, respec-

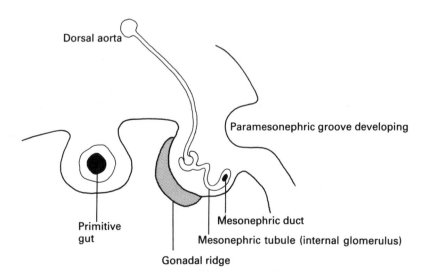

**Fig. 1.1** Development of the mesonephros

1

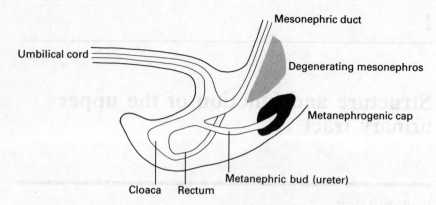

**Fig. 1.2** Development of kidney and ureter from metanephric blastema and bud

tively. At about the same time, a bud appears from the dorsal aspect of the lower end of the mesonephric duct, just above the cloaca. This grows dorsally and then turns caudally, to become the metanephric (*ureteric*) bud (Fig. 1.2).

A condensation of mesoderm (the *metanephrogenic cap*) appears at the tip of the ureteric bud in continuity with the lower part of the degenerating mesonephros; this condensation will become the parenchyma of the kidney. As the embryo develops further, the metanephrogenic cap moves caudally with its metanephric duct, partly as a result of continuing growth and partly because of unfolding of the embryo. The developing metanephros assumes a lobulated appearance (*fetal lobulation*) which may persist in the fully-developed adult kidney.

At its lower end, the developing ureter separates itself from the meso-nephric duct by differential growth to enter separately into the cloaca. At its upper end, the ureteric bud branches as it grows to form major and minor calyces with the final, fine branches forming the collecting tubules. The metanephrogenic cap develops into the renal parenchyma and the proximal portion of the nephrons. Numerous congenital anomalies may arise during the development of ureter and kidney and these are described in Chapter 5.

## THE KIDNEY

### Macroscopic anatomy

The kidneys are slightly lobulated organs approximately 11 cm long, 6 cm wide and 3 cm thick, weighing 135–150 g in adults. They lie on the posterior abdominal wall, with the right kidney normally slightly lower due to displacement by the liver (Fig. 1.3). For this reason, the lower pole of the right kidney may be palpable in a thin patient.

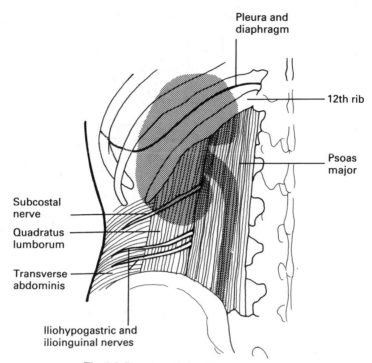

**Fig. 1.3** Posterior relationships of the kidney

Anteriorly (Fig. 1.4), the kidneys are covered by the peritoneum and the contents of the abdominal cavity. The adrenal glands lie superomedially on the upper pole of each kidney. The medial border of the kidney forms the hilum. This contains, from front to back, the renal vein, renal artery and renal pelvis. There is usually a posterior branch of the artery lying behind the renal pelvis which is important clinically in exposure of the renal pelvis from behind for stone removal. The hila of the kidneys lie at the level of $L_1$ (the *transpyloric plane of Addison*) and also contain nerves (mainly vaso-motor) and lymphatics.

The pelvis of the kidney divides within the hilum into two or three major calyces which, in turn, divide into a number of minor calyces. Each minor calyx is indented by a medullary pyramid onto which drain the collecting ducts. The kidney itself is ensheathed by a thin fatty envelope (perirenal fat) which extends into the hilum medially to surround the major calyces.

The adventitial tissue around the perirenal fat is condensed into a layer of perirenal fascia (*Gerota's fascia*). The anterior and posterior layers of this fascia fuse lateral to the kidney and blend medially with the fascia over the aorta and inferior vena cava; the fusion medially explains why perirenal collections of fluid do not cross the midline. They do, however, track down around the upper ureter, since the perirenal fascia is incomplete inferiorly.

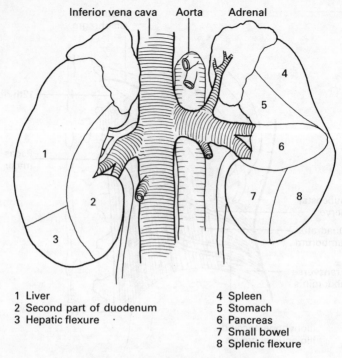

Inferior vena cava    Aorta    Adrenal

1 Liver
2 Second part of duodenum
3 Hepatic flexure
4 Spleen
5 Stomach
6 Pancreas
7 Small bowel
8 Splenic flexure

**Fig. 1.4** Anterior relationships of the kidneys

Although the renal fascia encloses the adrenal glands, these lie in a separate compartment from the kidneys and can, therefore, be preserved when a kidney is removed.

Blood supply to the kidney comes from the renal arteries, arising directly from the aorta on either side just below the superior mesenteric artery. The renal arteries give off twigs to the adrenal glands and upper ureter before dividing into lobar and interlobar arteries. These interlobar arteries divide into arcuate arteries which send branches into the renal medulla (interlobular arteries) and to the glomeruli (glomerular arteries). Aberrant renal arteries are common, usually arising directly from the aorta and penetrating the renal substance without entering the hilum: they usually supply the upper or lower pole of the kidney.

Venous drainage tends to be the reverse of this situation. However, the arterial supply to each lobe of the kidney does not communicate with that to its neighbouring lobe. As a result, segmental infarction of the kidney occurs when an interlobar or lobar artery is occluded. Venous drainage is not strictly segmental and shows some overlap between anatomical lobes of the kidney.

The left renal vein crosses in front of the aorta, receiving gonadal, lumbar and adrenal veins before entering the inferior vena cava. The right renal vein is shorter, drains directly into the vena cava and is not normally joined by a gonadal vein.

## Histology

Each kidney is packed with approximately 1 million nephrons (Fig. 1.5). The nephron consists of a Malpighian corpuscle in the renal cortex and a tubular system which delivers the urine formed by glomerular filtration to the collecting tubules. The Malpighian corpuscle is comprised of a tuft of blood vessels (the *glomerulus*) lying in the cup of a glomerular (*Bowman's*) capsule.

The glomerulus is a tuft of capillaries fed and drained by an afferent and efferent arteriole. The glomerular capsule is separated from the glomerular capillaries by a thin layer of flattened epithelial cells across which filtration takes place.

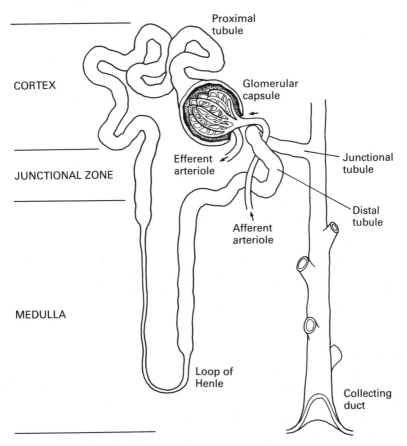

**Fig. 1.5** Diagrammatic representation of a nephron

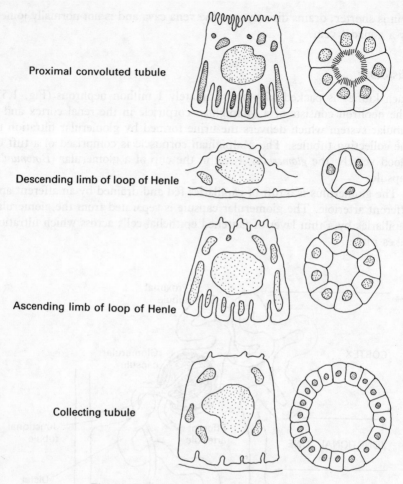

Proximal convoluted tubule

Descending limb of loop of Henle

Ascending limb of loop of Henle

Collecting tubule

Fig. 1.6 Epithelial characteristics of the nephron

The filtrate of plasma is then passed through a tubular system where it undergoes substantial modification by reabsorption and secretion, passing in turn through a proximal convoluted tubule, a U-shaped loop of Henle which dips into the renal medulla, a distal convoluted tubule, a junctional tubule and, finally, a collecting tubule (Fig. 1.6). The collecting tubules combine to form larger collecting ducts (*ducts of Bellini*) which open onto the tips of the renal pyramids.

The efferent glomerular arterioles continue after leaving Bowman's capsule as intertubular arteries which supply the distal and proximal tubules and send off branches deep into the medulla to supply the loop of Henle (*vasa recta*). This anatomical arrangement results in relatively concentrated blood coming into close contact with dilute urine in the renal medulla and forms the basis of the renal concentrating mechanism.

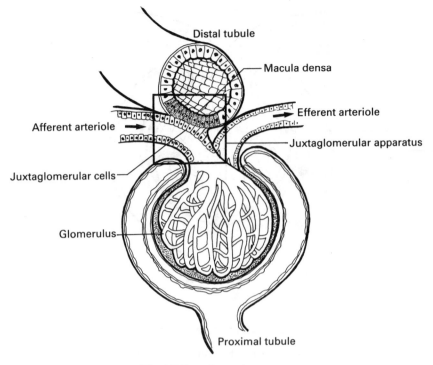

**Fig. 1.7** Juxtaglomerular apparatus

The distal convoluted tubule of each nephron lies close to its originating glomerulus, sited between the afferent and efferent glomerular arterioles. At this point, the cells in the media of the arterioles are atypical, forming a *juxtaglomerular apparatus* (Fig. 1.7) in combination with the densely packed distal tubular cells (*macula densa*). These atypical arterial cells contain secretory granules and this complex structure plays an important role in the regulation of blood pressure via the renin–angiotensin system.

## Physiology

The main functions of the kidney are excretion of waste products, maintenance of fluid, acid–base and electrolyte balance and the production of hormones. The functional unit of the kidney is the *nephron*.

### The function of individual components of the nephron

*Renal blood flow.* Between 20 and 25% of the cardiac output passes through the kidneys each minute, resulting in a renal blood flow of 300–400 ml/100 g of kidney/min (650 ml/min per kidney). The renal vasculature has very little resting tone, so that the normal blood flow

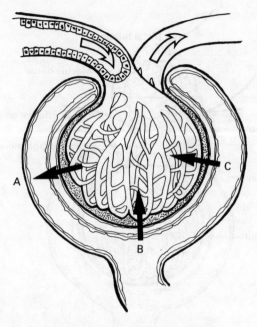

A   Glomerular blood pressure (60 mmHg)

B   Osmotic pressure of plasma proteins (32 mmHg)

C   Bowman's capsule pressure (18 mmHg)

NET FILTRATION PRESSURE   = A − (B + C)
                          = 10 mmHg

**Fig. 1.8** Filtration pressures in the glomerulus

through the kidneys is 80% of its maximal levels; in comparison, skeletal muscle has only 3% of its maximal blood flow when at rest.

Although overall oxygen consumption by the kidneys is high, the extraction rate of oxygen is low and this extraction rate does not change with alterations in renal blood flow. The renal blood pressure also remains remarkably constant despite profound changes in systemic blood pressure. This phenomenon is known as *autoregulation* and is brought about by changes in pre-glomerular vascular resistance. The underlying mechanism for this is thought to be the intrinsic myogenic tone of the renal blood vessels aided by prostaglandin release; autoregulation is not mediated by the renal sympathetic nerves.

*Glomerular filtration.* A total of 170–180 litres of plasma per day are filtered by the glomeruli at an overall rate of 125 ml/min (Fig. 1.8). The fluid in Bowman's capsule is, strictly, an ultrafiltrate of plasma. The glomerular membrane is impermeable to molecules larger than 4 nm diameter; this corresponds to a molecular weight of approximately 70 000. This large volume of filtrate is passed on to the tubular system of the nephron, where it undergoes substantial modification by reabsorption and secretion.

*Proximal tubular function.* The proximal tubule reduces the volume of glomerular filtrate by 75–80%. There is active reabsorption of glucose, phosphate, sodium, chloride, bicarbonate and potassium. Glucose is reabsorbed entirely from the proximal tubules unless the glucose load in the urine exceeds the tubular capacity for its absorption. Eighty per cent of the filtered sodium and 90% of bicarbonate are reabsorbed from the proximal tubules, sodium being pumped actively via $Na^+$–$H^+$ and $Na^+$–$K^+$ pumps. The filtrate in the proximal tubules, however, remains isosmotic throughout due to the simultaneous passive reabsorption of water and urea. Sulphates, amino acids and low molecular weight proteins are also reabsorbed, as is virtually all the filtered potassium.

*Loop of Henle function.* Sodium, chloride and water are reabsorbed passively from the loop of Henle. Water is reabsorbed from the more proximal part (descending limb) together with sodium, whilst the distal part (ascending limb) is impermeable to water but allows active sodium reabsorption. This selective reabsorption of sodium and water results in the development of a concentration gradient in the renal medulla and this is important in maintaining water balance. Diuretics which work on the loop of Henle (e.g frusemide) do so by inhibiting chloride and sodium reabsorption from the descending limb of the loop of Henle.

*Distal tubule and collecting duct function.* The filtrate is hypotonic as it leaves the loop of Henle and enters the distal tubules, where water reabsorption depends on the presence of antidiuretic hormone (ADH). Sodium is actively pumped out of the distal tubules, although reabsorption may be modified by aldosterone secretion.

The collecting tubules pass through the renal medulla. Reabsorption of water from the collecting tubules is independent of sodium reabsorption and is regulated by ADH secretion. Sodium is actively pumped out of the collecting tubules against a concentration gradient to maintain the hypertonicity of the renal medulla and this causes passive water reabsorption to a small degree. Large amounts of urea are also reabsorbed passively from the collecting tubules.

Many substances are secreted in the distal tubule. Potassium and hydrogen ions are secreted, as are many foreign agents (e.g drugs). Distal tubular secretion contributes 75% of the potassium content of urine; potassium secretion is intimately linked with sodium and hydrogen ion concentrations and is modified by aldosterone secretion. Hydrogen ion secretion occurs mostly in the distal tubules and occurs against a concentration gradient.

*Maintenance of water balance*

The osmolality of urine may vary from 50 mOsm/l to 1200 mOsm/l and

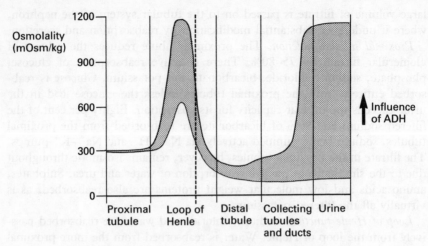

**Fig. 1.9** Osmolar concentrations at various points in the nephron

depends on the amount of water reabsorbed in the collecting tubules (Fig. 1.9). This, in turn, is dependent on the establishment of a corticomedullary osmotic gradient and on the permeability of the collecting ducts (governed by ADH).

Sodium and chloride are transported out of the ascending limb of the loop of Henle but are not accompanied by water. The sodium concentration in the ascending limb therefore falls progressively as the distal tubule is reached. The remainder of the loop of Henle remains in osmotic equilibrium with the renal interstitium.

As isosmolar filtrate reaches the bottom of the loop of Henle, the contents of the descending limb become more concentrated as a result of being 'pushed' into the hairpin bend before the ascending limb. This concentration is further increased by active sodium reabsorption in the ascending limb. This establishes an osmolar gradient in the renal medulla which can only be maintained if the medullary blood flow (in the vasa recta) is relatively low (Fig. 1.10).

Any increase in medullary blood flow (e.g as a result of haemodilution or volume expansion) results in dissipation of medullary osmolality, decreased water reabsorption and the production of large quantities of dilute urine. Dehydration, in contrast, results in release of ADH which increases the permeability of the distal nephron to water, resulting in increased water reabsorption.

Antidiuretic hormone (ADH) is released from the posterior lobe of the pituitary gland in response to raised plasma osmotic pressure, decreased plasma volume and afferent impulses from higher centres in the brain (Fig. 1.11).

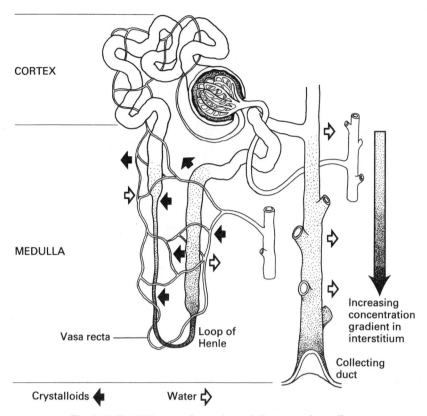

CORTEX

MEDULLA

Vasa recta —— Loop of Henle

Increasing concentration gradient in interstitium

Collecting duct

Crystalloids ◄    Water ⇨

**Fig. 1.10** Establishment of a corticomedullary osmotic gradient

The release of ADH is triggered by feedback from *osmoreceptors* close to the supraoptic nucleus which respond to sodium and chloride concentrations in the plasma. In addition, there are also *volume receptors* in the atria and great veins, supplied by the vagus nerve.

## Maintenance of acid–base balance

The kidney cannot excrete urine of pH less than 4.5. Acid–base balance is maintained by a complex series of buffer systems. In the proximal tubules, the predominant buffer system is dependent on $HCO_3^-/H_2CO_3$ whilst, in the distal tubules, the predominant buffer is $HPO_4^{2-}/H_2PO_4^-$. The weakest of the important buffers is the $NH_4^+$ system.

The phosphate buffer system is the most important during normal renal function. The $NH_4^+$ system, however, has the advantage that it allows the excretion of acid without the loss of metallic cations such as $Na^+$.

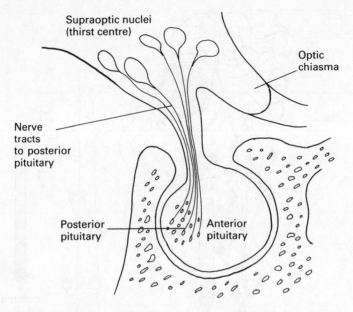

**Fig. 1.11** Hypothalamic control of ADH production

## Hormone production by the kidney

*Erythropoietin.* Erythropoietin is produced by the kidney in response to hypoxia, vasoconstriction, high circulating levels of the products of red cell destruction and a number of hormones. It is also produced by the plasma, liver and spleen. Erythropoietin results in an increase in nucleated red blood cells in haemopoietic tissue and a rise in red cell and reticulocyte counts in the peripheral blood.

*Prostaglandins.* The renal cortex and medulla can synthesise prostaglandins. The precursor for synthesis is phospholipid, which is converted to arachidonic acid and then to prostaglandins. The prostaglandins most commonly produced by the kidney are $PGI_2$, $PGE_2$, $PGF_2$ and thromboxane-$A_2$ ($TXA_2$). $PGE_2$ is a potent renal vasodilator, decreases sodium transport in the collecting tubules and antagonises ADH, whilst other prostaglandins have opposite actions. All the products of arachidonic acid breakdown are important in a number of disease states but their exact action during normal renal function is unclear.

*Renin–angiotensin.* Renin is released from juxtaglomerular cells in response to sympathetic nerve stimulation, a decrease in afferent arteriolar pressure and hyponatraemia. It acts upon circulating angiotensinogen to produce angiotensin I. This, in turn, is converted to circulating angiotensin II (Fig. 1.12).

Angiotensin II stimulates the zona glomerulosa of the adrenal gland to

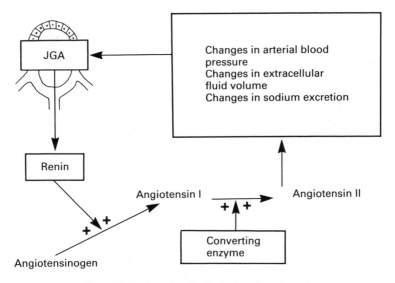

**Fig. 1.12** Renin-induced stimulation of angiotensin

produce aldosterone. This hormone increases sodium reabsorption by the kidneys as well as causing vasoconstriction and both these effects feed back to switch off renin secretion when homeostasis has been obtained.

*Other hormones.* Kallikrein is produced by the distal nephron and secreted in the urine. It acts upon other substrates to produce a variety of kinins. Some of these (e.g. bradykinin) are potent vasodilators and result in increased urine flow and sodium excretion. Other kinins may be involved in the activation of renin secreted by the juxtaglomerular cells.

The kidney is also involved intimately in calcium metabolism. 1α-hydroxylase is produced by the kidney as a result of low circulating levels of calcium. This enzyme converts 25-hydroxycholecalciferol into the potent metabolite 1,25-dihydroxycholecalciferol, which then stimulates calcium reabsorption from bone and decreases urinary calcium excretion.

## THE URETER AND RENAL PELVIS

### Macroscopic anatomy

The ureter is a hollow muscular tube, approximately 30 cm in length, commencing at the renal pelvis and finishing at its entry into the bladder. It can be divided, in anatomical terms, into abdominal, pelvic and intramural portions.

The abdominal portion lies on the psoas muscle posteriorly and is adherent to the posterior peritoneum anteriorly (an important point when trying to locate the ureter during surgery). It runs along the tips of the transverse processes of the lumbar vertebrae ($L_2$–$L_5$). The abdominal

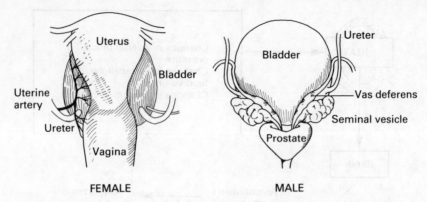

**Fig. 1.13** Relationships of the ureter at the bladder base (veiwed from behind)

ureter enters the pelvis as it crosses the bifurcation of the common iliac vessels. The right ureter is covered by duodenum in its upper part, lies just to the side of the inferior vena cava and is crossed obliquely by the gonadal vessels. The left ureter passes down behind the left colon and enters the pelvis behind the root of the sigmoid mesocolon.

The pelvic ureter runs along the lateral pelvic wall until it reaches the level of the ischial spine, where it turns medially and slightly upwards to enter the bladder wall. In the pelvis, the ureter runs just above the seminal vesicle in the male where it is crossed superficially by the vas deferens (Fig. 1.13).

In the female, the ureter lies below the broad ligament and uterine vessels just above the lateral vaginal fornix. It is at this point that large lower ureteric calculi can actually be felt (and removed) directly per vaginam. Upon entering the bladder wall, the ureter runs obliquely for 2 cm through the muscle before opening into the base of the bladder. This oblique intramural course provides a flutter-valve mechanism which prevents reflux of urine from bladder to kidneys. A knowledge of the course of the ureter is essential when assessing a plain abdominal film to look for stones in the kidney or ureter (Fig. 1.14).

Blood supply to the ureter is segmental, arising from aorta, renal, gonadal, internal iliac and inferior vesical arteries with corresponding venous drainage. The blood supply becomes more tenuous in the distal ureter and this has important implications in the healing of the lower ureter after surgery. Innervation is also segmental from the renal, aortic and hypogastric plexuses and is predominantly vasomotor or sensory.

### Histology

The ureter and renal pelvis consist of an inner layer of transitional epithelium with its supporting lamina propria, a thick muscle layer and an outer

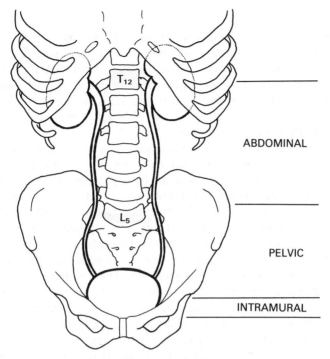

**Fig. 1.14** The course of the ureter

adventitial layer of connective tissue. In the renal pelvis, the muscle bundles lie in various directions, mostly in a circular orientation and are continuous with the muscle at the pelviureteric junction. There are morphologically and histochemically atypical muscle cells lying in the region of the minor calyces, deep to the more typical muscle layer. It has been suggested that these groups of cells have a 'pacemaker' function in initiating ureteric peristalsis.

The muscle bundles in the ureter do not spiral as is normally described but form a complex syncitium of interconnecting bundles. The longitudinal and circular layers are difficult to distinguish separately. However, in the upper ureter, the outer fibres do tend to be circular or oblique whilst the inner fibres are longitudinal. Lower down the ureter, outer longitudinal fibres become more apparent until, at the ureterovesical junction, the muscle is arranged in predominantly longitudinally orientated bundles.

The ureter has a rich innervation of autonomic nerve fibres. Most of these are vasomotor but a small number lie free between muscle bundles although there are no intramural ganglion cells in the ureter. The lower ureter does contain a few ganglion cells which are anatomically continuous with those in the bladder wall. It seems most likely that these nerves modify the contraction waves in the ureter although they do not initiate them.

## Physiology

Although the exact mechanism of ureteric peristalsis is still not clear, initiation of a ureteric contraction wave seems to take place in the minor calyces. The specialised muscle cells in the walls of the minor calyces probably initiate contraction waves which are propagated into the walls of the minor calyx and then into the renal pelvis. Each successive contraction is initiated by a different minor calyx although the same calyx does occasionally fire twice in succession.

The fact that pacemaker cells occur very close to the renal parenchyma suggests that propagation of the peristaltic wave is always away from the kidney, thus protecting the parenchyma from pressure rises. At high urine flow rates, each pacemaker firing initiates a contraction wave which is propagated down the ureter. At lower flow rates, not all impulses are propagated. This suggests that the pelviureteric junction acts as a 'gate' mechanism to regulate the rate of ureteric peristalsis.

Subsequent propagation down the ureter is dependent on the formation of a bolus of urine by myogenic contraction. The first bolus is formed just above the pelviureteric junction by strong circular contraction of the pelvis with relaxation of the pelviureteric junction distally. Longitudinal muscle contraction then pulls the ureter up over the formed bolus of urine and the process continues down the ureter. Peristalsis, therefore, is dependent on the ability of the circular muscle to coapt the ureteric walls. The pressure generated within a bolus is greater than that in the ureter or renal pelvis above it: coaption stops this pressure being transmitted to the kidney.

At the ureteric orifice, contraction of circular muscle pushes the bolus downwards whilst longitudinal muscle contraction allows the intramural ureter and ureteric orifice to open and urine to pass into the bladder. The oblique course of entry of the ureter through the bladder wall prevents reflux of urine from bladder to ureter during bladder filling or voiding.

# 2

# Structure and function of the lower urinary tract and male genital tract

## EMBRYOLOGY

In the early embryo, the lower urinary tract and the hindgut share a common origin from the cloaca, whose external surface is covered by the cloacal membrane. During the 4th week of gestation, the cloaca divides by caudal migration of the urorectal fold; this results in the formation of a urogenital sinus anteriorly and the rectum posteriorly.

The urogenital sinus receives the paired mesonephric (Wolffian), metanephric and Mullerian (paramesonephric) ducts; the Mullerian ducts fuse at their lower ends to form a single cavity (Fig. 2.1). The urogenital sinus communicates cranially with the allantois. The cranial portion of the sinus differentiates into the bladder, whilst the caudal portion develops into the urethra. As the sinus enlarges, the mesonephric and metanephric ducts migrate so that the metanephric ducts (ureters) come to empty into the bladder while the mesonephric ducts grow towards the proximal urethra.

By the 4th month, the fetal bladder begins to assume its adult shape with smooth muscle cells in its wall. The allantois becomes the *urachus* whose lumen is normally obliterated late in intrauterine life to become the *median umbilical ligament*.

Subsequent development of the caudal portion of the urogenital sinus and associated Mullerian and Wolffian ducts differs according to the sex of the fetus. In the male, this area forms the prostatic, membranous and penile parts of the urethra. The prostate gland develops by budding from the proximal urethra and the mesonephric ducts become the vasa deferentia. A dorsal diverticulum from each mesonephric duct develops into the seminal vesicle. The paramesonephric ducts degenerate, leaving a small vestige (the *utriculus masculinus*) in the posterior wall of the prostatic urethra.

In the female fetus, the caudal urogenital sinus develops into the urethra, vestibule and lower vagina. The fused paramesonephric ducts develop into the upper vagina, uterus and fallopian tubes whilst the mesonephric ducts largely degenerate. Numerous congenital anomalies may occur during this complicated sequence of development and these are outlined in Chapter 6.

17

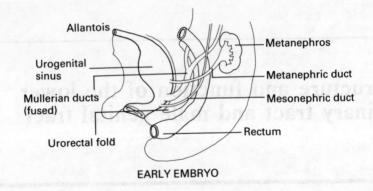

EARLY EMBRYO

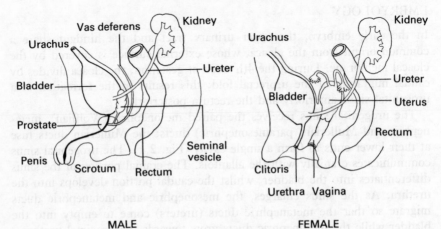

MALE                                    FEMALE

**Fig. 2.1** Embryological development of the bladder

The testis develops from the urogenital ridge in the early embryo. The cortex is derived from coelomic epithelium and the medulla from mesenchymal cells which proliferate to form sex cords. Primordial germ cells migrate into the sex cords from their site of origin in the yolk sac; the mesenchymal cells differentiate into the supporting Sertoli cells and the hormone-producing Leydig cells. The medial part of the primary sex cords develops into the rete testis which then connects with the mesonephric tubules to form the epididymis and feeds into the vas deferens (Fig. 2.2).

In late intrauterine life, the testis descends through the inguinal canal into the scrotum guided by a mesenchymal structure known as the *gubernaculum*. As the testis descends it takes with it a sleeve of peritoneum (*processus vaginalis*) which later forms the visceral and parietal layers of the tunica vaginalis. In the normal male fetus, this becomes separated from the peritoneal cavity around birth.

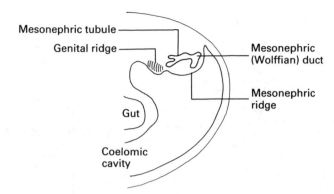

A. EARLY EMBRYONIC DEVELOPMENT

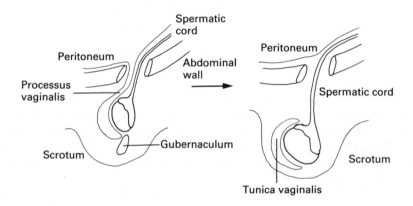

B. DESCENT OF THE TESTIS AND FORMATION OF THE TUNICA VAGINALIS

**Fig. 2.2** Embryology of the testis

## THE BLADDER

### Macroscopic anatomy

The bladder lies in the anterior half of the pelvis, bordered in front by the pubic bone and laterally by the diverging walls of the pelvis. The superior surface of the bladder is covered by peritoneum, which is reflected anteriorly onto the abdominal wall and peels upwards as the bladder rises out of the pelvis on filling. It is possible, therefore, to approach the anterior wall of the bladder through the retropubic space (*cave of Retzius*) without entering the peritoneal cavity.

In the male, the vasa deferentia and seminal vesicles lie against the bladder base (Fig. 2.3). Behind them lies the rectum, separated from the

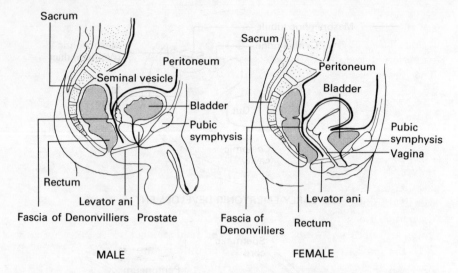

**Fig. 2.3** Anatomical relationships of the bladder

bladder by the *fascia of Denonvilliers*. This fascia is derived from the fused peritoneal layers of the rectovesical pouch; its tough nature produces a barrier to invasion of the rectum by tumours of the bladder or prostate and provides a plane of surgical cleavage between bladder and rectum. In the female, the vagina and cervix lie posteriorly, separated from the bladder by a thin layer of pelvic fascia.

Inferiorly, the prostate gland is attached to the bladder base in males and the urethra traverses the prostate before piercing the pelvic floor. In females, the bladder rests on the muscles of the pelvic floor (levator ani and coccygeus) and the urethra pierces the muscles anteriorly.

Blood supply to the bladder is from the anterior branch of the internal iliac artery via two main vessels, the superior and inferior vesical arteries. Venous drainage is to the internal iliac veins. Lymphatic drainage of the bladder is along the vesical blood vessels to internal iliac nodes and thence to para-aortic nodes.

## Histology

The ureters enter the posterior wall of the bladder near its base and run obliquely through the muscle and mucosal layers for 1.5–2 cm, terminating at the ureteric orifices. A prominent transverse ridge (the *interureteric bar*) runs between the ureteric orifices. The triangular area bounded by the ureteric orifices and the internal urethral meatus is known as the *trigone*. The trigone is relatively fixed and, unlike the remainder of the bladder, undergoes little change in size during bladder filling.

The remainder of the bladder is highly distensible and its wall is made up of a network of smooth muscle bundles (*detrusor muscle*). These bundles are interlaced throughout the bladder wall and not arranged in discrete layers. The detrusor muscle is innervated chiefly by cholinergic parasympathetic nerves, although a few adrenergic sympathetic nerves are present. The lumen of the bladder is lined by *transitional epithelium* supported by a layer of loose subepithelial connective tissue.

The anatomical nature of the bladder neck (proximal) sphincter is poorly understood and differs between the sexes. In the male, there is a circular collar of smooth muscle at the bladder neck which merges distally with the prostatic capsule and is richly innervated by noradrenergic sympathetic nerves. These nerves instigate contraction of the bladder neck during ejaculation to prevent retrograde passage of semen into the bladder. The role of this muscle in maintaining continence is less clear and it seems likely that other mechanisms such as the presence of circularly orientated elastic fibres are more important in keeping the bladder neck closed at rest.

In the female there is no such circular muscle ring. Instead, the smooth muscle bundles run in a longitudinal or oblique direction into the urethral wall and are innervated by cholinergic nerves. Despite the apparent absence of a proximal sphincter in women, the bladder neck remains closed at rest. It seems likely that circular elastic fibres and the valvular effect of the vascular urethral mucosa are involved in the closure of the bladder neck in women.


## THE URETHRA

### The male urethra and distal sphincter mechanism

The male urethra is divided into prostatic, membranous and spongiose parts. It is lined by transitional epithelium proximally and by squamous epithelium near the external meatus (*navicular fossa*).

The *prostatic urethra* is 3–4 cm long and receives the prostatic ducts on its posterior surface. A prominence on its posterior wall (the *verumontanum*) near the apex of the prostate provides an important landmark in transurethral prostatic surgery. Prostatic resection kept proximal to the verumontanum avoids injury to the sphincter mechanism in the adjacent membranous urethra. The ejaculatory ducts open on either side of the verumontanum and the utriculus masculinus opens on its apex.

The *membranous urethra* is the site of sphincteric activity in the male urethra. It is about 2 cm in length and extends from the apex of the prostate through the levator ani muscle to the bulb of the penis.

The *spongiose urethra* is surrounded by the corpus spongiosum, part of the erectile tissue of the penis, which expands distally to form the glans penis. The spongiose urethra receives the ducts of numerous glands including those of the paired Cowper's glands. Its proximal part is surrounded by the bulbospongiosus muscle and is commonly known as the *bulb of the urethra.* Contraction of the bulbospongiosus muscle assists in emptying of the urethra at the end of voiding and aids emission of semen during ejaculation. Dorsal to the spongiose urethra lie the paired corpora cavernosa, the main erectile structures of the penis, which pass from the ischiopubic rami and converge to lie side by side extending just beyond the corona of the glans penis.

Sphincteric activity in the male urethra is traditionally attributed to a sphincter derived from fibres of the levator ani which surrounds the membranous urethra as it penetrates the pelvic floor. Recent anatomical studies, however, have shown that, although fibres from the levator ani form a periurethral sling, this does not constitute a complete muscle ring.

The main contribution to the distal sphincter mechanism is from muscle within the urethral wall itself. In addition to an inner layer of smooth muscle, the intrinsic urethral musculature has an outer circular layer of striated muscle fibres (the *rhabdosphincter*); these fibres are designed for prolonged tonic contraction (*slow-twitch fibres*). The rhabdosphincter is innervated by somatic nerves from $S_2$ and $S_3$.

Although the periurethral sling of pelvic floor muscle is not capable of sustained contraction, it can contract rapidly to constrict the urethra for short periods (*fast-twitch fibres*). This may contribute to continence during the sudden rises in intravesical pressure seen, for example, with coughing or straining. The distal sphincter mechanism exerts a higher closure pressure than the bladder neck and is a more potent sphincter in terms of maintaining continence.

## The female urethra and distal sphincter mechanism

The female urethra is approximately 4 cm long. It passes through the levator ani anterior to the vagina and its external meatus opens 2.5 cm behind the clitoris. It is lined by transitional epithelium proximally and by squamous epithelium nearer the external meatus. In some women, squamous epithelium extends along the entire length of the urethra to the bladder neck and sometimes even onto the trigone. Numerous mucus-secreting glands drain into the urethral lumen.

As in men, urethral closure in women is largely dependent on an intrinsic urethral sphincter. The urethral musculature consists of an inner longitudinal layer of smooth muscle and an outer, circular slow-twitch rhabdosphincter. The rhabdosphincter extends from bladder neck to external meatus but is most pronounced in the middle third of the urethra. The muscle is thickest anteriorly and is thinner posteriorly where it is separated from the vagina by only a thin layer of fascia. The periurethral muscle sling (*fast-twitch fibres*) derived from the levator ani provides closure against sudden episodes of high bladder pressure, as it does in men, but the rhabdosphincter is the main protection against incontinence.

## THE PHYSIOLOGY OF MICTURITION

### Peripheral innervation of the bladder, urethra and sphincters

The bladder and urethra function as a single complex unit for storage and expulsion of urine. These functions are controlled by somatic and autonomic nerves with complex central connections allowing voluntary control over micturition.

Sensory nerves from the bladder and urethra pass in the pelvic parasympathetic nerves ($S_2$–$S_4$) to the spinal cord. From there, fibres ascend in the lateral spinothalamic tracts to micturition centres in the pons and cerebral cortex (Fig. 2.4). However, sacral nerve blockade does not abolish bladder sensation completely because some sensory fibres accompany the sympathetic nerves to the hypogastric plexus.

Detrusor contractions are mediated by parasympathetic cholinergic nerves ($S_2$–$S_4$). These travel in the pelvic nerves (*nervi erigentes*) to the pelvic ganglia from where numerous fibres are distributed to the bladder. Sympathetic nerves ($T_{10}$–$L_2$) travel to the bladder via the hypogastric nerves and the pelvic plexus. They are largely vasomotor but some sympathetic fibres synapse with parasympathetic nerves in the pelvic ganglia and produce inhibition of detrusor contractions.

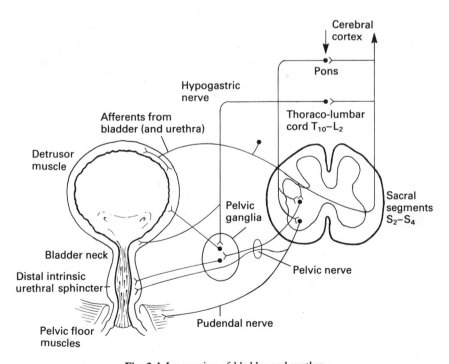

**Fig. 2.4** Innervation of bladder and urethra

The rhabdosphincter is innervated by somatic fibres from $S_2$ and $S_3$ which travel with autonomic fibres in the nervi erigentes; the autonomic fibres supply the inner smooth muscle of the urethra. The periurethral muscle sling is also supplied by somatic fibres from $S_2$ and $S_3$ but these fibres travel in the pudendal nerve.

## Central connections and the control of micturition

During storage of urine in the bladder, the detrusor is inhibited from contracting and its intrinsic properties allow filling with little or no rise in intravesical pressure. Continence is maintained by closure of the bladder neck and by the distal sphincter mechanism. For voiding to occur, contraction of the detrusor muscle must be accompanied by opening of the bladder neck and relaxation of the distal sphincter mechanism (Fig. 2.5).

The traditional belief that a simple spinal reflex arc controls micturition is no longer tenable. It is now recognised that a spino-pontine-spinal reflex involving a micturition centre in the pons is essential for co-ordinating detrusor contraction with sphincter relaxation. Influences from higher centres also impinge on the pontine micturition centre to bring this reflex under voluntary control.

The anterior portion of the frontal lobe is the cortical area primarily responsible for voluntary control of micturition. During bladder filling, afferent proprioceptive impulses from stretch receptors in the detrusor muscle pass via the posterior roots of $S_2$–$S_4$ and the lateral spinothalamic tracts to the frontal cortex. These impulses register the desire to void and this desire is suppressed by the frontal cortex until a suitable time and place for micturition have been selected. When it is appropriate to pass urine, there is cortical facilitation of the micturition reflex.

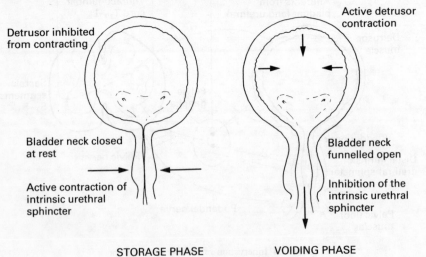

Detrusor inhibited from contracting

Active detrusor contraction

Bladder neck closed at rest

Bladder neck funnelled open

Active contraction of intrinsic urethral sphincter

Inhibition of the intrinsic urethral sphincter

STORAGE PHASE        VOIDING PHASE

**Fig. 2.5** The micturition cycle

During voluntary micturition, relaxation of the urethral sphincter precedes detrusor contraction and produces a marked fall in intra-urethral pressure. There is simultaneous relaxation of the pelvic floor muscles and funnelling of the bladder neck. Parasympathetic activity then initiates detrusor contraction and urine flow commences. The presence of urine in the urethra produces reflex facilitation of the detrusor which helps to sustain its contraction until the bladder is empty.

At the end of micturition, urine flow ceases, the intravesical pressure falls and the urethral sphincter voluntarily contracts. As the proximal urethra closes, its intrinsic muscle contracts in a retrograde fashion and 'milks' any trapped urine back into the bladder. Once these events are complete, inhibition of the micturition reflex is reapplied from higher centres so that the bladder is ready to enter the next filling cycle.

## THE TESTIS AND EPIDIDYMIS (Fig. 2.6)

The testis is responsible for production of spermatozoa which pass into the epididymis and along the vas deferens to be stored in the ampulla of the vas in preparation for ejaculation. The testis also produces the male sex hormone *testosterone* (see Ch. 24).

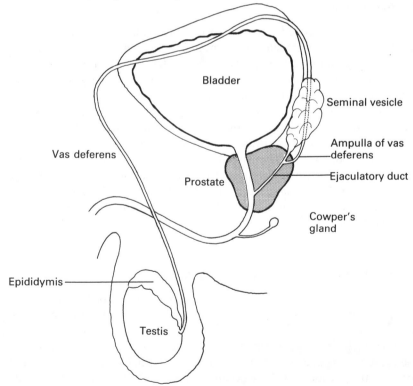

**Fig. 2.6** The male genital tract

## Macroscopic anatomy

The testis lies anteriorly in the scrotum and has the epididymis attached to its posterior surface. Each testis has a thick fibrous capsule (*tunica albuginea*) and is covered on its anterior and lateral surfaces by the tunica vaginalis; there is normally a small amount of serous fluid between the parietal and visceral layers of the tunica vaginalis.

Blood supply to the testis is via the testicular artery, which arises directly from the abdominal aorta, reflecting the embryological origin of the testis from the posterior abdominal wall. Venous drainage is via a venous plexus in the spermatic cord (*pampiniform plexus*) to the testicular vein. On the right, the testicular vein passes directly into the inferior vena cava, whilst on the left it drains into the left renal vein. Lymphatic drainage follows the arterial supply passing to para-aortic lymph nodes; there is no drainage of testicular lymph to inguinal nodes.

The epididymis consists of a head, body and tail applied to the back of the testis. The head of the epididymis is connected to the testis by the vasa efferentia whilst the tail gives rise to the vas deferens. Blood supply is from intrascrotal branches of the testicular artery.

## Histology (Fig. 2.7)

Each testis is composed of approximately 600 coiled seminiferous tubules. Each tubule has a basement membrane and contains several layers of developing germinal cells supported by Sertoli cells. The basal layer of germ cells consists of spermatogonia which divide to form primary spermatocytes. These undergo meiotic division to form secondary spermatocytes and these, in turn, divide to form spermatids which eventually mature into spermatozoa. Between the seminiferous tubules lie the interstitial (*Leydig*) cells which are responsible for testosterone production.

The head of the epididymis contains a number of coiled tubes (*lobules*) which receive spermatozoa from the testis via the vasa efferentia. The lobules merge into a single convoluted duct to form the body and tail of the epididymis and this duct expands near the tail of the epididymis to become the vas deferens.

## THE VAS DEFERENS AND SEMINAL VESICLE

The vas deferens is a small calibre muscular tube, approximately 45 cm long, which arises from the tail of the epididymis and passes upwards to traverse the scrotum and inguinal canal in the spermatic cord. It enters the pelvis via the internal inguinal ring and runs along the lateral pelvic wall before turning medially at the level of the ischial tuberosity towards the base of the bladder. Here it becomes sacculated and convoluted (*ampulla of the vas*) before joining the more laterally placed seminal vesicle to form

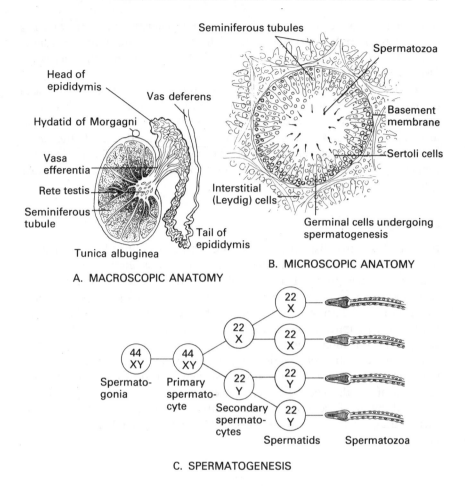

**Fig. 2.7** Structure of testes and the sequence of spermatogenesis

the ejaculatory duct. The ejaculatory duct pierces the prostate and opens into the urethra by the side of the verumontanum.

The seminal vesicle is a coiled, sacculated, muscular tube which lies extraperitoneally at the bladder base. Each vesicle can hold 1.5–2.5 ml of seminal fluid. This fluid makes up 80% of the volume of the ejaculate and contains nutrients (such as fructose) for the sperm together with enzymes that dissolve cervical mucus. Muscular contraction of the vas deferens and seminal vesicles occurs during ejaculation and emission of semen.

## THE PROSTATE

### Macroscopic anatomy

The prostate surrounds the urethra just below the bladder neck and its apex rests on the muscles of the pelvic floor. The majority of the prostate lies on the lateral and posterior aspects of the urethra; there is little prostatic tissue anteriorly. It is separated from the rectum by the fascia of Denonvilliers.

Arterial blood supply to the prostate comes from the inferior vesical artery and venous drainage is to an extracapsular plexus of veins. This plexus is joined by the dorsal vein of the penis and drains into the internal iliac vein. Some venous blood from the prostate passes directly to the valve-less prevertebral venous plexus of Batson and this might explain the propensity of prostatic carcinoma to spread at an early stage to the lumbar spine.

### Histology

In the embryo, five distinct prostatic lobes can be identified but this distinction is lost as the prostate develops. Embedded in a fibromuscular stroma there is an inner group of mucosal glands derived from endoderm (*central zone*) and an outer group of mesodermally-derived glands (*peripheral zone*). The glands of the central zone drain via short ducts into the urethra, whilst those of the peripheral zone drain into ducts which enter the urethral sinus close to the verumontanum (Fig. 2.8).

This subdivision is of practical importance because the majority of prostatic carcinomas arise in the peripheral zone whilst benign hypertrophy tends to affect the central zone. In benign hypertrophy, the prostate is moulded by its false capsule (the compressed peripheral zone) and by surrounding structures into the 'surgical' lobes (two lateral and one middle lobe).

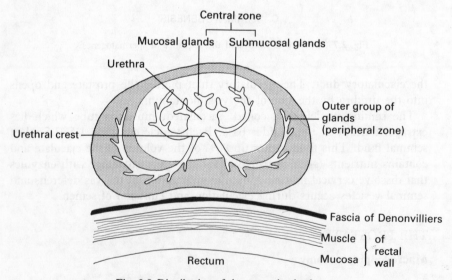

**Fig. 2.8** Distribution of the prostatic glands

## Physiology

Prostatic secretion is under the control of androgens and provides 10–20% of the volume of the ejaculate. Its precise function is poorly understood but certain substances contained in prostatic fluid (e.g. sialic acid) are thought to be important in penetration and fertilization of the ovum. Other constituents include prostaglandins and the enzyme acid phosphatase. Prostatic secretion also has antibacterial activity and this may help to prevent urinary infection in men.

# 3

# Urological history and examination

A well-taken history and thorough clinical examination are vital factors in the assessment of any urological patient. A few minutes spent taking a careful story and, above all, listening to what the patient has to say, are worth many hours of expensive investigations. Once a good history has been taken and a clinical examination performed, it usually becomes obvious in which direction further investigations should proceed.

When taking a history from a patient with a urological complaint, it is important to remember that many such patients are elderly with multi-system disease, many are taking drugs which may affect kidney or bladder function and that the general health of such patients may be poor. For these reasons, non-specific enquiries must be made about general health as well as asking questions specific to the presenting urological symptoms.

## HISTORY TAKING

### General information in urological patients

The occupation of the patient may be important, since some patients come into contact with carcinogens during their work. In particular, workers in the dye, rubber, cable or sewage industries are at risk of developing urothelial cancer as a result of occupational exposure to carcinogens. It may prove valuable in patients who have retired from work to determine whether they have ever been in such high-risk occupations at any time during their working lives because there is a long latent period (15–20 years) between exposure and the development of bladder cancer.

In women, a brief obstetric history is important, with particular reference to prolonged labour (resulting in lax perineal musculature), perineal tears during delivery and the number of Caesarean sections performed. A long history of pelvic inflammatory disease may be relevant in women with symptoms referred to the lower urinary tract. In addition, a full menstrual history is useful, especially if urinary symptoms appear to be related to a woman's periods. Also, it is important to prevent a woman from being exposed to the potential danger of X-rays during the early stages of pregnancy.

A full past medical history should be obtained routinely, since it is one factor in determining general fitness. However, it may reveal clues to the cause of urological symptoms. Periods of time spent in hot climates or bilharzial areas, a history of previous venereal disease or tuberculosis and past trauma or surgery to the urinary tract may all be relevant to the presenting complaint.

Smoking habits should be determined and it is always worth asking, if a patient does not smoke, whether he has smoked in the past and, if so, when he stopped. Components of cigarette smoke have been implicated in the production of urothelial tumours.

The possibility of allergies should always be borne in mind to avoid prescribing the patient drugs to which he or she is sensitive. Some allergic reactions can produce interstitial damage to the kidneys which may be relevant to the presenting symptoms. Occasionally, patients may be discovered to be asthmatic; such patients run a risk of developing acute bronchospasm after injection of intravenous contrast media. Similarly, a history of iodine allergy is significant if there is any chance of iodine-containing contrast media being administered to the patient during radiological investigations.

It is useful to enquire how well the patient sleeps. Whilst nocturia (waking at night to pass urine) is a common symptom of urological disease, a poor sleeper may relate that he has to void many times during the night. In fact, such patients void because they wake rather than wake to void and are often suffering from a sleep problem based on anxiety or depression rather than a primary urological problem.

Although some patients may interpret recent weight loss as a sign of malignant disease, it is not always so and is simply a useful indicator of general ill-health. Bowel function may be disturbed in urological patients and some symptoms such as pneumaturia or faeces in the urine suggest a primary bowel pathology which has also affected the urinary tract. A few elderly patients have concomitant large bowel neoplasms causing a change in bowel habit and it is a tragedy to ignore such symptoms whilst concentrating on a urological complaint.

### Review of specific systems

A full system enquiry should be undertaken as an assessment of general fitness. There are, however, certain generalised symptoms which may be associated with urological disease and specific questions should be asked about these (Table 3.1).

### Drug consumption

Many drugs may affect the urinary tract directly by actions on the kidney and bladder or indirectly by producing ureteric obstruction. Although most

**Table 3.1** Systemic symptoms associated with urological disease

Headaches and visual disturbances
Deafness and impairment of the sense of smell
Tremor, fits, cramps and pruritus
Sweating attacks, fever and rigors
Peripheral oedema, orthopnoea and dyspnoea
Chest pain and symptoms of peripheral vascular disease
Cough, haemoptysis and production of sputum
General malaise, anorexia, nausea and vomiting
Back pain and localised skeletal pain

of these are prescribed by medical practitioners, patients often take pro-
prietary preparations bought over the chemist's counter. Some of these preparations (e.g. cough linctuses) contain substances which affect the urinary
tract. Herbal remedies often contain dyes which may colour the urine (see
Fig. 3.1 for examples).

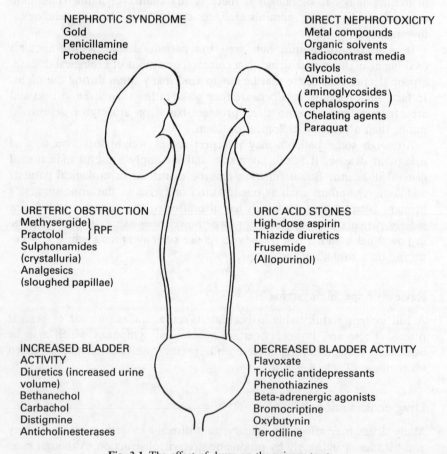

NEPHROTIC SYNDROME
Gold
Penicillamine
Probenecid

DIRECT NEPHROTOXICITY
Metal compounds
Organic solvents
Radiocontrast media
Glycols
Antibiotics
(aminoglycosides
cephalosporins)
Chelating agents
Paraquat

URETERIC OBSTRUCTION
Methysergide}
Practolol      }RPF
Sulphonamides
(crystalluria)
Analgesics
(sloughed papillae)

URIC ACID STONES
High-dose aspirin
Thiazide diuretics
Frusemide
(Allopurinol)

INCREASED BLADDER
ACTIVITY
Diuretics (increased urine
volume)
Bethanechol
Carbachol
Distigmine
Anticholinesterases

DECREASED BLADDER ACTIVITY
Flavoxate
Tricyclic antidepressants
Phenothiazines
Beta-adrenergic agonists
Bromocriptine
Oxybutynin
Terodiline

**Fig. 3.1** The effect of drugs on the urinary tract

## Voiding pattern

In determining how often patients void and how much urine is passed on each occasion, frequency/volume charts may be useful. The patient simply records, for a period of 1–2 weeks prior to assessment, the time of each void both by day and night and the voided volume on each occasion. The resulting figures give a useful indication of the incapacity the patient is experiencing from urinary symptoms but must be related to fluid intake over the same period. In the event of frequency of voiding being volunteered, it is useful to know if this is associated with urgency (an overwhelming desire to pass urine immediately), urge incontinence (wetting when voiding cannot be instituted quickly enough) or nocturia (frequent passage of urine during the night). Most important, however, is to determine how such symptoms differ from *what is normal for the patient*.

Patients with bladder outflow obstruction often need to strain to void. This is especially noticeable during the night or at the first void in the morning. This may be associated with *hesitancy* where the patient has to stand and wait for the urine flow to start, sometimes for several minutes. An uncontrollable and often painful desire to pass urine which results in little or no urine being voided is known as *strangury* and is often a feature of bladder or lower ureteric calculi.

Outflow obstruction usually results in a urinary stream of reduced force and increased duration. The stream may stop and start or may simply be a dribble. Typically, it is difficult for the patient to cut off the stream after voiding and *terminal dribbling* results. Dribbling may occur several minutes after cessation of voiding (*post-micturition dribbling*), usually as a result of trapping of urine in the urethra. Obstruction may also be associated with a sense of incomplete bladder emptying and the desire to return to the toilet shortly afterwards to void again (*pis-en-deux*). Hesitancy, a reduced urinary stream and terminal dribbling are the hallmarks of bladder outflow obstruction. Frequency, nocturia, urgency and urge incontinence may occur in the absence of outflow obstruction but are often seen in patients with obstruction and secondary bladder instability.

*Spraying or 'forking'* of the urinary stream suggests the possibility of a urethral or meatal stricture which is disrupting the 'rifling' effect of the normal urethra, although it may also be caused by stones or foreign bodies impacted in the distal urethra. Post-micturition dribbling is also common with such urethral lesions due to pooling of urine behind the stricture after voiding.

## Incontinence

Patients who wet themselves may do so for a number of reasons. The pattern of wetting often gives a clue to the underlying problem. *Stress incontinence* is usually seen in women with bladder neck or sphincter incompetence, although it may be seen in men after prostatectomy. *Urge incon-*

*tinence* has already been described and is usually caused by bladder (detrusor) instability. *Overflow incontinence* is usually seen in chronic retention of urine. It causes involuntary leakage at any time, although typically it is worse at night, often resulting in bed-wetting. One rare but special case is incontinence of urine both by day and night in girls which may be due to an ectopic ureter opening into the urethra or vagina (i.e. distal to the normal sphincter mechanism).

### Nature of the urine passed

The voided volume is of some importance and is best determined from a frequency/volume chart. Frequent passage of small volumes of urine suggests a functional or anatomical reduction in bladder capacity or an irritative lesion in the lower urinary tract.

It is helpful to know whether the urine is frothy, smelly, turbid or thick and what its colour is. The presence of calculi in the urine may be obvious to the patient and these may cause pain as they are passed. Bubbles of gas (*pneumaturia*) and faecal particles in the urine (*faecuria*) are an indication that there is a pathological connection between the bowel and the bladder. This is usually caused by bowel disease (diverticulitis, carcinoma of the colon, Crohn's disease) although rarely it may result from bladder carcinoma. The presence of gas alone in the urine may occasionally be the result of gas-fermenting organisms in the bladder; this is most likely to occur in the sugar-laden urine of diabetics.

The symptom of blood in the urine (*haematuria*) is dealt with elsewhere but it may be possible to determine the source of bleeding from the history. Bleeding occurring at the end of the stream, or even spontaneous bleeding from the urethra independent of voiding, suggests an origin in the bladder neck or urethra. Bleeding mixed throughout the stream may come from any source. Heavy bleeding from any source will result in the passage of clots and may cause *clot retention* but, if these clots are long, thin and worm-like, they are likely to have arisen in the upper urinary tract and have been shaped by passage down the ureter. The association of pain with the haematuria is important, since the bleeding caused by urothelial tumours is most commonly painless whilst painful haematuria is more suggestive of an inflammatory or calculous lesion.

With the current vogue for jogging and marathon-running, increasing numbers of patients are seen with haematuria after exertion. Such '*exercise haematuria*' does not normally last for more than a few hours after cessation of activity and, if it does, should alert the surgeon to the possibility of another cause and the need for further investigation. Very occasionally, a patient presents with red urine occurring only at night: whilst this should be fully investigated, it may be due simply to paroxysmal nocturnal haemoglobinuria. Beetroot and some drugs (e.g. pyridium, rifampicin, phenindione, phenolphthalein) may also colour the urine.

### Haemospermia (blood in the semen)

This is an unusual and alarming symptom. The first step is to establish that the blood is, in fact, in the semen of the male partner and not arising from the vagina of the female partner. Haemospermia may be confirmed by masturbation, or by ejaculation into a condom. The association of pain on ejaculation or testicular discomfort with haemospermia often suggests an inflammatory cause, usually in the prostate gland. Haemospermia in more elderly patients, however, should raise the possibility of a prostatic tumour.

### Pain

Pain is a common feature of urological disease and the nature of the pain may be useful in determining the site of origin. Whilst pain in the upper back has many causes, loin pain usually arises from the kidney. The patient often indicates this with a characteristic pressing of the hand into the loin (Fig. 3.2).

Ureteric pain normally radiates from the loin down towards the scrotum or labia, often extending into the genitalia and perineum. The pain of renal or ureteric distension is typically colicky in nature but is usually super-imposed on a constant background pain. Fixed renal pain tends to be constant and does not radiate to the groin. If the pain is severe, it is worth enquiring whether it doubles the patient up and induces a feeling of nausea or causes vomiting; such symptoms are typical of ureteric colic. The pain of ureteric colic is said by mothers who have experienced it to be worse than that of uterine contractions during childbirth.

Pain may radiate to the testicle from other sites (e.g. ureteric colic, lumbar disc disease, inguinal hernia pressing on the ilioinguinal nerve) or

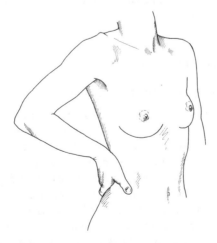

Fig. 3.2 The characteristic gesture of loin pain

the testicular pain may be the direct result of a lesion in the scrotum. Inflammatory conditions in the scrotum may produce pain in the lower abdomen or iliac fossae and this pain can radiate into the thighs. Lower abdominal and iliac fossa pain are often the first symptoms in torsion of the testis. The association of testicular, perineal, groin and back pain is very suggestive of inflammation in the prostate gland (*prostatitis*).

Pain on voiding is usually termed *dysuria*. Its causes are many but it often helps to determine whether the pain occurs before, during or after voiding. Post-voiding pain is very suggestive of a urethral origin.

Chest, back or bone pain may be a sign of bony metastatic spread from a primary tumour of the urinary tract, although there are many other causes of pain at these sites which are unrelated to urological problems.

### Testicular swelling

It is useful to know whether testicular swelling appeared suddenly or whether its onset was gradual. Sudden swelling is suggestive of an inflammatory condition or torsion of the testis, whilst slowly-progressive swelling is more often seen with cystic lesions or testicular tumours. An association with urinary symptoms may be important in infective disorders of the scrotum. A swelling in the scrotum which varies in size during the day is suggestive of an inguino-scrotal hernia (in adults) or a patent processus vaginalis (in children).

### Features specific to individual problems

In conditions such as impotence, incontinence and infertility, specific questions need to be asked to help in determining the cause of the problems. This disease-specific information can be found in the appropriate sections elsewhere in this volume.

## CLINICAL EXAMINATION

### General examination of the urological patient

The first general impression of the patient is important and may be gained simply by observation. It does not require specific training in medicine to determine whether a patient looks well, is in pain, seems anxious or depressed, has skeletal deformities or smells of urine.

Since many patients presenting to the urologist are elderly and generally unfit, a brief but careful examination of the cardiovascular, respiratory, alimentary, nervous and locomotor systems is essential. Examination should always include a recording of the patient's blood pressure.

Special attention should be paid to skin pigmentation, stature, body hair and fat distribution. The optic fundi should be examined if diabetes or hypertension are suspected. In patients with lower urinary tract symptoms, it is important to examine the spine and to assess the power, tone, sensation and reflexes in all the limbs. Sacral sensation and reflexes should also be tested, since these are good indicators of whether bladder innervation is intact.

### Examination of the abdomen

It goes without saying that the abdomen should be examined gently with warm hands in a warm room with the patient lying supine on a comfortable couch. After a visual inspection for any abnormal swellings, gentle palpation may reveal unsuspected abdominal tenderness. If this is sufficient to produce guarding, it is cruel to elicit rebound tenderness. It is far kinder to the patient, and just as useful to the surgeon, to percuss the abdomen gently as one would the chest. Any tenderness on gentle percussion is highly suggestive of peritoneal irritation.

Once areas of tenderness have been noted, deeper palpation may commence to detect intra-abdominal masses (Fig. 3.3). Most abdominal signs in urology are related either to enlarged kidneys or to a palpable bladder. An enlarged kidney may be felt anteriorly in the subcostal region on deep inspiration, although it should be remembered that, in thin patients, the lower pole of a normal right kidney is often palpable at the height of inspiration. Characteristically, a renal mass arises from the loin, is palpable bimanually and ballottable and moves with respiration. It has colon overlying it which is resonant to percussion. It is usually possible to 'get above' an enlarged kidney (in contrast to an enlarged spleen or liver).

Firm palpation in the loin may reveal tenderness in the costovertebral angle from a painful kidney. The notorious 'kidney punch' to elicit renal tenderness is an unnecessarily painful means of finding what can usually be elicited by more gentle palpation. It is useful to listen with a stethoscope

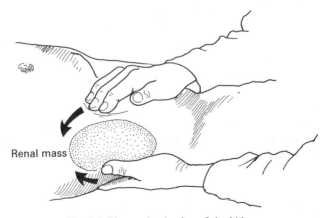

Renal mass

**Fig. 3.3** Bimanual palpation of the kidney

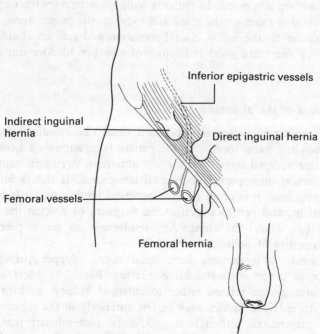

**Fig. 3.4** Inguinal and femoral hernia

both anteriorly above the umbilicus and in the loin for a vascular bruit which may be associated with renal artery stenosis or an arteriovenous malformation in the kidney.

An enlarged bladder may be palpable as a cystic mass arising from the pelvis. It is not, however, always palpable in more obese patients; here percussion may reveal suprapubic dullness suggestive of bladder enlargement. Percussion for an enlarged bladder should commence well above the umbilicus, progressing downwards from a resonant area into a dull one. Tenderness of a distended bladder helps to distinguish painful acute retention from the more insidious and generally painless chronic retention. It is worth bearing in mind that the bladder does not always rise symmetrically from the pelvis, so a mass arising above the pubis which is not in the midline may be an enlarged bladder. If a pelvic mass is an enlarged bladder, it will, of course, disappear when the bladder is catheterised and the urine drained from it.

The inguinal and femoral canals should be examined for the presence of hernias with the patient lying and standing. Hernias are usually made more obvious by asking the patient to cough (Fig. 3.4).

### Examination of the external genitalia

Each side of the scrotal sac should be carefully examined. A conscious effort must be made to examine each structure in turn (cord, vas deferens, epididymis and testis) for shape, size and consistency. Any swellings should, if possible, be related to these structures. It is useful, diagnostically, to describe scrotal swellings as inflammatory, solid or cystic.

If a swelling is present in the scrotal sac, the first step is to determine whether one can 'get above it'. If this is possible, the swelling is truly scrotal; if not, the swelling is inguino-scrotal and probably an inguinal hernia. Scrotal swellings should be transilluminated with a pen-torch in a darkened room; transillumination is the hallmark of fluid-filled scrotal lesions. If the swelling is not cystic, it is probably solid and likely to be a testicular tumour. Examination of the scrotum with the patient standing may unmask a varicocele which was not visible when the patient was supine. Typically, there are distended veins above the testis (usually on the left) which transmit a cough impulse and are described as 'a bag of worms'.

The penis, foreskin, glans and external urethral meatus should be examined carefully. If the patient is uncircumcised, the foreskin should be gently retracted to enable the glans and urethra to be seen. It is important in patients with a history of penile pain, erectile deformity or impotence to feel the shaft of the penis carefully for plaques of fibrosis (*Peyronie's disease*) and to inspect the frenulum for shortening or scarring.

## Rectal examination

Rectal examination forms a vital part of the urological assessment. In addition to allowing palpation of the prostate, it may detect a previously unsuspected rectal tumour; 70% of rectal tumours are within reach of the examining finger. Reassurance, explanation and the gentle insertion of a well-lubricated gloved examining finger are the essentials of successful rectal examination. The procedure is best performed with the patient in the left lateral position although the kneeling ('knee-elbow') position may be used.

The prostate gland should be assessed for size. The normal prostate weighs about 15 g and is the size of a chestnut. Any enlargement should be noted and an approximate estimate of size given. In the presence of retention of urine, the bladder often presses the prostate down towards the examining finger, giving a false impression of gross prostatic enlargement; a more reliable estimate of prostatic size is obtained after catheterisation of the bladder. If there is a clinical suspicion of bladder enlargement on abdominal examination, this can often be confirmed in men by bimanual assessment during rectal examination.

The contour and consistency of the prostate are important. A firm or hard gland should raise the suspicion of prostatic carcinoma, as should extension of the induration beyond the apparent confines of the gland. Loss of mobility of the rectal mucosa over the surface of the prostate may also be a sign of malignancy within the gland. Nodules in the prostate should suggest the possibility of carcinoma of the prostate although only 50% of prostatic nodules are, in fact, malignant.

Tenderness of the prostate with a feeling of 'bogginess' and oedema is suggestive of prostatic inflammation. Pressure on, or massage of, the prostate in this situation may give rise to *expressed prostatic secretions* which can be swabbed and sent for bacteriological or Chlamydial culture.

The seminal vesicles, if diseased, may be enlarged and palpable above the prostate but normal vesicles cannot generally be detected. Enlargement of the seminal vesicles is usually due to chronic inflammation (e.g tuberculosis) or local invasion by a bladder or prostatic tumour.

## Pelvic assessment in women

Vaginal examination is an important adjunct to rectal examination in women. The urethra and introitus should be inspected for abnormalities and atrophic changes. Any vaginal discharge should be swabbed for culture and, if possible, a cervical smear taken. A cystocele or rectocele may be obvious on inspection; asking the patient to cough may accentuate any prolapse and demonstrate stress incontinence. The uterus and vaginal fornices should be examined bimanually for masses and tenderness; a stone in the lower ureter may be palpable in a woman through the lateral vaginal fornix. Careful bimanual examination will usually confirm the nature and origin of an abdominal swelling arising from the pelvis.

## Sacral reflexes

Testing the innervation of the bladder is a technique which is poorly documented. Although loss of perianal sensation may be a useful indicator of bladder denervation when combined with neurological signs in the lower limbs, it is better to test the integrity of the sacral reflex arc formally (see Ch. 18).

# 4

# Investigation of urological symptoms

Although it is often possible to arrive at an accurate diagnosis from the clinical history and examination alone, a number of ancillary techniques are available to help in evaluating the urinary tract. Appropriate investigations will usually allow a diagnosis to be reached and management to be planned.

## LABORATORY INVESTIGATIONS

### Urine analysis

This is best performed on a mid-stream specimen of urine (MSU) to obtain a sample representative of bladder urine. After cleansing the external urethral meatus, the first 20 ml or so of urine (containing bacteria and cells from the urethra) are discarded before collecting the next part of the voided urine in a sterile container.

### Chemical tests

Simple analysis is carried out using 'dipstix', a strip coated with chemicals for measuring the urine pH and for detecting the presence of glucose, protein or blood; bilirubin, urobilinogen, ketones and nitrites can also be detected.

The urine pH varies between 4.5 and 8.0 but a persistently alkaline urine (pH > 8.0) suggests infection with urea-splitting organisms such as *Proteus mirabilis*. Very acid urine is typically found in uric acid stone formers and in aminoaciduria.

The amount of protein in the urine is normally less than 100 mg/24 h. Dipstix will only detect levels greater than 0.3 g/l. The presence of a small amount of protein in the urine may be innocent or may be caused by disorders such as glomerulonephritis, hypertension or infection. Whilst transient proteinuria is seen in some disorders (e.g. infection), only persistent proteinuria need be fully investigated.

Glycosuria usually indicates diabetes mellitus. This should be confirmed with a fasting blood sugar, since glycosuria may be found in the presence of a normal blood glucose (*renal glycosuria*); this is due either to an inherited defect which causes a low renal threshold for glucose or to certain tubular disorders.                                         *protein 300mg/litre*

The dipstix is a very sensitive indicator of blood in the urine and can detect as few as 5–10 red cells/$\mu$l of urine. The test actually detects haemoglobin, whether free or in erythrocytes, so microscopy must be used to confirm the presence of red cells following a positive result.

In patients with stone disease, additional biochemical studies are performed to detect any metabolic predisposition to stone formation (e.g. increased urinary calcium, urate or cystine excretion).

*Microscopy* (Fig. 4.1)

The urine can be examined directly or the urinary sediment studied after centrifugation. Microscopy may show red or white blood cells, casts from glomerular disorders (hyaline or cellular), crystals related to stone disease (e.g. calcium oxalate) or bacteria; ova may be seen in schistosomiasis.

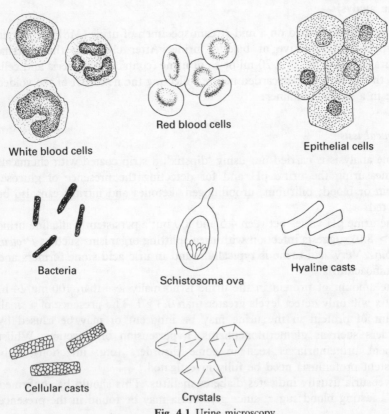

White blood cells

Red blood cells

Epithelial cells

Bacteria

Schistosoma ova

Hyaline casts

Cellular casts

Crystals

**Fig. 4.1** Urine microscopy

If bacteria are present, a Gram stain should be performed; if tuberculosis is suspected, the urinary sediment should be stained using the Ziehl-Neelsen method.

Urine cytology may be helpful in showing malignant cells in the urine after staining the sediment with Papanicolaou stain.

### Culture

The specimen should be plated out promptly or refrigerated until processing to prevent multiplication of bacteria after voiding. Standard bacteriological techniques are used for culture and identification of organisms, and a quantitative estimate of the number of organisms per ml of urine obtained from the number of colonies produced. Significant infection is present if there are more than 100 000 organisms/ml, whilst counts less than 10 000/ml suggest contamination. Antibiotic sensitivities are determined using culture plates with antibiotic discs that inhibit the growth of susceptible organisms.

If tuberculosis is suspected, three early morning samples of urine (EMU) are taken and cultured on Lowenstein–Jensen medium.

## Blood tests

### Renal function studies

Basic evaluation of renal function includes measurement of the plasma urea (normal range 2.3–6.9 mmol/l) and creatinine (normal range 50–120 $\mu$mol/l). Significant renal damage can occur, however, before the plasma urea and creatinine rise, so a more accurate guide to renal function is the creatinine clearance (normally 100–140 ml/min), which closely approximates to the glomerular filtration rate (GFR). This can be determined from measurements of urine volume (V), plasma creatinine (Pcreat) and urine creatinine concentrations (Ucreat); the clearance is calculated from the formula, Ucreat $\times$ V/Pcreat.

An alternative method of determining GFR is to measure the plasma clearance of $^{51}$Cr-labelled ethylenediamine tetra-acetic acid (EDTA). After an intravenous bolus of the isotope, serial blood samples are taken and the GFR is calculated from the rate of decline of radioactivity in the blood as the isotope is excreted by the kidneys. This technique has the advantages that no urine collection is required and that it is more accurate than creatinine clearance when renal function is poor.

### Haematology

A full blood count allows the detection of anaemia (due either to blood loss or renal impairment) and polycythaemia (which may cause raised urate levels). The white blood cell count may be raised in infections and the ESR is elevated in certain disorders (e.g renal adenocarcinoma, retroperitoneal fibrosis).

*Other tests*

Other biochemical tests may be required in certain circumstances. For example, serum calcium and urate are measured in patients with stone disease, acid phosphatase in prostatic carcinoma and liver function tests in suspected hepatic metastases from any malignancy.

## DIAGNOSTIC IMAGING

### Plain abdominal X-ray (KUB)

The KUB (a plain X-ray to include the kidneys, ureters and bladder) is useful to detect soft tissue masses in the renal areas or pelvis. Urinary calculi can normally be seen (90% are radio-opaque) unless they overlie areas of the bony skeleton; other causes of calcification include gallstones (10% are radio-opaque), pelvic phleboliths and calcified lymph nodes. It is important to look for bony abnormalities such as sclerotic deposits in prostatic carcinoma or spinal defects in patients with neuropathic bladder.

### Intravenous urogram (IVU) (Fig. 4.2)

This is the most frequently used radiological technique in urological disorders. After a plain film, iodine-containing contrast medium is injected intravenously and serial films are taken to follow its excretion by the kidneys. Facilities for tomography should be available to allow accurate imaging of the kidneys unimpeded by overlying bowel gas.

On the initial film 1–3 minutes after injection, contrast medium is in the glomeruli and proximal tubules so that a clear image of the renal outline is obtained (the *nephrogram*); any irregularity of the renal outline should be noted, as should space-occupying lesions (e.g. tumours or cysts).

Subsequent excretion of contrast medium outlines the collecting systems, renal pelvis, ureters and bladder, showing any structural abnormalities or filling defects. In the normal individual, the whole urinary tract should be visualised after 20 minutes; the patient is then asked to pass urine and a final post-micturition film taken to assess bladder emptying and detect any residual urine.

The procedure may have to be modified according to individual circumstances; for example, delayed films may be required when upper tract obstruction or slow opacification of the collecting system is present and frusemide is sometimes given to assess clearance of contrast medium in cases of equivocal pelviureteric junction obstruction.

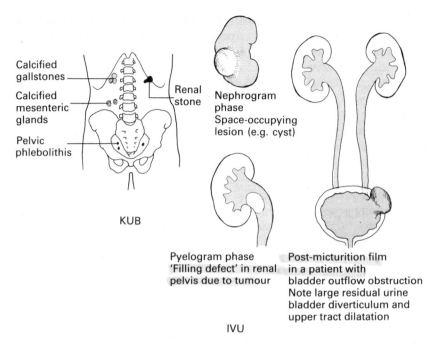

Calcified gallstones

Calcified mesenteric glands

Pelvic phlebolithis

Renal stone

KUB

Nephrogram phase
Space-occupying lesion (e.g. cyst)

Pyelogram phase
'Filling defect' in renal pelvis due to tumour

Post-micturition film in a patient with bladder outflow obstruction Note large residual urine bladder diverticulum and upper tract dilatation

IVU

**Fig. 4.2** The IVU sequence

In order to improve the concentration of contrast medium in the urine, the patient is usually deprived of fluid for 4–6 hours before an IVU. Care should be taken, however, if the patient has impaired renal function; in view of their inability to concentrate urine, such patients must not be dehydrated beforehand.

The procedure may be complicated by allergic reactions to the contrast medium, ranging in severity from a mild urticarial rash (that responds to antihistamines) to anaphylactic shock requiring intravenous hydrocortisone and circulatory support. There is a mortality rate of 1 per 100 000 urograms, so adequate resuscitation equipment should always be at hand. Newer non-ionic contrast media are now being more widely used because of their low morbidity and mortality.

### Ultrasound

This involves the passage of high-frequency sound waves from a transducer through the patient's body; this sound beam is then reflected, deflected or absorbed depending on the tissue it encounters. From the reflected signals picked up by the transducer, a sonic picture of the tissues is obtained. With modern grey-scale ultrasound, good anatomical detail can be displayed in a non-invasive manner.

*size of kidney*
*cortex thick or thin*

Ultrasound imaging has proved of particular value in distinguishing between solid and cystic lesions (especially in the kidney) and in assessing obstruction in the urinary tract (e.g hydronephrosis, residual bladder urine). It is the investigation of choice in assessing the urinary tract in pregnant women, to avoid the risk of radiation to the fetus, and is also useful in patients who require regular monitoring for evidence of upper tract dilatation.

Other uses of ultrasound are in the evaluation of scrotal masses and in the assessment of prostatic disease (using a transducer within the rectum).

### Computed tomography (CT scanning)

In CT scanning, an X-ray beam is rotated around the body and its absorption at different angles measured by multiple detectors. From the differences in tissue density, a computer then reconstructs two-dimensional cross-sectional images of the body with a remarkable degree of anatomical detail.

Iodine-containing contrast medium can be given during CT scanning to help display the renal pelvis and ureters. The technique is especially useful in the diagnosis of renal and retroperitoneal masses, when it allows differentiation between fluid-filled and solid lesions. In renal tumours, local extension of the disease, nodal metastases and involvement of the renal vein or inferior vena cava can also be assessed. CT scanning is now the investigation of choice for staging testicular tumours and is also useful in planning radiotherapy or radical surgery for prostatic or bladder carcinoma.

### Arteriography

This involves the injection of contrast medium directly into an artery to look at normal and pathological vascular anatomy. The two main applications in urology are renal and iliac arteriography, which can be performed via a femoral artery puncture. Renal arteriography is used in the diagnosis of renal vascular disorders, renal tumours and renal trauma; therapeutic embolisation of the renal artery can be performed at the same time to control bleeding from the kidney. Iliac arteriography is useful for assessing pelvic tumours or trauma and therapeutic embolisation of the internal iliac artery is occasionally used for uncontrollable bladder haemorrhage and priapism.

### Other radiological techniques

In the upper urinary tract, antegrade pyelography can be useful in the diagnosis of obstruction, contrast medium being injected via a small-bore needle passed into the collecting system under local anaesthetic (Fig. 4.3). An ascending ureterogram, using a catheter inserted into the ureteric orifice

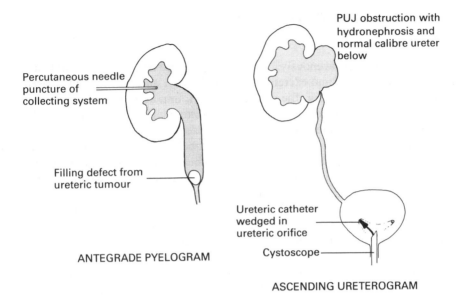

**Fig. 4.3** Antegrade pyelogram and ascending ureterogram

at cystoscopy, is often used to outline the ureter and collecting system in patients with upper tract obstruction or tumours.

In the lower urinary tract, urethrography is indicated for evaluation of urethral strictures before surgery and for urethral trauma; contrast medium is instilled directly into the urethra via a small Foley balloon catheter or a specially-designed (*Knutsson's*) clamp. A micturating cystogram is useful to demonstrate vesicoureteric reflux; contrast medium is instilled into the bladder via a catheter and ureteric filling screened during passive bladder filling and voiding (after the catheter has been removed).

Lymphography following injection of contrast medium into a lymphatic in the foot is used to demonstrate the iliac and para-aortic nodes in pelvic malignancy; nowadays, it has largely been replaced by CT scanning.

Other specific procedures (e.g. vasography, cavernosography) are discussed elsewhere.

## Magnetic resonance imaging (MRI)

This is rapidly emerging as a valuable technique in diseases of the central nervous system and is likely to have applications in the urinary tract. In addition to imaging, MRI spectroscopy gives information about the metabolism of normal and abnormal tissues; this may prove useful in assessing tissue physiology in, for example, renal transplants.

## RADIONUCLIDE STUDIES

### Renal scintigraphy

When injected intravenously, certain radioisotope-labelled compounds are selectively taken up and excreted by the kidneys. Using an externally placed scintillation counter (e.g. the gamma camera), important information about renal function can be obtained. Different isotopes are used to study specific aspects of kidney function.

In the static renal scan, $^{99m}$technetium-labelled dimercaptosuccinic acid (DMSA) is taken up by the renal tubules; this allows assessment of the size and position of the kidneys, their differential function and any parenchymal defects such as scars, cysts or tumours.

In dynamic scintigraphy, $^{99m}$technetium-labelled diethylenetriamine penta-acetic acid (DTPA) or $^{131}$iodine-labelled hippuran are taken up by the kidney and excreted in the urine. This process can be divided into three phases: the *vascular phase* is due to arrival of isotope in the kidney from the bloodstream, with a rapidly-rising curve of activity lasting about 30 seconds. The rate of rise then slows as isotope is concentrated and passed into the collecting system (*filtration phase*). A peak is then reached as isotope passes down the ureter as fast as it is arriving in the collecting system, after which activity falls as isotope is no longer being delivered to the kidney but continues to be transported down the ureter (*excretion phase*) (Fig. 4.4).

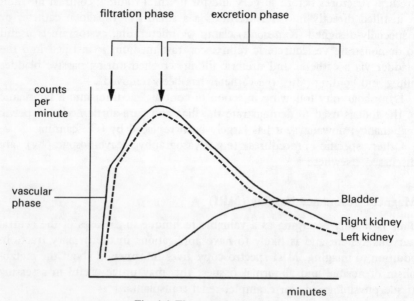

**Fig. 4.4** The normal renogram

Alterations to this pattern occur in certain disorders. For example, in renal artery stenosis there is impairment of the vascular phase so that there is a slowly-rising curve. In obstruction of the upper urinary tract, there is a prolonged excretory phase and frusemide may help to determine whether this is due to obstruction or simple stasis.

The study can be modified in patients with suspected vesicoureteric reflux to detect increased activity in the upper tracts after voiding.

### Bone scintigraphy

$^{99m}$Technetium-labelled methylene diphosphonate (MDP) is taken up from the circulation into areas of bone where there is increased osteoblastic activity, as may occur at the site of tumour metastases. The sites of increased uptake can then be detected with the gamma camera. The technique is very sensitive and may detect metastases as small as 1 cm diameter before they are visible on conventional X-rays.

The technique is most widely used in the detection of bony metastases from prostatic carcinoma, but also detects spread from other sites (e.g. renal or bladder tumours).

## URODYNAMIC STUDIES

Most of the investigations described provide information only about anatomy of the urinary tract. Several specialised tests are available for assessing disorders of function and these are collectively known as *urodynamic studies*.

### Lower urinary tract

The bladder and urethra act as a functional unit for storage and expulsion of urine, and both should be assessed when dealing with voiding disorders.

### *Voiding urinary flow rate* (Fig. 4.5)

The flow rate is the volume of urine passed in a certain time and is expressed as ml per second; it can be measured electronically using a number of different types of equipment. The flow rate in the normal individual rises rapidly to a peak which is maintained until the bladder is nearly empty before subsiding. The flow rate is reduced when only small volumes are passed and at least 200 ml should be voided for the test to be meaningful. Information can be gained not only from the flow rate itself but also from the voiding pattern (e.g. prolonged curve, intermittent voiding). The peak urinary flow rate varies with age and between the sexes.

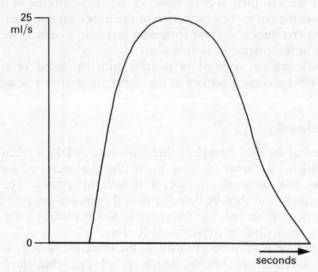

A. NORMAL URINE FLOW TRACE

B. VARIATION OF NORMAL URINE FLOW RATE WITH AGE

| Age (years) | Male (ml/s) | Female (ml/s) |
|---|---|---|
| 16–45 | >25 | >30 |
| 46–55 | >15 | >25 |
| 56–80 | >12 | >15 |

**Fig. 4.5** Urine flow studies

## Cystometry (Fig. 4.6)

This involves measurement of the intravesical pressure during changes in bladder volume and is recorded as a tracing (*cystometrogram*). Two fine urethral catheters are passed into the bladder, one to fill the bladder and the other to measure the intravesical pressure. The total pressure in the bladder is the sum of the pressure produced by the bladder wall itself (*detrusor pressure*) and the intra-abdominal pressure. The intra-abdominal presure is measured simultaneously via a fluid filled catheter in the rectum or vagina and is electronically subtracted from the total pressure to determine the detrusor pressure.

Detrusor function can be evaluated during bladder filling and during voiding when the urine flow rate is also recorded. Using contrast medium to fill the bladder, bladder and urethral activity can be seen on fluoroscopy; the X-ray images can be recorded alongside the pressure tracings on video-tape to give a permanent record (*videocystourethrography*).

The normal bladder is characterised by little change in pressure during filling, the pressure only rising by 5–10 cm of water up to a normal capacity

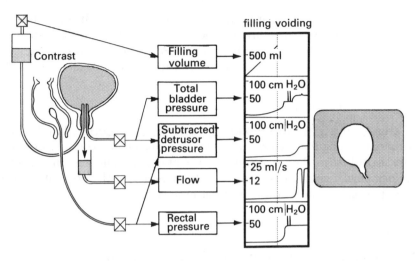

**Fig. 4.6** Diagrammatic representation of combined pressure-flow cystourethrography

of 400–500 ml in the adult. Even on provocation by coughing straining or changing posture, the detrusor does not contract until the individual voluntarily initiates voiding. This behaviour is referred to as a *stable bladder* (Fig. 4.7).

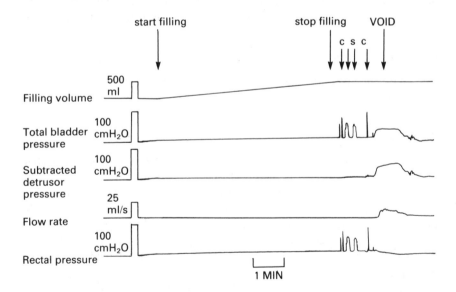

Stable bladder on filling
No detrusor contraction on provocation by coughing (c) or straining (s)
Voiding by voluntary detrusor contraction

**Fig. 4.7** Normal urodynamic study

When voiding is voluntarily initiated in the normal individual, the detrusor pressure rises smoothly to a peak and is then maintained until the bladder is empty before subsiding; a further rise in intravesical pressure (*the after-contraction*) is occasionally seen in the normal bladder.

### Urethral pressure profile

If a fine catheter with side openings near its tip is perfused and slowly withdrawn along the urethra, the pressure to maintain a constant flow will vary according to the activity of the urethral wall. This test (the *urethral pressure profile*) gives an assessment of the function of the urethral muscles from the bladder neck to the external meatus.

### Electromyography

Further information about the activity of the urethral sphincter can be obtained by electromyography (EMG). A fine needle electrode is inserted into the periurethral striated muscle or an electrode mounted on a probe is inserted into the rectum to record electrical activity from the pelvic floor muscles. Normally, electrical activity increases gradually as the bladder fills and then ceases as the sphincter relaxes during voiding. The main disadvantage with this technique is that only one of the muscle groups involved in urethral closure is sampled and the activity of other groups, chiefly the intrinsic urethral sphincter, cannot necessarily be inferred from the results.

## Upper urinary tract

The main value of upper tract urodynamics is in the diagnosis of upper tract obstruction.

### Antegrade perfusion studies (Whitaker test) (Fig. 4.8)

This involves insertion of a needle percutaneously into the collecting system of the kidney; the kidney is then perfused with fluid at a rate of 10 ml/min and the intrapelvic pressure measured through a side-arm channel. The intravesical pressure is also measured via a urethral catheter and the pressure difference between renal pelvis and bladder recorded (*relative pressure*). The bladder is normally kept empty during the procedure, but it can be allowed to fill to study the effect of abnormal bladder function on upper tract pressures.

On perfusion, any rise in intrapelvic pressure is recorded. Perfusion is continued until an equilibrated pressure is reached or the pressure becomes excessively raised. Antegrade contrast studies are usually performed at the same time to give anatomical information.

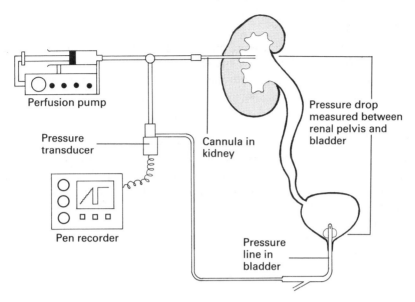

**Fig. 4.8** Antegrade perfusion study (Whitaker test)

In the unobstructed kidney, there is little or no pressure rise during perfusion, a plateau pressure is quickly reached and the relative pressure between kidney and bladder remains less than 15 cm of water. In obstruction, there is a marked rise in relative pressure, usually to more than 22 cm of water but there is an equivocal range between 15 and 22 cm of water.

When this technique is combined with frusemide renography, clear evidence on the presence or absence of upper tract obstruction is provided in over 90% of patients.

## ENDOSCOPIC INVESTIGATIONS

### Cystoscopy

In many disorders of the lower urinary tract, direct examination of the urethra and bladder using a cystoscope is required. The urethra should be examined as the instrument is passed into the bladder under direct vision; this is particularly important in the male to exclude a urethral stricture or tumour. The inside of the bladder is then carefully inspected and biopsies can be taken for histological examination.

Cystoscopy can also be used to introduce catheters into the ureteric orifices. This may be performed to obtain samples of urine from each kidney (e.g. to localise infection, to allow cytological analysis) or to instill contrast medium to take X-rays of the upper urinary tracts (*ascending ureteropyelography*).

## Ureteroscopy

The ureteroscope is a narrow-bore instrument which can be introduced into the ureter after dilatation of the ureteric orifice. The instrument can then be passed under direct vision into the ureter and even into the renal pelvis to allow removal of stones, biopsy of tumours and dilatation of strictures.

## Nephroscopy

The interior of the kidney can be inspected with a modified cystoscope (*nephroscope*) introduced either through an incision in the renal pelvis at open operation or via a percutaneous tract dilated to a sufficient diameter to accomodate the instrument. This is usually performed to remove renal calculi.

# 5

# Congenital anomalies of the upper urinary tract

Although, by definition, congenital anomalies are present at birth, it is surprising how many become manifest only in the older child or adult. Some of these anomalies may be associated with obstruction or infection and it is reasonable to assume that renal function may deteriorate if the anomaly is left untreated or undetected. Therefore the emphasis is now on early diagnosis and treatment.

Young children with upper tract anomalies present with symptoms of urinary infection, with a mass in the abdomen or with the systemic effects of bilateral renal obstruction. Older children complain of pain which they may localise sufficiently to indicate which upper tract is diseased. Haematuria may be the only symptom in a child with upper tract obstruction. Intrauterine diagnosis is now possible using ultrasound antenatally.

## ANOMALIES OF THE KIDNEY

### Unilateral renal agenesis

The incidence of unilateral renal agenesis is between 1 in 500 and 1 in 1000 of the population. There is usually no ureter and the appropriate half of the trigone of the bladder is missing. In 10% of patients the adrenal gland is also absent.

The solitary kidney shows compensatory hypertrophy but is also frequently abnormal with ectopia, malrotation or hydronephrosis which cause half these children to present in the first few years of life.

In boys the ipsilateral seminal tract and testis may be absent. Girls may have absence of the tube and ovary, anomalies of the uterus (unicornuate or bicornuate), or aplasia of the vagina. Imperforate anus and anomalies of the vertebrae or cardiovascular system may also coexist.

An absent kidney may also be discovered by chance whilst a child is being investigated for a urinary infection or for suspected renal trauma with non-excretion of one kidney on a urogram.

The diagnosis is made by ultrasound which fails to locate a kidney, a cystoscopy which usually shows an absent hemitrigone, and a high index of suspicion when associated anomalies are present. CT scanning may be needed if doubt still exists but aortography is now rarely necessary.

Treatment is limited to the management of associated anomalies and disease of the solitary kidney. Dangerous body-contact sports, such as judo, should be avoided but children should not be overprotected because they have unilateral renal agenesis.

### Bilateral renal agenesis

The risk of a child being born with no kidneys is probably less than 1 in 3000 and such a child may survive for a few days. The ureters, bladder and urethra are either underdeveloped or absent, and other anomalies are frequent.

The absence of fetal urine leads to oligohydramnios which, in turn, is associated with hypoplastic lungs and the Potter facies of low set ears, flattened nose and wide set eyes.

Treatment is not appropriate as, even if renal transplantation was possible, the hypoplastic lungs are incompatible with life.

### Malrotation

During development and ascent of the kidney the renal pelvis comes to face more medially. The most usual anomaly is for the renal pelvis to face forwards; the more ectopically placed the kidney, the more severe is the rotation.

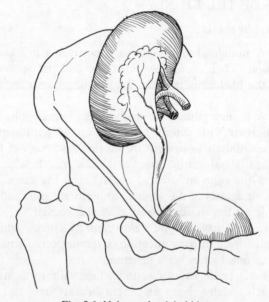

**Fig. 5.1** Malrotated pelvic kidney

Malrotation is best seen on an IVU, where the calyces point in unusual directions and the ureter emerges more laterally from the forward facing pelvis (Fig. 5.1). Hydronephrosis may occur in a malrotated kidney but the condition should not be overdiagnosed because of the unusual appearances.

No treatment is necessary for the uncomplicated case of malrotation.

### Renal ectopia

A kidney that has incompletely ascended and remains lower than normal in the abdomen is ectopic. Occasionally, the kidney from one side is located on the opposite side (crossed ectopia) (Fig. 5.2). The incidence of ectopia is approximately 1 in 800. In general, the lower the kidney the more abnormal it is.

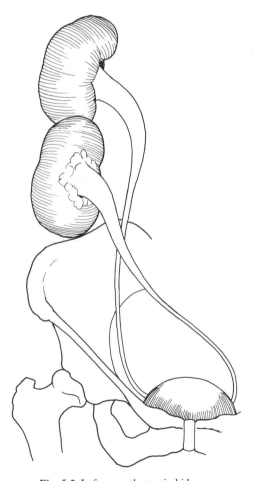

Fig. 5.2 Left crossed ectopic kidney

Symptoms are produced by associated vesicoureteric reflux or pelvi-ureteric obstruction. Some low lying kidneys may be discovered during the investigation of a palpable adominal mass, whilst other ectopic kidneys are found by chance during the investigation of a child with a urinary infection.

Diagnosis of renal ectopia is made with an IVU but malrotation or poor function, associated with scarring or obstruction, may make the urographic appearances difficult to interpret. Reflux, as shown on a cystogram, may locate a small scarred kidney in an abnormal position and nuclear imaging may be necessary to define function, drainage and scarring. Treatment is directed at the anomalies of the ectopic or contralateral kidney.

## Fused kidneys

If both kidneys are low they may be joined as a single mass of renal tissue, usually drained by two ureters, that lies at or below the pelvic brim.

*Horseshoe kidney* (Fig. 5.3) occurs with an incidence of between 1 in 600 and 1 in 1800. It is more common in males. The two kidneys are joined across the midline, usually at their lower poles, by renal tissue of varying thickness, or by a fibrous band. The conjoined kidney is low lying as its full ascent has been limited by the inferior mesenteric artery. The blood supply is anomalous and the renal pelves are rotated anteriorly with the ureters passing down over the isthmus. The lower poles of the two halves are also rotated medially.

Although a horseshoe kidney may be found in an infant with other multiple anomalies, they often present later in life with the complications of reflux, obstruction or stone formation although they may be asymptomatic.

An IVU shows the characteristic medially pointing calyces and the isthmus may be seen. In children with infections, reflux should be excluded

A. LEFT PELVIURETERIC
   JUNCTION OBSTRUCTION

B. DIVISION OF ISTHMUS TO
   ENABLE PYELOPLASTY

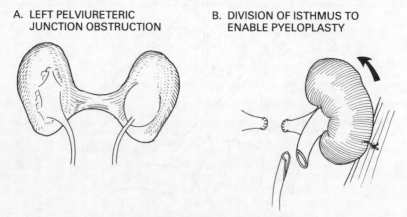

Fig. 5.3 Horseshoe kidney

with a cystogram and renal damage documented with a $^{99m}$Tc-dimercaptosuccinic acid (DMSA) scan.

## CALYCEAL ABNORMALITIES

### Hydrocalyx and hydrocalycosis

These terms describe the structural change in a calyx or calyces that have been subjected to raised pressure (Fig. 5.4). If all the calyces are dilated, it is likely that high pressure has resulted from such problems as pelviureteric obstruction or obstructed megaureter. If a single calyx or group of calyces are dilated the cause is probably a local lesion such as a congenital infundibular stenosis, extrinsic compression from a vessel or tumour, intrinsic pressure from a stone or local infection from tuberculosis.

Antibiotic therapy and appropriate drainage may be necessary before definitive treatment is instituted. Persistent symptoms may be relieved by a partial nephrectomy.

### Megacalycosis

This is a congenital maldevelopment of the kidney, usually unilateral, in which the calyces are uniformly 'dilated' on urography. In fact, they look more like calyces that have previously been dilated from obstruction and this has led to a theory that this condition may be a burnt-out obstruction, perhaps from the obstructive effects of fetal folds in utero.

There is often a fullness of the renal pelvis but no obstruction is present and the importance of the condition is that pyeloplasty is not necessary. The

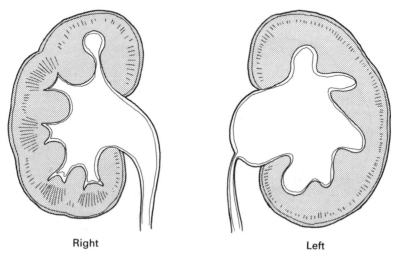

Right    Left

**Fig. 5.4** Isolated right hydrocalyx. Diffuse left hydrocalycosis due to pelviureteric obstruction

associated stasis, however, can lead to infection and stone formation which may need treatment in their own right.

### Calyceal diverticulum

This is a cavity within the renal parenchyma that communicates with a calyx, usually via a narrow neck. It is probably a congenital malformation and occurs most often in the upper pole of the kidney. The majority of these diverticula are asymptomatic but stasis can lead to infection and stone formation. Only occasionally is an operation needed and it may amount to a partial nephrectomy.

## PELVIURETERIC JUNCTION OBSTRUCTION (Fig. 5.5)

Obstruction at the junction of the renal pelvis and upper ureter is a common congenital form of urinary obstruction that causes morbidity in all ages, despite the fact that the tendency to obstruct is almost certainly present from birth.

The cause of obstruction is still not known but a feature common to all theories is an abrupt change in shape between the pelvis and the ureter so that the usual peristaltic conduction of a bolus is interrupted.

Kinks, adhesions and valves have all been implicated, as have lower polar blood vessels that cross or press against the area in question. However, common though these vessels are, they are rarely the prime cause of the obstruction; more often they aggravate an intrinsic obstruction that is already present.

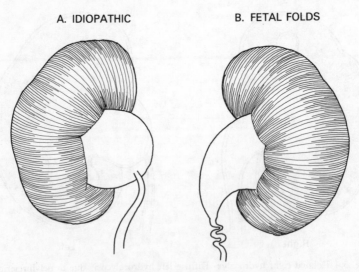

A. IDIOPATHIC        B. FETAL FOLDS

**Fig. 5.5** Pelviureteric junction obstruction

Fetal folds (invaginations of the muscle and mucosa) are often present in the upper ureter in infants but rarely seen in older children or adults, so that the natural history is probably one of disappearance. Persistence of these folds, however, can produce a true obstruction.

## Types of pelviureteric junction obstruction

### Chronically obstructed hydronephrosis

There is fixed dilatation of the calyces and renal pelvis, usually with loss of parenchyma. There may be almost complete destruction of the kidney, particularly in neonates who present with an abdominal mass or a hydronephrosis that is found on a fetal ultrasound.

Haematuria, a mass or failure to thrive are the typical symptoms in a small child whilst, in older children or adults, loin pain or non-specific abdominal pain is more usual.

### Intermittently obstructed hydronephrosis

Sometimes the pelviureteric junction only obstructs intermittently, precipitated by factors such as a high fluid load, lying on one side in bed or a stressful situation. Between attacks the IVU can be deceptively normal but during the attack there are all the signs of acute, severe obstruction, such as dilated calyces, delayed nephrogram and delayed excretion. The attack, which can cause severe pain and vomiting, usually lasts for hours or days.

Although diuresis renography and pressure flow studies can be helpful, the best method of diagnosing an intermittent obstruction is with an IVU during an attack of pain.

### Reflux induced hydronephrosis (Fig. 5.6)

Marked vesicoureteric reflux can overdistend the renal pelvis and prevent efficient drainage, leading to a true secondary pelviureteric obstruction. The condition is usually symptomless unless associated with a urinary infection, but occasionally loin pain may be experienced at the height of voiding. If the pelvis is not distended on an IVU then reimplantation of the ureter is needed and not pyeloplasty.

### Equivocally obstructed hydronephrosis

This category is mentioned to emphasise the need to be certain that a true obstruction is present before suggesting an operation.

## Diagnosis

An IVU remains the best way of demonstrating a hydronephrotic kidney.

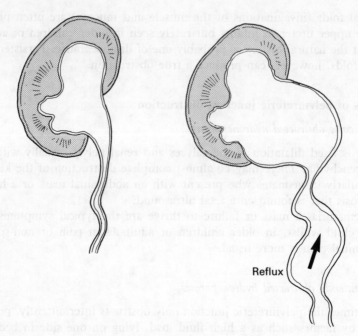

Reflux

**Fig. 5.6** Reflux-induced hydronephrosis

If the obstruction is severe with delay in appearance and disappearance of the contrast then a urogram may be all that is needed. However, in some patients the diagnosis of obstruction is still not clear and delayed X-rays or the use of a diuretic during an IVU may help to stimulate an acute obstruction.

Other tests may also be needed. Diuresis renography can be helpful but may be misleading in a very dilated or poorly functioning kidney that cannot respond adequately to a diuretic. In these difficult cases a percutaneous pressure flow study can usually be relied upon to give a definitive answer.

A cystogram is indicated if there is any suspicion of reflux and retrograde ureterography, performed just before surgery, is useful to demonstrate the ureter.

### Associated anomalies

Hydronephrosis may be associated with almost any other abnormality of the genitourinary or other system. The opposite kidney may also be abnormal in 10–15% of patients with a similar hydronephrosis or another abnormality such as a multicystic kidney.

## Complications

A large hydronephrosis is easily damaged by minor injury and this is a common mode of presentation. Any child who has haematuria after even a minor abdominal injury should have an IVU. Stones or a pyonephrosis can occur in an infected kidney. The hypertension that is seen occasionally in association with hydronephrosis can sometimes by cured by a pyeloplasty.

## Management

The standard surgical treatment of a kidney with a proven obstruction is a pyeloplasty. Although there are several types of pyeloplasty they all aim to produce a gradually tapering pelviureteric junction that allows the transmission of a peristaltic wave and bolus formation.

Very occasionally, it may be justified to perform an operation simply to lessen the size of the pelvis with the aim of reducing the stasis and hence avoiding the risk of urinary infection. Such a decision must be tempered by the knowledge that an obstruction may be introduced when none was present before.

In a patient with an acutely obstructed hydronephrosis it is sensible to drain the kidney by percutaneous puncture as a temporary measure. Even after temporary relief of the obstruction it may become apparent, either from analysis of the urine that is produced by the diseased kidney or from a DMSA scan, that the kidney is not worth preserving. If the kidney is only a thin shell with less than 10% of overall function, in the presence of a normal kidney on the other side, it is probably not worthy of preservation. In young children, however, the kidney should always be preserved, if possible, since a remarkable degree of recovery can be seen.

Pyeloplasty is generally a most successful operation but complications include leakage of urine via the wound drain, haemorrhage (usually associated with the placement of a nephrostomy tube) and stenosis of the anastomosis. Most of these can be avoided with good surgical technique. A follow-up ultrasound at 1 month is useful, with an IVU at 3–6 months.

## DYSPLASTIC, HYPOPLASTIC AND CYSTIC DISEASES OF THE KIDNEY

### Renal dysplasia

This is a histological diagnosis in which primitive glomeruli, tubules, ducts and cartilage are seen as a focal or diffuse change. Although more obvious dysplastic changes occur in the presence of obstruction (posterior urethral valves or multicystic kidney with atretic ureter), dysplasia may be seen in its absence (prune belly syndrome or reflux).

### Multicystic kidney (Fig. 5.7)

This is a good example of severe renal dysplasia. The kidney is composed of a mass of cysts loosely held together by a fibrous stroma. It is occasionally bilateral and then incompatible with life. Most multicystic kidneys are now diagnosed on a prenatal ultrasound scan and are often palpable in the newborn period. The ultrasound appearances of non-communicating cystic spaces together with no function on a DMSA scan are diagnostic.

There is usually atresia of the ureter in association with a multicystic kidney and other genitourinary anomalies are common.

The natural history of multicystic kidney remains unclear. They are only occasionally found in adults, so they probably become smaller or even disappear over the years. There has been a tendency to remove these kidneys because of an uncertainty in diagnosis and the risk of urinary infection, malignancy or hypertension, but this is no longer justified unless the mass is particularly large.

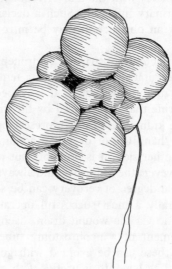

Fig. 5.7 Multicystic kidney

### Renal hypoplasia

This term describes a small kidney with normal renal tissue, no dysplasia and a normal ureter. It is usually associated with gross abnormalities of the opposite kidney, resulting in renal insufficiency.

### Infantile polycystic disease

This is a rare autosomal recessive condition in which neonates present with gross enlargment of both kidneys and, over a few days, show evidence of renal failure with rising levels of blood urea and creatinine. Both sexes are equally involved. Urography shows large kidneys with a diffuse radial streaking of contrast, quite unlike the pattern in Wilms' tumour, mesoblastic nephroma or renal vein thrombosis which are amongst the differential diagnoses. Ultrasound gives a characteristic appearance and rapidly distinguishes the condition from hydronephrosis and multicystic kidney.

The children tend to die from renal or respiratory failure in the first few days or weeks of life. A proportion of children do survive for several years, only to develop portal hypertension due to hepatic involvement later.

Treatment is directed towards the management of the renal failure, hypertension and respiratory problems.

## Adult polycystic disease

This is an autosomal dominant condition which typically presents in the 3rd and 4th decades with hypertension, renal impairment or large palpable kidneys. Cysts may also be found in the liver but without changes in hepatic function.

Urography shows large kidneys with calyceal distortion caused by the enlarging cysts throughout the kidneys. Treatment is directed to the management of the hypertension and renal failure. It is no longer believed that local treatment such as drainage of the cysts is wise unless performed early in the disease process.

## Multilocular cystic kidney

This rare cystic condition can be considered more as a tumour than as a localised cystic change. A multilocular cyst is a large developmental lesion with a definite capsule that compresses the normal renal tissue around it. The cystic nature is only revealed when the lesion is cut open and a mass of cysts of varying sizes are seen containing clear or yellowish fluid.

Smaller cysts may extend into the renal pelvis and prolapse into the pelviureteric junction to give an acute obstruction with sudden enlargement of the kidney.

They may occur equally in either sex. The lesion presents as a mass, vague abdominal symptoms or occasionally with haematuria. Ultrasound, urography and CT findings are similar to those of cystic Wilms' tumours but the diagnosis is made most commonly when the lesion is sectioned after nephrectomy.

## Medullary sponge kidney

In this condition there is dilatation and cyst formation of the distal collecting tubules that gives the characteristic urographic appearance of a streaky blush extending into the medulla from the involved calyces. It may be limited to part of one kidney or involve the whole of both kidneys. In adults there is nephrocalcinosis in the typical distribution of the papillae.

It is rarely diagnosed in children, but usually presents in patients 30–40 years old with the symptoms of infection or stone formation that is secondary to stasis. The stones are usually small and, considering the number that are produced in some patients, it is surprising how rarely surgery is necessary. Infection can usually be controlled by antibiotics. Partial nephrectomy can sometimes be appropriate if the disease is limited to a small area of one kidney. Hemihypertrophy of the body has been well documented in medullary sponge kidney.

## Simple cysts

Simple cysts are rarely seen in children and yet they are extremely common in older patients, suggesting that they are an acquired disease. They occasionally produce symptoms of fullness or even a mass in the loin, but more usually they are chance findings. The diagnosis is confirmed by ultrasound and puncture, when clear fluid is aspirated. If there is blood staining of the fluid, cytology should be undertaken.

## CONGENITAL ANOMALIES OF THE URETER

### Duplications of the upper urinary tract

Duplications can present at any age but the clinical and radiological findings are usually most dramatic in children. Urography and cystography provide the diagnosis in all but a few cases and cystoscopy, particularly in children, has only a small part to play. Most duplications are commoner in girls and are frequently bilateral. If the kidney is drained by two separate ureters the upper pole ureter drains the upper group of calyces and the lower ureter the middle and lower calyces.

### Simple partial duplication (Fig. 5.8)

The two ureters can join anywhere to give little more than a bifid pelvis or two ureters meeting just outside the bladder. Such partial duplications rarely give symptoms, although the 'yo-yo' movement of urine between the two ureters can lead to stasis and infection. An IVU with fluoroscopy or a renogram will confirm this abnormal drainage and, if symptoms are persistent, an operation can be performed to reduce stasis. The upper ureter can be anastomosed to the renal pelvis of the lower half of the kidney and the lower part of the upper pole ureter then excised. If one half of the kidney, usually the upper half, has been severely damaged it is occasionally necessary to perform a partial nephrectomy.

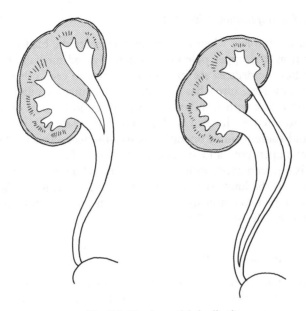

**Fig. 5.8** Simple partial duplication

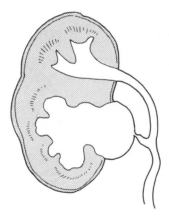

**Fig. 5.9** Lower moiety pelviureteric junction obstruction

A pelviureteric obstruction is sometimes seen in the lower pelvis (Fig. 5.9), requiring a pyeloplasty, but such a lesion is almost never seen in the upper pole. Reflux of urine from the bladder into the common stem can occur and should be treated in its own right.

In the absence of infection, simple partial duplication is unimportant and symptoms should not be attributed to it.

*Simple complete duplication* (Fig. 5.10)

Duplication is complete when the two ureters enter the bladder separately. The ureter from the upper pole opens inferiorly and medially to the lower pole ureter but the orifices are in close proximity to each other. The lower pole ureter, however, often has a more direct course through the bladder wall and may reflux with resultant scarring of the lower pole of the kidney.

Reflux associated with such a duplication is less likely to stop spontaneously and some form of operation is usually necessary. In the presence of a normal upper pole and normal contralateral kidney a badly scarred lower pole is best removed, with excision of the refluxing ureter as far down as is practical. If the lower pole is satisfactory, a reimplant is indicated. The two ureters are in a common sheath so that both ureters can be reimplanted together in a double-barrelled fashion.

*Duplications with ectopic ureter*

As the upper pole ureter becomes ectopic it inserts more distally towards the bladder neck or beyond. The further away it inserts, the more dilated is the ectopic ureter and the more dysplastic the upper pole of the kidney above it.

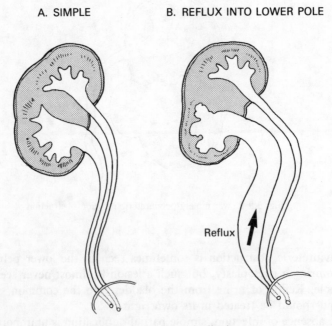

A. SIMPLE          B. REFLUX INTO LOWER POLE

Reflux

**Fig. 5.10** Complete duplication

*Ectopic ureter opening low on trigone or at bladder neck*

The ectopic ureter opens lower and more medially than the lower pole ureter either on the trigone, at the bladder neck or within the proximal urethra. Reflux may occur into the ectopic ureter or there may be obstruction from a terminal atretic segment. The lower pole is normal (Fig. 5.11).

Pain and fever may indicate a urinary infection. An IVU shows either a normal lower pole or calyces that are displaced downwards by the dilated upper pole to give the classical 'drooping-flower' appearance. The upper pole is usually poorly excreting. If reflux is present it will be shown on a cystogram. If there is no reflux and the situation is not clear on a urogram then ultrasound or CT scanning will confirm the diagnosis. The upper pole is rarely worth saving and the treatment should be an upper pole partial nephroureterectomy with excision of as much of the refluxing ureter as is practical.

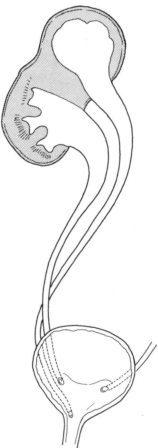

Fig. 5.11 Ectopic ureter opening at bladder neck

*Ectopic ureterocele*

The ectopic ureter may end as a bulbous dilatation in the base of the bladder extending to a variable extent down the urethra, with its narrowed orifice just inside the bladder neck (Fig. 5.12).

The ureterocele may be large or small and may encroach upon the ipsilateral and contralateral ureteric orifices to cause obstruction or reflux. It may impact into the bladder neck to give outflow obstruction or, in girls, it may prolapse and appear externally as a plum-coloured swelling.

Symptoms may be due to infection or outflow obstruction. Ectopic ureteroceles are seven times more common in females and 10% are bilateral. In most there are other duplex anomalies of the opposite system.

An IVU shows the same appearances as an ectopic ureter at the bladder neck but, in addition, there is a smooth, circular filling defect in the base of the bladder that does not opacify. A cystogram is needed to document reflux into the other ureters.

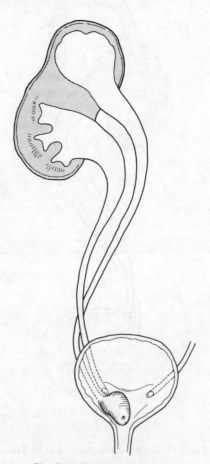

Fig. 5.12 Ectopic ureterocele

Treatment is complex and difficult involving upper pole partial nephro-ureterectomy with excision of the ureterocele, including its extension into the upper urethra, and repair of the bladder wall. In addition, reimplantation of the other ureters may be needed. Some urologists now perform an upper pole partial nephrectomy only, leaving the lower ureter and ureterocele in the hope that they will collapse and give no further trouble. This lesser operation is successful in 80% of patients but, in the remainder, a further procedure is necessary at a later date to remove the lower ureter and ureterocele.

*Ectopic ureter opening elsewhere* (Fig. 5.13)

*Female.* In females the ureter may open into the urethra below the sphincter to give continuous wetting despite normal voiding. This never happens in boys. Alternatively, the ureter may open into the vagina, or

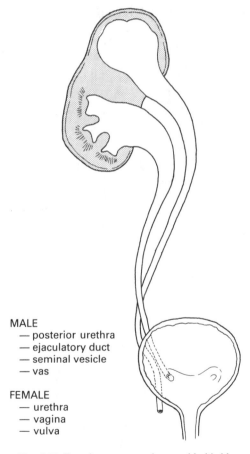

MALE
  — posterior urethra
  — ejaculatory duct
  — seminal vesicle
  — vas

FEMALE
  — urethra
  — vagina
  — vulva

**Fig. 5.13** Ectopic ureter opening outside bladder

vulva near the external urethral opening. Incontinence, infection and vaginal discharge are the typical features.

*Male.* If the ureter opens into the posterior urethra it is always above the sphincters so that continuous wetting from an ectopic ureter in boys does not occur. Epididymitis in a prepubertal boy should raise the possibility of an ectopic ureter inserting into the seminal vesicle or ejaculatory duct. This is usually associated with a multiloculated mass which can be felt per rectum.

The condition is cured in both sexes by partial nephrectomy. It is unwise and unnecessary to try to remove the lowest part of the ectopic ureter, or the multiloculated mass in boys, for risk of damaging the sphincters or ejaculatory mechanisms.

### Simple ureterocele

This is a bulging dilatation of the submucosal portion of a single ureter which is situated in the position of a normal orifice on the lateral end of the trigone (Fig. 5.14). It is not infrequently bilateral. The size of the

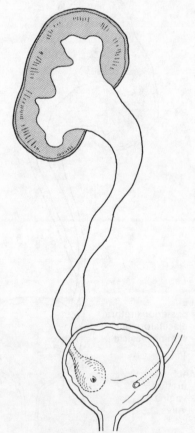

Fig. 5.14 Simple ureterocele

ureteric orifice determines whether it is a lax structure that collapses on bladder filling, or whether it remains tense at all times and is then associated with ureteric dilatation and/or renal impairment.

Pain and other symptoms of infection are the usual presenting features but ureteroceles are sometimes diagnosed by chance during a urogram for other reasons. If renal function is preserved, the ureterocele opacifies with a thin black halo around it resembling a cobra's head; if not, it remains as a negative shadow in the contrast filled bladder.

Treatment is best achieved by excising the ureterocele and reimplanting the ureter but a cure can be obtained endoscopically, without inducing reflux, with a small 'smile' incision along the lower edge of the ureterocele using a diathermy needle.

## Retrocaval ureter

Abnormal development of the vena cava causes the right ureter, in its upper third, to pass behind the vena cava and emerge between it and the aorta before resuming its normal course (Fig. 5.15).

It can be diagnosed or suspected on an IVU and confirmed by performing an ascending or descending ureterogram. Treatment is only necessary if there is significant obstruction of the upper tract above the anomaly and consists of division of the ureter and reanastomosis lateral to the cava.

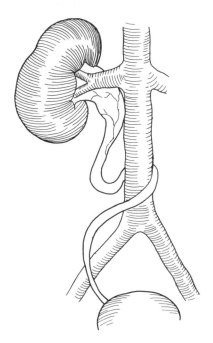

Fig. 5.15 Retrocaval ureter

## Megaureter (Fig. 5.16)

Any ureter so wide that effective transport of urine by peristaltic activity cannot occur throughout its length is a megaureter. If, in addition, there is definite obstruction then it is an obstructed megaureter. This implies, rightly, that some megaureters are not obstructed and this is important to bear in mind, as operations for megaureter are not always straightforward and a non-obstructed megaureter can all too easily be converted to an obstructed megaureter by inappropriate surgery.

In general, megaureters that are obstructed have muscular activity which cannot coapt the ureteric walls. However, once the obstruction is relieved, coaption may be possible and normal peristaltic activity returns. Non-obstructed wide ureters have poor muscle activity so that inappropriate operative intervention is doomed to failure.

Any wide ureter, particularly if bilateral, may be due to the secondary effect of bladder outflow obstruction and this should always be excluded on a cystogram which will also exclude reflux. If reflux is seen in an obstructed megaureter, operation is necessary.

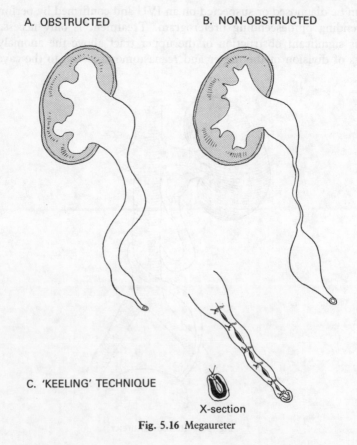

A. OBSTRUCTED                    B. NON-OBSTRUCTED

C. 'KEELING' TECHNIQUE

X-section

**Fig. 5.16** Megaureter

Megaureters are four times more common in males. Non-specific abdominal pain, loin pain, haematuria or symptoms of a urinary infection are the usual features that lead to investigation. An IVU gives a considerable amount of information. A wide ureter in which there are areas of good occlusion, usually in the midureter, is almost certainly not obstructed, especially if the calyces are normal. The converse is not true; a full ureter from top to bottom is not necessarily obstructed; diuresis renography and pressure flow studies may be needed to elucidate the true situation. If the anatomy is in doubt it is best displayed with an antegrade pyelogram.

Surgery is necessary for ureters with proven obstruction. Reimplantation is performed, often with tapering or 'keeling' of the lowest part of the ureter to facilitate the formation of the submucosal tunnel. A non-functioning system is best removed, but a period of nephrostomy drainage may be necessary to show that recovery has not occurred.

If no obstruction is present, the symptoms of urinary infection can usually be controlled with antibiotics. Occasionally it may be justified to operate to lessen the stasis and to improve the ureteric transport down such a non-obstructed megaureter in a patient with persistent urinary infection.

# 6

# Congenital anomalies of the lower urinary tract

## ANOMALIES OF THE BLADDER

### Bladder exstrophy

Exstrophy of the bladder (ectopia vesicae) is part of a spectrum of defects in which there is failure of fusion of the lower abdomen, genitalia and pelvic bones. The defects range from isolated epispadias to complex anomalies involving the bladder and intestine. Bladder exstrophy occurs in 1 in 10–40 000 live births and is twice as common in male infants.

The bladder mucosa lies exposed on the lower abdominal wall with the bladder neck and urethra laid open. Secondary inflammatory changes are common with squamous metaplasia, cystitis cystica, cystitis glandularis and, eventually, fibrosis of the bladder wall. There is an increased risk of adenocarcinoma of the bladder occurring after the 3rd decade of life and this risk is not eliminated by closure of the bladder.

The prostate and testes are normally developed. The penis is short and wide with upward chordee and a prepuce that is all on the ventral side. Girls have a bifid clitoris, often a short vagina and variable anomalies of the uterus. However, affected children of both sexes may have normal fertility in adult life. The pubic bones are separated and the recti lie apart.

For the first half of this century, the treatment of exstrophy was cystectomy and diversion of urine into the bowel by ureterosigmoidostomy. This, or an ileal loop diversion, remains the treatment of choice in the child with a small bladder in whom bladder reconstruction is impossible. In children with larger bladders, successful reconstruction of the bladder, sphincters and urethra can be accomplished in approximately half. This usually involves reimplantation of the ureters (which usually reflux) to provide more room for bladder neck reconstruction. Closure is best performed in the 1st year of life to make tissue approximation easier and to avoid the secondary changes that occur in the bladder wall. Surgical correction of the genitalia can be deferred until the child is older and is usually performed in stages.

## Epispadias

As an isolated anomaly in boys, epispadias can vary in its severity according to the site of the urinary meatus. The more severe the deformity the more likely the child is to be incontinent: in girls incontinence is the rule. Reconstruction is similar to that for the epispadias associated with exstrophy and needs staged procedures.

## Anomalies of urachal origin (Fig. 6.1)

Urachal problems are extremely rare, occurring in 1 in 300 000 births. Urachal anomalies may be associated with bladder outflow obstruction or an atretic urethra (occasionally seen in boys with the prune belly syndrome), and are more common in boys.

### Patent urachus

This is easily diagnosed by cystography. The differential diagnosis of fluid discharging from the umbilicus is a patent vitello-intestinal duct in which instillation of contrast shows a connection with the small bowel. Treatment of a patent urachus is excision of the whole tract from umbilicus to bladder.

### Urachal cyst

This usually develops in the lower third of the urachus and is found when the upper and lower portions close off, leaving a cystic area between them. Infection or a mass may lead to investigation, and although the lesion may be suspected on ultrasound, it can only be confirmed by exploration and excision.

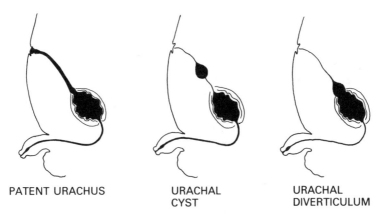

PATENT URACHUS          URACHAL          URACHAL
                        CYST             DIVERTICULUM

**Fig. 6.1** Urachal anomalies

### Urachal diverticulum

This occurs when the lower portion of the urachus remains patent and forms a diverticulum extending from the vault of the bladder. If it has a wide neck and is symptomless, no treatment is necessary. If infective complications occur, the diverticulum should be excised.

## Bladder diverticulum (Fig. 6.2)

A diverticulum is a protrusion through a weak point in the bladder muscle and embryologically this is more likely to occur close to the ureterovesical junction. Although commonly associated with bladder outflow obstruction, diverticula can occur in the absence of a high bladder pressure.

### Congenital bladder diverticulum

This condition usually occurs in boys, is commonly solitary and may be any size. There are no signs of obstruction at cystoscopy or cystography. The diverticulum is usually situated 1–2 cm above and lateral to the ureteric orifice. There is little or no muscle in the wall of these diverticula and therefore they enlarge as they are stretched with each bladder contraction.

Such a diverticulum may cause stasis, urinary tract infection and even stone formation. Occasionally, it is so large that it extends down behind the bladder neck, pushing it forwards to give secondary bladder outflow obstruction. This in turn leads to expansion of the diverticulum and worsening of the outflow obstruction.

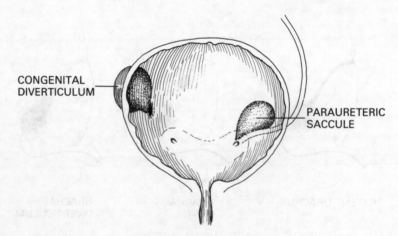

CONGENITAL
DIVERTICULUM

PARAURETERIC
SACCULE

**Fig. 6.2** Bladder diverticulum

*Paraureteric saccule*

This is associated with the ureteric orifice, is often bilateral and may occur in either sex. There is a tendency for the orifice to become incorporated into the saccule as growth continues and this results in reflux. Later, with increasing involvement of the orifice, the saccule can obstruct the lower ureter. In boys these paraureteric saccules usually require surgical attention, whilst in girls there is a tendency for them to disappear spontaneously with maturation of the bladder base. Excision of a saccule that is closely associated with the lower ureter usually involves reimplanting the ureter.

Although diverticula may be seen on an IVU, they are best demonstrated on a voiding cystogram with oblique views. The smooth outline of the diverticulum contrasts with the appearance of the rest of the bladder. However, the exact relationship with the lower ureter may only be seen at cystoscopy.

Diverticula associated with bladder outflow obstruction pose a slightly different problem. The first priority is to deal with the outflow obstruction and only later should the diverticulum be considered in its own right.

## Bladder neck obstruction

Primary bladder neck obstruction is extremely rare and yet 30 years ago it was commonly diagnosed and many children underwent bladder neck surgery on the erroneous assumption that it was the cause of reflux. Other more common causes of bladder neck hypertrophy must be excluded before accepting a diagnosis of primary bladder neck obstruction. These include neuropathic dysfunction, posterior urethral valves and ectopic ureterocele.

An unequivocal diagnosis requires the findings of a thickened trabeculated bladder which empties poorly with urodynamically proven high pressure voiding. Urinary tract infection, difficult voiding and a palpable bladder might be expected as presenting symptoms and signs.

The diagnosis must be fully substantiated before surgery is contemplated since bladder neck incision may lead to retrograde ejaculation, incontinence and even fistula formation.

## ANOMALIES OF THE URETHRA

### Posterior urethral valve

This is the most common form of outflow obstruction in boys and represents one of the most challenging aspects of paediatric urology. Obstruction is due to a diaphragm which extends across the urethra at the apex of the prostate (Fig. 6.3). It has a slit-like opening posteriorly, the edges of which attach to each side of the lower margin of the verumontanum. The lowest part of the valve extends down into that part of the urethra which is

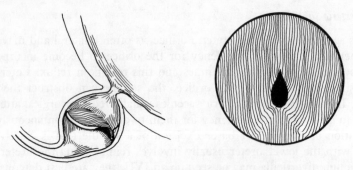

**Fig. 6.3** Posterior urethral valve

surrounded by the external sphincter complex and it can distort this structure so that even after the valve has been destroyed the sphincter may not function normally.

Above the valve there is dilatation of the prostatic urethra and this dilatation undermines the already hypertrophied bladder neck. The bladder is thickened, trabeculated and usually sacculated from the long-standing, severe obstruction. The upper tracts are dilated and the kidneys damaged to a variable degree. Reflux into one or both ureters occurs in approximately half these boys and, if unilateral, is usually associated with severe dysplasia or non-function of the kidney.

Severe obstruction from the valve usually results in presentation in the neonatal period, with a distended bladder and kidneys and impaired renal function. Dribbling, vomiting and failure to thrive are also common. Half the boys present under the age of 1 year. With lesser degrees of obstruction the signs are not so obvious and presentation may be delayed until the child notices a poor stream, haematuria or incontinence.

A baby boy with a palpable bladder should have a small infant feeding tube passed urethrally to drain the bladder and a cystogram performed. Cystography shows a thick, sacculated bladder and the posterior urethra dilated with characteristic appearances. The valve is best seen on a lateral voiding film and the presence of vesicoureteric reflux should be determined. The kidneys are best demonstrated by DMSA (dimercaptosuccinic acid) scintigraphy, since the immature neonatal kidneys handle contrast medium poorly. In older boys an IVU is more helpful but the diagnosis of a valve is primarily made by voiding cystourethrography.

Bladder drainage, correction of dehydration and electrolyte imbalance with treatment of any urinary infection are the initial priorities. When the boy is fit enough the valve should be destroyed. In infants with a narrow urethra this can be performed without anaesthesia using a thin insulated diathermy hook under X-ray control. In older boys the same procedure is applicable but the valve can be destroyed cystoscopically under direct vision using diathermy. Catheterisation before and after the valve ablation should be minimised to avoid urethral damage and urinary infection.

In boys in whom renal function does not improve on drainage it may be necessary to consider temporary nephrostomy or ureterostomy drainage. There may be temporary obstruction at the ureterovesical junction as the thick-walled bladder contracts down onto it. This improves with time and rarely is there a true, lasting obstruction at this level.

In the vast majority of boys, simple valve ablation is all that is needed. In boys with unilateral reflux and a non-functioning kidney, it is best to perform a nephroureterectomy. Careful follow-up is needed to monitor renal function and to ensure that the valve has been adequately destroyed. Reflux stops spontaneously in half the patients after relief of the valve obstruction. Associated bladder neck obstruction is rare and the bladder neck should never be incised or resected unless unequivocal obstruction has been proven, because of the risk of producing incontinence. Continence often improves spontaneously at puberty but can be helped by imipramine (Tofranil). Proteinuria is a bad prognostic sign, as all boys who develop it eventually suffer renal failure. Provided that the bladder functions adequately, these boys can be considered for dialysis and renal transplantation.

## Urethral diverticulum (Fig. 6.4)

### Posterior (bulbar) urethral diverticulum

This condition occurs in boys and is rare. It may cause persistent urinary tract infection or obstruction, and stone formation is not uncommon. The diverticulum has a narrow neck and should be excised if causing persistent problems. A diverticulum must be distinguished from a vagina or utricular cyst in a patient with an intersex disorder.

### Anterior urethral diverticulum

This may have a wide or narrow neck and probably represents incomplete reduplication of the urethra. Infection or post-micturition dribbling are presenting features.

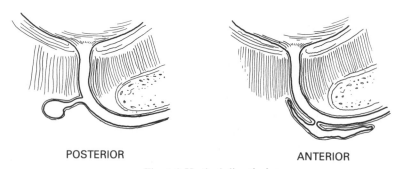

POSTERIOR                    ANTERIOR

Fig. 6.4 Urethral diverticulum

*Anterior urethral valve*

This is caused by occlusion of the urethra by the distal edge of an anterior urethral diverticulum. It can cause severe urethral obstruction in the neonate or chronic problems in the older patient. The leading edge of the valve or diverticulum can be incised endoscopically with diathermy, to relieve the obstruction and allow the whole diverticulum to drain into the urethra. Alternatively, a two-stage urethroplasty may be performed.

## Urethral polyp

A single pedunculated polyp may arise from the verumontanum and be of sufficient size to prolapse down the urethra and obstruct it. The lesion is seen on a cystogram and can be removed endoscopically.

## Urethral stricture

Short diaphragmatic bulbar strictures are occasionally seen without any history of trauma or infection. They are easily dilated or cut with a urethrotome but occasionally a urethroplasty may be necessary.

## Atresia of the urethra

This may be seen in association with the prune belly syndrome when there is also a patent urachus. There are usually other severe anomalies of the kidneys and the prognosis is poor.

## Megalourethra

Absence of the corpus spongiosum leads to a urethra with no support. The penis may look normal but the defect becomes obvious on voiding when dilatation of the urethra is seen. The defect is confirmed by urethrography, voiding cystography and cystoscopy. It is frequently seen in the prune and pseudo prune belly syndromes (q.v.). No specific treatment is needed.

## Urethral duplications (Fig. 6.5)

The two urethras can lie side by side or one in front of the other, the latter arrangement being more common.

Symptoms from the epispadiac type may be due to the associated upward chordee of the penis, incontinence via the accessory channel or to discharge from the sinus. If symptomatic, the extra urethra should be excised.

In the Y-duplication, the normally sited urethra is usually atretic in its distal portion and staged reconstruction is necessary. Bladder and ureteric anomalies are commonly seen in association with this type of severe abnormality.

A. EPISPADIAC                          B. HYPOSPADIAC

                                C. Y-DUPLICATION

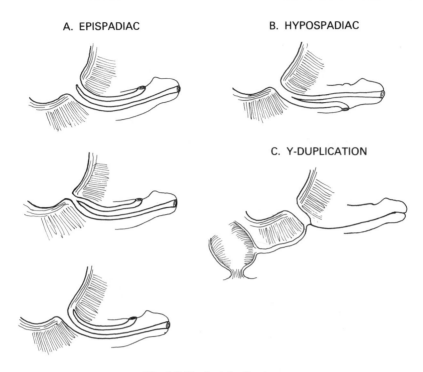

**Fig. 6.5** Urethral duplications

## ANOMALIES OF THE PENIS

### Hypospadias (Fig. 6.6)

This is a common genital anomaly occurring in approximately 1 in 400 live male births and often runs in families. The meatus opens ventrally anywhere from a few millimetres below the normal site to as far back as the perineum and is associated with a hooded (ventrally-deficient) prepuce. In general, the more abnormally sited the meatus, the more likely is there to be a downward curvature of the penis on erection (ventral chordee). However, it is possible to have marked chordee with a normal meatus or, conversely, moderately severe hypospadias with minimal chordee. Chordee is due to a combination of deficiency of the ventral skin, shortness of the urethra and the presence of tight fibrous thickening on the ventral aspect of the tunica albuginea. Other anomalies of the urinary tract can sometimes be found with hypospadias but a routine IVU is not necessary.

  The aim of treatment is to allow the patient to void with a forward pointing stream and to have a penis which is straight on erection and outwardly normal in appearance. However, it is not vital that the meatus be sited on the tip of the glans, as some of the worst complications are encountered when trying to achieve this.

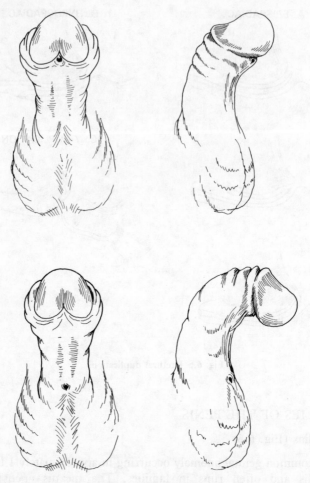

**Fig. 6.6** Hypospadias

The optimum age for operative correction is before the age of 2. This permits good maternal bonding but completes treatment before the onset of genital awareness and before the child needs to stand to void at school. It remains to be seen if late results of chordee correction are satisfactory beyond puberty.

In 70% of patients with hypospadias, the meatus is coronal or glanular so that a simple procedure can give an excellent cosmetic and functional result. The MAGPI procedure is now popular and effective. For more significant degrees of hypospadias there is a move towards one-stage procedures that correct the chordee and advance the meatus to a terminal position in a single operation. The operations that give the most consistently good results are those that use the well-vascularised inner preputial skin to reconstruct the new distal urethra.

However, even in the best hands, complications such as stricture, fistula and breakdown of the distal urethra are still seen. These are mostly due to infection, tension, overlapping suture lines and skin flap ischaemia.

### Chordee with normal meatus

The penis may have chordee with a normally placed meatus for two reasons. First, the ventral penile skin and tunica albuginea may be restrictive. In this group, it is usually possible to release the various constituents of the chordee and swing skin around from the dorsal aspect.

Second, a *congenital short urethra* may be present which can only occasionally be corrected without dividing the urethra and reconstructing it by a two-stage urethroplasty.

### Webbed penis

This is a term used when the scrotal skin extends along the ventral aspect of the penis so that, on erection, the scrotal skin is pulled up. Treatment is either to incise the web and drop the scrotal skin back or to perform a circumcision, leaving proportionally more skin on the ventral aspect.

### Parameatal cyst

This is a harmless, fluid-filled cyst on the lateral edge of the urethral meatus. Parents find it unsightly and it is easily excised.

### Buried or concealed penis

The penis can appear very short in boys with a marked fat pad in front of the pubis but, when the fat is pushed back, a normal sized penis is revealed. In addition, the skin may be inadequately attached to the penis. Surgery to attach the skin to the penis or to remove the fat pad often gives poor results. Firm reassurance whilst the child is young is probably the best management and surgery can be considered later if necessary.

### Torsion of the penis

This condition in which the penis is twisted, usually pointing to the patient's left, is seen with hypospadias and can easily be corrected at the time of the repair by modifications of the usual techniques.

### Micropenis

A micropenis is a normally formed penis that is smaller than normal but not associated with an intersex state. It is a result of lack of fetal stimulation by androgens due to testicular or hypophyseal failure. It is only rarely an end-organ response failure.

Full endocrine investigations are necessary, including an HCG stimulation test, as micropenis may be associated with some of the known syndromes of hypopituitary hypogonadism. Chromosome analysis shows a 46XY karyotype. Testosterone cream 5% should be applied to the penis daily and usually results in a rapid increase in penile size. The cream works as a result of systemic absorption so intramuscular testosterone is equally effective and more easily controlled. A surprising amount of penile growth is achieved but it is debatable if these boys ever attain normal penile size. In the unlikely event of treatment failure, consideration should be given to gender reassignment.

## MISCELLANEOUS CONDITIONS AFFECTING THE URINARY TRACT

### Prune belly syndrome (Fig. 6.7)

The components of this syndrome are absence of the abdominal wall muscles, undescended testes and general maldevelopment of the urinary

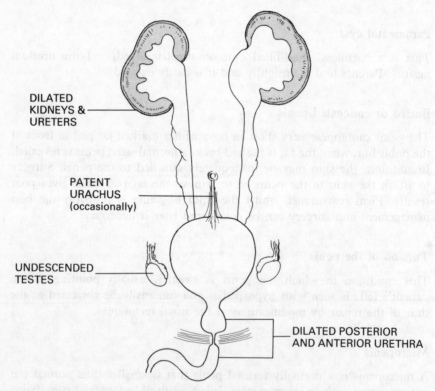

DILATED KIDNEYS & URETERS

PATENT URACHUS (occasionally)

UNDESCENDED TESTES

DILATED POSTERIOR AND ANTERIOR URETHRA

**Fig. 6.7** Prune belly syndrome

tract. The term prune belly is apt, as the abdominal wall is lax and wrinkled. In the older child, the lack of support for the abdominal contents leads to a distensible and protuberant abdomen. The true syndrome only occurs in boys.

The urinary tract defects include dysplastic kidneys, gross dilatation of the ureters and bladder, vesicoureteric reflux, dilatation of the prostatic urethra, urethral atresia, patent urachus and megalourethra. The most severe defects are incompatible with life and, overall, 50% of affected children die within 2 years. Associated gastrointestinal and cardiovascular abnormalities are common.

In less severely affected boys, the gross dilatation is not usually associated with obstruction, but stasis and inefficient drainage lead to recurrent urinary infections. Infection may be introduced at the time of cystoscopy or cystography and such investigations should only be performed if essential to exclude obstruction. The large bladder empties poorly, either because of its hypotonicity and associated gross reflux or because of posterior urethral narrowing. Long-term survival is dependent on the degree of renal dysplasia and the clinician's ability to keep the urine sterile.

Management options range from urinary diversion or total urinary tract reconstruction to a policy of non-intervention and antibiotics when necessary. The abdominal wall can be functionally and cosmetically improved by surgery but such operations are rarely performed. Orchidopexies are necessary and are best performed at a young age.

There is undoubtedly a spectrum of anomalies with some features in common with the prune belly syndrome; these are encompassed by the term *pseudo prune belly syndrome*. The abdominal wall muscles are often normal and the testes may be descended but the urinary tract is grossly dilated and dysplastic, often with a dilated posterior urethra or megalourethra. Reflux is common but not necessarily helped by reimplantation, since the contractility of the ureteric muscle is poor. Conservative treatment with high fluid intake and antibiotics, as necessary, is the best management. The differential diagnosis lies between diabetes insipidus, neuropathic bladder and bladder outflow obstruction.

## UROLOGICAL PROBLEMS ASSOCIATED WITH IMPERFORATE ANUS

Problems in the urinary tract may be part of the original anomaly or they may arise after the correction of the rectal abnormality. Thus, in any child with a lower bowel problem of this nature, an IVU is essential as part of the initial assessment.

In boys with *high rectal atresia* there is usually a fistula between the end of the bowel and the posterior urethra (Fig. 6.8).

Meconium and flatus may be passed urethrally. A colostomy is essential

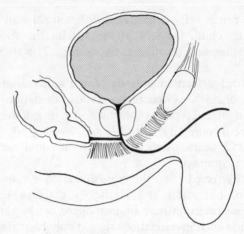

**Fig. 6.8** High anorectal agenesis

and, later, a pull-through operation for the bowel is needed, at which time the fistula is ligated.

In *low rectal atresia* the bowel may end in the bulbar urethra. This can be dealt with via a perineal approach.

In girls the high lesion results in a *high rectovaginal fistula* or a much more complex cloacal problem where there is confluence of the urethra, vagina and rectum. The low anomaly in girls is a *low vaginal or covered anus*. This can be corrected surgically via the perineum.

In the high lesions, half the infants have associated urinary tract anomalies including absence, malrotation or ectopia of the kidney, ureteric duplication, megaureter, ureterocele and hypospadias. Such lesions should be treated on their own merits. Associated defects of the vertebral column, such as hemivertebrae or missing sacral segments, may lead to a neuropathic bladder with all its problems.

Corrective surgery for the rectal anomaly may damage pelvic nerves, resulting in disturbed bladder function. Other complications include incomplete excision of the fistula with subsequent infection and stone formation, or recurrent colo-urethral fistula.

## ANOMALIES OF THE TESTIS AND SPERMATIC CORD

### Infantile hernia

Persistent patency of the upper end of the processus vaginalis in young children leaves a peritoneal sac into which bowel or omentum can prolapse (Fig. 6.9). The sac may be small or may extend into the scrotum. The neck of the sac is often tight and there is a risk of an incarcerated hernia which needs urgent surgery.

Herniation of abdominal contents is often intermittent, so that the typical

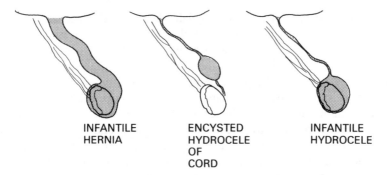

INFANTILE          ENCYSTED          INFANTILE
HERNIA             HYDROCELE         HYDROCELE
                   OF
                   CORD

**Fig. 6.9** Anomalies of processus vaginalis

bulge in the groin may not be apparent on examination. Because of the risk of incarceration it is best to explore the groin at the earliest opportunity and, if there is the slightest suggestion of a bilateral problem, the opposite groin should also be explored.

### Encysted hydrocele of the cord

This is a cystic lesion that forms in the processus vaginalis when its upper and lower parts close off. It is found in the groin or upper scrotum and is firm, irreducible and transilluminable. If there is no associated hernia, the lesion is harmless but probably best operated upon when the child is old enough for safe elective anaesthesia.

### Infantile hydrocele

If a processus vaginalis remains open as a narrow tract, it results in a hydrocele. The tract may be wide and the hydrocele fluid may be reduced by squeezing it back into the abdomen; it will then have a cough and cry impulse. This wide type of patent processus is unlikely to close off spontaneously and is best ligated at the internal ring as an elective procedure, leaving the distal sac around the testis alone. Great care should be taken to avoid disturbing the cord any more than necessary to prevent damage to the vas deferens and scarring in this region which may cause a secondary undescended testis.

A very narrow processus may close off spontaneously up to the age of 3 years and, if a hernia has been excluded, a conservative approach may be justified for the first few years.

### Varicocele in children

A varicocele is a dilatation of the pampiniform plexus of the left testis, caused by the failure of the venous valve system in the testicular vein. It is rarely seen before puberty, after which it is reported to occur in over 15% of males. The question of early varicocele ligation to avoid testicular damage and consequent subfertility is a difficult one. The left testicle below the varicocele may already be smaller than the right and it is tempting to believe that this is because of the presence of the varicocele.

The best compromise is to ligate a varicocele above the inguinal canal if it is large or if the testis is already smaller than the contralateral one. In older boys, it is possible to perform semen analysis and use the quality and quantity of sperm as a guide. The boy and his parents should, however, be warned that the success rate of surgery for varicocele is only 80–90% because secondary veins open up either in or above the inguinal canal.

## Undescended testis (Fig. 6.10)

### Classification of undescent

A testis that is not in the scrotum may either be retractile, ectopic, truly undescended or absent. To be normal, but retractile, it must reach to the bottom of the scrotum. An ectopic testis is one which has left the normal path of descent, is found in the perineum, upper thigh, base of the penis or in the superficial inguinal pouch and cannot be pushed down into the scrotum. If it *can* be pushed into the scrotum then it is not strictly ectopic.

The possible positions for a truly undescended testis (one that has stopped in the normal path of descent) are intra-abdominal, inguinal, emergent, high scrotal and mid-scrotal. Testes in the last three positions can easily swing up into the superficial inguinal pouch and be confused with an ectopic testis. Five per cent of testes that are not palpable are absent.

### Incidence

There is a 20% incidence of testicular undescent in premature boys, a 2% incidence in full term boys and a 1% incidence at 1 year. There is little evidence that testes descend spontaneously after this age. Late descent probably occurs so rarely that it should not influence clinical management. Late ascent (a testis that was in the scrotum subsequently going back into the groin) is now recognised as a more frequent event than was previously supposed. It probably does not occur to a testis that reaches right to the bottom of the scrotum. The clinical implication of this is that all testes that are not perfect should be followed up until puberty.

### Optimal age for surgery

For the reasons shown in Table 6.1, surgery should be performed by the age of 2 years. Children referred after this age should undergo operation

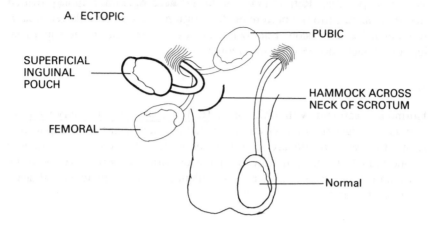

A. ECTOPIC

SUPERFICIAL INGUINAL POUCH

PUBIC

HAMMOCK ACROSS NECK OF SCROTUM

FEMORAL

Normal

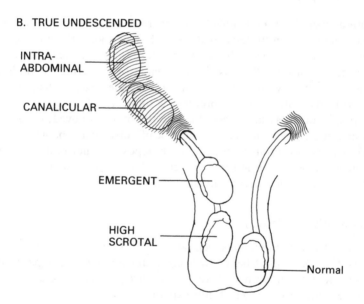

B. TRUE UNDESCENDED

INTRA-ABDOMINAL

CANALICULAR

EMERGENT

HIGH SCROTAL

Normal

**Fig. 6.10** Undescended testis

**Table 6.1** The advantages of early orchidopexy

1. Deals with the hernia (present in 90%)
2. Lessens the risk of trauma
3. Lessens the risk of torsion and makes the diagnosis easier
4. Reduces the psychological trauma
5. Increases the chances of fertility
6. *May* lessen the risk of malignancy

as soon as possible. Retractile testes do not need operating upon provided that they do reach to the bottom of the scrotum. Testes that only reach half-way down by persuasion, but spend the rest of the time in the superficial inguinal pouch, do need an orchidopexy.

### Hormone treatment

Hormone treatment with HCG or LHRH has success rates varying from 5 to 90%, suggesting that selection of patients is important. The implication is that the better results are seen with retractile testes. Use of hormones is an individual choice, but they cannot deal with the hernial sac or bring down an ectopic testis and there is a tendency for the testis to ascend again when treatment ceases.

### Malignancy risk

There is overwhelming evidence that there is a 20–30 times increased risk of malignancy in an undescended testis. Furthermore, the life-time risk for an adult of developing malignancy in a testis that remains undescended is in the region of 1 in 30. This risk is negated by removing the undescended testis after puberty and any 16-year-old, or older, should have the undescended testis removed if the problem is unilateral. If bilateral, one should be brought down as far as possible and the other removed, even though it remains uncertain if this halves the risk of subsequent malignancy.

Testes that are brought down at orchidopexy are not immune from later malignancy, but there is some evidence that the risk is reduced if orchidopexy is performed before the age of 8 years.

### INTERSEX (Table 6.2)

Severe forms of ambiguous genitalia occur in perhaps 1 in 10 000 live births, the commonest being virilising congenital adrenal hyperplasia. The management of children with these complex problems should be confined to those with special interest and experience.

In the neonatal period there should be as little delay as possible in arriving at an accurate diagnosis and plan of management, but initially it will be necessary to tell the parents that the sex of the child cannot be assigned until the results of tests are available.

A buccal smear may be misleading in the immediate neonatal period and so a chromosome analysis is performed as soon as possible, together with plasma estimations of LH, FSH, testosterone and 17-hydroxyprogesterone. Ultrasound and contrast studies of the genital sinus may help to delineate the internal organs. The decision on the sex of rearing depends not so much on the gonadal or genetic sex but more on the size of the phallus and the likelihood of it being an efficient erectile organ.

**Table 6.2**  Classification of intersex disorders

|  | Karyotype | Gonad | Genitalia | Clinical notes/treatment |
|---|---|---|---|---|
| *Gonadal dysgenesis* | | | | |
| Turner's syndrome | 45XO or variant | Streaks | Female | Sexual infantilism, short stature, primary amenorrhoea, various inconsistent physical features. |
| Klinefelter's syndrome | XXY | Seminiferous tubule dysgenesis | Male | Small, firm testes, aspermic, tall (long legs), gynaecomastia in 50%, may have mental and emotional difficulties. |
| True hermaphroditism | 46XX, 46XY, or mosaic | Ovary and testis or ovotestis | Ambig. or male | Variable int. and ext. organs, phallus, bifid scrotum, hypospadias. Surgery according to sex of rearing. |
| Mixed gonadal dysgenesis | Mosaic (XO/XY) | Streak + UDT | Ambig. or female | Short stature, mixed int. organs. Us. rear as female. Gonadectomy for cancer risk and virilisation. |
| Pure gonadal dysgenesis | 46XY | Streak | Female | Variable clitoral hypertrophy, failure of sexual development, primary amenorrhoea, gonadal cancer risk. |
|  | 46XX | Streak | Female | No clitoral hypertrophy, no gonadal cancer risk. |
| 46XX male | 46XX | Testes | Male or ambig. | Infertility, hypospadias, UDT, short stature. Genital surgery needed. Rare |
| *Male pseudo-hermaphroditism* | | | | |
| Complete androgen resistance syndrome (testicular feminisation) | 46XY | Testes (UDT) | Female | Female ext. organs, short vagina, no uterus, breasts at puberty, gonad cancer risk. Due to defective end-organ response. |
| Incomplete androgen resistance syndrome (incomplete testicular feminisation) | 46XY | Testes (UDT) | Ambig. | Small phallus, variable labioscrotal fusion and virilisation, gynaecomastia. Due to defective end-organ response. |

**Table 6.2** (contd)

| | Karyotype | Gonad | Genitalia | Clinical notes/treatment |
|---|---|---|---|---|
| Testosterone biosynthetic defects, e.g 17-ketosteroid reductase deficiency | 46XY | Testes | Ambig. (UDT) | Male int. organs, severe hypospadias, short, blind vagina, variable virilisation at puberty, variable breast development. |
| 5-alpha reductase deficiency | 46XY | Testes | Ambig. | Virilise at puberty. Failure to convert T to DHT in androgen sensitive cells. |
| Hernia uteri inguinale (persistent Mullerian structures) | 46XY | Testes (UDT) | Male | Normal phallus, uterus and tubes (may be in inguinal hernia), poor sperm and hormone production, gonad cancer risk. Can be familial. Presumed failure of MIF production. Rare. |

*Female pseudo-hermaphroditism*

| | Karyotype | Gonad | Genitalia | Clinical notes/treatment |
|---|---|---|---|---|
| Virilising congenital adrenal hyperplasia (e.g. 21-hydroxylase deficiency) | 46XX | Ovaries | Ambig. | Virilised, salt loss in 50%, uterus and upper vagina present, clitoral hypertrophy. Excess fetal androgen, raised plasma hydroxyprogesterone. Autosomal recessive. 1: 10 000 live births. |
| Transplacental androgen | 46XX | Ovaries | Ambig. | Virilised. Exogenous androgen, or from virilising tumour in mother. Rare. |

# 7

# Genitourinary tract trauma

Many patients are admitted to hospital each year as a result of trauma but only a small proportion have genitourinary tract injuries. In most cases, injuries to other systems take precedence. However, it is worth remembering that 10–15% of all patients with abdominal injuries have associated injuries to the urinary tract. Failure to recognise this in the early stages may be a major source of long-term problems for the patient.

It must be stressed that, in any badly injured patient, the priorities are establishment of an adequate airway, arrest of haemorrhage, restoration of organ circulation and assessment of central nervous system status. Only after these have been attended to should any attempt be made to assess the patients for injury to the genitourinary tract.

The clinical history with particular reference to the type and site of injury may be helpful in determining the likelihood of damage to the genitourinary tract. Injuries particularly likely to produce damage are trauma to the loin or lower ribs, trauma to the pelvis and direct blows to the perineum or genitalia. Blunt trauma is, in the UK, the commonest source of injury and usually results from road traffic accidents or sporting injuries. The possibility of penetrating injury is usually clear from gunshot or knife wounds, although the injured organ(s) may be remote from the site of penetration.

Careful examination after initial resuscitation should include a search for crepitus or fractured ribs, deformities of the pelvis, superficial bruising in the abdomen, loins or perineum and obvious swelling, deformity or tissue loss in the genital region. Rectal examination should be performed if the patient's condition permits, especially if urethral rupture is suspected. Penetrating wounds should be examined for urine leakage.

The most important indicator of urinary tract trauma is the presence of *blood in the urine* which should be inspected at the earliest possible opportunity. Urine for analysis should be obtained, if possible, by spontaneous voiding but may be collected by catheterisation of the bladder, except when there is visible blood at the urethral meatus suggesting urethral rupture. The presence of even a trace of blood in the urine suggests that there has been a significant injury to the urinary tract, but the amount of bleeding does not correlate with the severity of the injury. Blood is present in the

urine of 60–70% of patients with renal injuries and in all patients with
bladder or urethral injuries.

## RENAL INJURIES

### Mechanism of injury (Fig. 7.1)

Injury to the kidney is caused by blunt trauma in 70–80% of cases, the
remainder being due to penetrating wounds. Eighty per cent of penetrating
renal injuries, usually those produced by gunshot, are associated with injury
to other abdominal organs, whereas this is seen in only 40% of patients with
blunt renal trauma.

Blunt trauma probably causes its damage by crushing the relatively
immobile kidney between the mobile anterior ends of the lower ribs and
the upper lumbar spine. This is often associated with bruising in the flank,
signs of a retroperitoneal haematoma and fractures of the lower ribs or
transverse processes of the lumbar vertebrae.

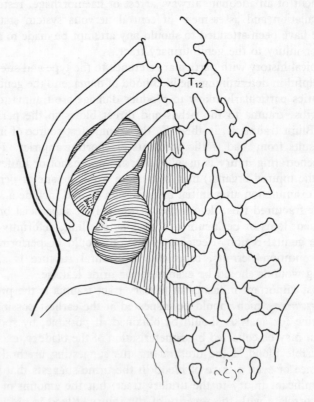

**Fig. 7.1** Mechanism of renal injury

### Clinical assessment and investigation

After the initial clinical assessment, the first step in a suspected renal injury is to perform an intravenous urogram (IVU). This is to display the extent of any injury and, perhaps more importantly, to determine the presence of a normal contralateral kidney. It should also be remembered that 10% of patients who develop haematuria after even a minor blow to the loin have an underlying abnormality of the kidney which has made it more prone to trauma than a normal kidney.

An absent nephrogram on an IVU may suggest congenital agenesis of the kidney but, more seriously, may be a sign of severe injury to the renal vasculature (e.g. renal pedicle avulsion, traumatic renal artery thrombosis). With lesser degrees of renal injury, the IVU may reveal cortical tears, extravasation of contrast medium or areas of the kidney which are not opacified (Fig. 7.2). If the IVU raises the possibility of vascular injury or shows a non-functioning kidney, then arteriography is the next step to clarify the situation but only after immediate facilities for surgery have been organised. Radionuclide studies may also give useful information about blood flow to the kidney.

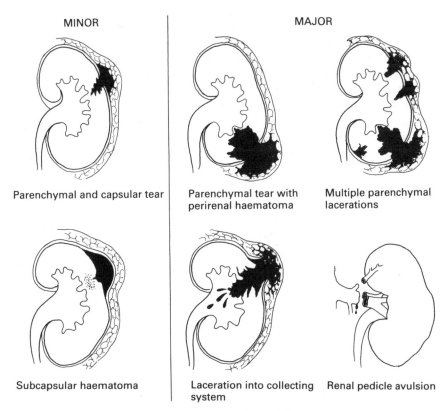

MINOR

MAJOR

Parenchymal and capsular tear

Parenchymal tear with perirenal haematoma

Multiple parenchymal lacerations

Subcapsular haematoma

Laceration into collecting system

Renal pedicle avulsion

**Fig. 7.2** Types of renal injury

In recent years, CT scanning has become popular as a means of assessing renal injuries but is not immediately available in all centres. Ultrasound is of little value in the acute phase, although it may help to follow the progress of fluid or blood collections in the longer term. Retrograde ureterography should be mentioned only to condemn it because of the risk of introducing infection into the extravasated collections of blood and urine.

## Management of renal trauma

The main aims of management are to preserve renal function and to minimise blood loss. In most cases, this can be accomplished by conservative means. Minor degrees of renal injury can be managed without surgery, as can deeper lacerations with minor degrees of urine extravasation. More major injuries require surgery only in the event of delayed or persistent bleeding.

Complete bed rest and sedation, if necessary, are prerequisites of conservative management. Blood should be taken for grouping and routine measurement of haemoglobin, urea, electrolytes and creatinine. All urine is tested for blood and, if possible, a representative sample kept for comparison with urine produced later. Regular routine observations are performed, including abdominal girth measurements if there are signs suggestive of a retroperitoneal haematoma. Fluids must be given intravenously in patients with major renal injury and oral intake restricted, since retroperitoneal haematoma is a potent stimulator of paralytic ileus. Indeed, the absence of bowel sounds is a sensitive indicator of the degree of intra-abdominal injury. In more minor degrees of injury, oral intake is permissible provided bowel sounds are normal. Antibiotics should be given to patients with any evidence of extravasation. In the presence of minor injury or of major injury with minimal urine leakage, a conservative policy results in only 10% of patients coming to operation (Table 7.1).

If surgical exploration is needed, it should be performed through an abdominal incision to allow a full laparotomy with inspection of all intra-abdominal viscera. However, it is worth remembering that laparotomy to look at a traumatised kidney frequently results in nephrectomy. Preliminary control of both renal pedicles is mandatory before exploration of a retroperitoneal haematoma. Occasionally, such a haematoma will be found unexpectedly at laparotomy for injury to other organs. In this case, an 'on-

**Table 7.1** Indications for surgery in renal trauma

Expanding retroperitoneal haematoma with signs of progressive blood loss
Severe urinary extravasation on IVU
Proven renal pedicle or arterial injury
Penetrating renal trauma (high probability of multiple organ damage)

table' IVU should be performed and the haematoma only explored if the IVU indicates severe injury requiring surgery.

Devitalised areas of kidney should be excised, whilst lacerations can usually be sutured directly with appropriate attention to bleeding vessels in the edges of the laceration. It is important to close the collecting system carefully to prevent further urinary leakage, and this may be helped by using the omentum to provide vascular and lymphatic support for the kidney. Vascular injuries may require delicate arterial reconstruction or, more likely, nephrectomy.

Postoperative care is exactly as it would be for any major abdominal operation. A drain is normally left in the renal bed after nephrectomy and should be removed when drainage is minimal.

### Prognosis and follow-up

Hypertension is occasionally seen after renal injury and may occur at an early stage. This is usually renin mediated and often transient. However, it may persist in the presence of renal arterial damage or ischaemic renal segments, and surgery may then be required to remove the kidney. An arteriovenous fistula is common after penetrating renal injury and can nowadays be embolised under X-ray control without the need for surgical exploration. Long-term follow-up of all renal injuries is essential: patients should have renal scintigraphy periodically and should have regular blood pressure measurements.

## URETERIC INJURIES

Injuries to the ureter are uncommon. They may be due to external trauma, usually a penetrating injury, or may occasionally result from closed hyper-extension injuries of the spine. The commonest cause, however, is iatro-genic damage during the course of intra-abdominal surgery.

### Surgical injury to the ureter

There is evidence that, when rectifying surgical injuries to the ureter, the best results are obtained if the injury is recognised at the time of surgery and dealt with immediately. In this situation, the rate of nephrectomy may be as low as 4.5% whereas, if the injury is not recognised immediately, nearly a third of patients subsequently require nephrectomy. Delayed recognition usually results either in obstruction to the ureter with loin pain or the development of a fistula between ureter and vagina, rectum, peritoneal cavity or skin.

Inadvertent ligature or clamping of the ureter may be dealt with by releasing the ligature. However, ligation usually renders a portion of the

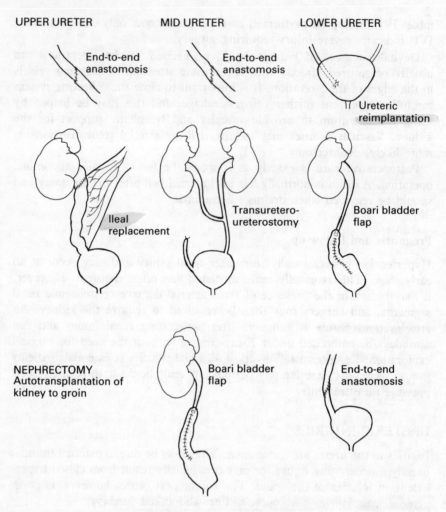

UPPER URETER    MID URETER    LOWER URETER

End-to-end anastomosis

End-to-end anastomosis

Ureteric reimplantation

Ileal replacement

Transuretero-ureterostomy

Boari bladder flap

NEPHRECTOMY
Autotransplantation of kidney to groin

Boari bladder flap

End-to-end anastomosis

**Fig. 7.3** Repair of ureteric injuries

ureteric wall ischaemic and it is best to splint the ureter for 4 weeks afterwards using a ureteric stent. If a ureteric stricture develops subsequently, it is dealt with by the methods described below.

Division of the ureter may be dealt with by a variety of means, the exact method depending on the site of the division (Fig. 7.3). Primary direct repair should only be attempted if the ureter has a good blood supply, if it has not been previously irradiated, if the patient's condition is stable and if repair can be effected without tension or obstruction. All repairs need internal splintage and external drainage, the former for at least 10 days and the latter until the risk of anastomotic leakage has passed.

Delayed presentation is uncommon and usually requires both an IVU and retrograde ureterogram to clarify the situation regarding the site and type of damage. Vital dyes such as methylene blue have also been used to colour the urine and detect sources of leakage. Such dyes are most useful in distinguishing between vesicovaginal and ureterovaginal fistulae.

One special form of injury is that produced by irradiation for malignant disease of the pelvis (e.g cervix, bladder or prostate). In this situation, primary local repair is usually doomed to failure and higher diversion is the treatment of choice.

### Congenital ureteric anomalies and trauma

It is a tribute to surgical skill that the ureter is not injured more often during pelvic operations. However, it is especially likely to undergo damage when there are unrecognised anomalies of the ureter, particularly ureteric duplication. If there is any doubt about the ureters being at risk during planned surgery or being involved by the underlying disease, then a pre-operative IVU is essential before embarking upon surgery. It may also be helpful to pass ureteric catheters cystoscopically before the procedure to aid identification of the ureters.

### Penetrating ureteric trauma

Penetrating injuries of the ureter are uncommon in this country. They are frequently associated with other injuries, especially to the duodenum, colon and major vessels. High velocity missile injuries may produce no immediate damage to the ureter but cause devitalisation with later development of a urinary fistula.

The principles for surgical repair are the same as those applied to operative ureteric injuries, except that radical excision of devitalised tissue is essential. The association of other injuries often means that this involves external diversion of intestinal contents as well as urine.

## BLADDER INJURIES

It is a function peculiar to the bladder that it can alter its shape and size radically to accommodate a large volume of urine. This is achieved by the bladder base being relatively fixed, whilst the dome of the bladder is very mobile and thin, supported only by peritoneum (Fig. 7.4).

At its fundus the bladder is so poorly supplied with muscle that it is possible under certain circumstances to get spontaneous rupture of the bladder. This tends to occur when the bladder is overdistended, as it is after a period of alcohol intake, and may be precipitated by straining at stool, childbirth or protracted vomiting.

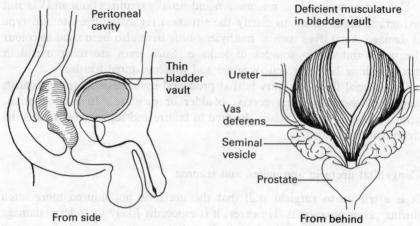

Fig. 7.4 The weak area of the bladder

## Intraperitoneal rupture of the bladder

Until the days of catheters and safer surgery, intraperitoneal rupture of the bladder was universally fatal. Typically, it occurs when a full bladder is compressed by an external force e.g. a seat belt during a motor accident or a direct blow to the lower abdomen. Less commonly, it may occur as a result of a penetrating suprapubic injury piercing a full bladder. Rupture may also be produced by a surgeon working endoscopically within the bladder, e.g. during resection of a urothelial tumour in the fundus of the bladder.

Initially, there may be no abnormal signs with intraperitoneal bladder rupture. However, it soon becomes clear that the patient is unable to void. What urine is present on bladder catheterisation is usually bloodstained and the abdomen becomes progressively distended with loss of bowel sounds. If there is blood in the urine and some doubt about the possibility of bladder damage, an IVU should be performed. This may demonstrate leakage of urine into the peritoneal cavity but the final diagnosis of intraperitoneal rupture can be confirmed by a cystogram.

Immediate surgical repair is indicated if rupture is found. This entails a full laparotomy, evacuation of all blood and urine from the peritoneal cavity and suture of the rupture in the dome of the bladder. It is probably best to give antibiotics in the perioperative period to prevent generalised peritoneal infection. The peritoneal cavity and prevesical space should be drained and the bladder drained with a urethral catheter.

## Extraperitoneal rupture of the bladder

This is usually associated with fractures of the pelvis. However, only 10% of pelvic fractures result in bladder damage, probably due to the fact that the empty bladder is rarely injured. Extraperitoneal rupture may also result from endoscopic perforations of the bladder wall or prostatic cavity as well as from 'bursting' of the bladder during Helmstein balloon distension of the bladder for interstitial cystitis, detrusor instability or bladder carcinoma.

Extravasation in extraperitoneal rupture results in blood and urine tracking up the anterior abdominal wall between the transversalis fascia and the peritoneum to cause suprapubic swelling and induration. If neglected, this becomes painful, red and tender and is associated with signs of toxaemia.

Minor degrees of extravasation can often be treated simply by urethral catheterisation for a week or so. The rupture usually seals itself off rapidly and is not associated with long-term problems. More major ruptures, usually those associated with extensive disruption of the pelvis by fractures, need exploration and drainage. The perivesical space should be exposed and drained, without opening the peritoneum, and a urethral catheter inserted into the bladder for a minimum period of 10 days.

When there are large defects in the bladder as a result of gross disruption of the pelvic ring, it may be necessary to make some attempt to reduce and fix internally the pelvic fractures to try and minimise the distraction forces being placed on the bladder. It may even be necessary to construct flaps from the dome of the bladder to cover up any defects after reconstruction of the pelvis.

Early recognition and treatment of bladder rupture are crucial. Untreated, major perforations of the bladder are associated with 100% mortality. If recognised and treated within 24 hours the mortality falls to 55% and, if within 12 hours, to 11%.


## URETHRAL INJURIES

Injuries to the female urethra are very rare; only injuries to the male urethra will be considered here.


### Injuries to the anterior urethra

By contrast with other injuries to the urinary tract, anterior urethral injuries are usually solitary and are frequently caused by instrumentation with cystoscopes, sounds, dilators or catheters. Recognition of the injury is not difficult, with extravasation of blood and urine confined to the penis and scrotum.

Diagnosis can be confirmed either by urethroscopy or urethrography using water-soluble contrast medium. Minor injuries can be treated by simple urethral catheterisation for a week. More major injuries can be treated by immediate repair of the damaged urethra, provided extensive debridement of devitalised tissue is not required. If primary repair is not possible, a suprapubic catheter should be inserted and the damage repaired at a later date when the local conditions are more favourable.

### Rupture of the bulbar urethra (Fig. 7.5)

This has traditionally been attributed to the 'straddle injury' typified by the mythical fall astride a manhole cover. Nowadays, it is far more likely to occur as a result of a direct kick to the perineum or a fall astride a bicycle crossbar.

Typically, there is bruising in the perineum and scrotum with blood visible at the urethral meatus. An ascending urethrogram using water-soluble contrast medium is useful to assess the site and extent of the rupture. If contrast medium passes readily into the bladder with a small amount of extravasation, it is permissible to pass a well-lubricated urethral catheter to try and cross the injury site. If this fails, it is best to insert a suprapubic catheter and summon expert urological help.

If the rupture seems to be complete on urethrography, there is much to be gained from primary repair, provided the tissues are reasonably healthy and the operator is experienced. A spatulated end-to-end anastomosis may produce a normal urethra without any subsequent stricturing, although further surgery may be required at a later date if a stricture does develop.

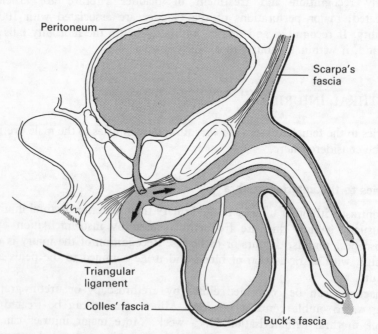

**Fig. 7.5** The anatomy of bulbar urethral rupture

In the absence of urological help, it is safest simply to insert a suprapubic catheter.

### Rupture of the prostatomembranous urethra (Fig. 7.6)

Like extraperitoneal rupture of the bladder, rupture of the membranous urethra is usually associated with fractures and gross disruption of the pelvic ring. It is therefore usually seen with other serious skeletal injuries. Such trauma almost invariably damages the pelvic nerve plexuses as well as the urethra and this often results in the patient becoming impotent in the long term.

Typically, the patient has a fractured pelvis, is bleeding from the urethral meatus and cannot pass urine. An IVU is mandatory in this situation to exclude other injuries to the urinary tract and usually shows a 'teardrop' bladder displaced upwards in the pelvis and compressed at its base by haematoma. A further clue to the diagnosis of complete rupture is on rectal examination, where the prostate is impalpable, having swung upwards and forwards.

There is some controversy about the best form of treatment for prostatomembranous urethral rupture. Those of conservative opinion recommend that a suprapubic catheter should be inserted and no other surgery performed: any subsequent stricture can then be treated at a later date.

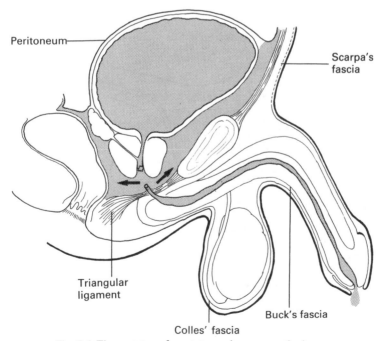

**Fig. 7.6** The anatomy of prostatomembranous urethral rupture

A more aggressive approach, however, is usually justified. A urethrogram performed under full sterile conditions with water-soluble contrast medium should reveal whether there is complete urethral disruption or whether there is continuity with only a little extravasation. If the latter is true, a well-lubricated urethral catheter may be passed with little risk of turning a partial rupture into a complete one.

If there is complete disruption on urethrography, primary anastomotic repair is doomed to failure. It is, however, well worth trying to approximate the base of the bladder and the urethra. In the past, the recommended method of accomplishing this was to apply traction on a urethral catheter. It is now realised that this can damage the bladder neck by pressure necrosis, rendering the patient permanently incontinent. It is better to explore the retropubic space, evacuate the haematoma and 'railroad' a urethral catheter into the bladder. A traction suture is then inserted through the anterior prostatic capsule and this is brought out through the perineum. Continuous low-grade traction on this suture reduces the displacement of the prostate and may prevent a stricture developing (Fig. 7.7).

If a stricture does develop as a result of an untreated prostatomembranous rupture, simple treatment of the stricture may be ineffective and complicated repair then becomes necessary. Correct treatment at the time of the initial injury often means that any subsequent stricture is relatively easy to deal with.

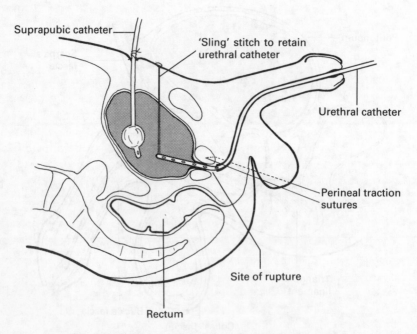

Fig. 7.7 Primary treatment of prostatomembranous rupture

## INJURIES TO THE PENIS

Simple cutaneous injuries to the penis such as the typical 'zipper' injury to the foreskin can usually be managed conservatively, although circumcision may occasionally be necessary. A torn frenulum is a common cause of penile pain and bleeding after intercourse and is readily dealt with by simple elongation of the frenulum (*frenuloplasty*) (Fig. 7.8). However, if there is any real foreskin tightness, a circumcision is better. More radical skin loss over the penis such as that caused by 'vacuum cleaner' injuries may require either skin grafts or burying of the penis in scrotal skin to provide skin cover which can, at a later date, be reconstructed into a penile tube.

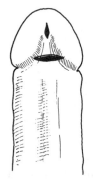 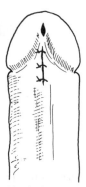

Transverse incision
across frenulum

Vertical suture

**Fig. 7.8** Frenuloplasty

Seventy per cent of penile shaft injuries occur as a result of coitus or other sexual practices. The commonest of these is 'fracture' of the penis. In this condition, the erect penis is bent acutely during intercourse. Fracture may be associated with an audible crack as the tunica albuginea ruptures. There is immediate detumescence and swelling of the penis, often with a visible deformity. Treatment is immediate exploration and repair of the defect in the tunica albuginea. Although conservative treatment may be effective in some cases, the least degree of long-term deformity and the most rapid return to normal sexual function are seen after surgical repair.

Non-disruptive coital injuries are less common. Acute bending of the penis downwards during penetration may result in rupture of the suspensory ligament of the penis (*dislocated penis*). Injury to the erectile tissue can occur without disruption of the tunica albuginea. This results in a condition known as *traumatic cavernous fibrosis* causing either impotence or deformity of the penis on erection. The treatment is to straighten the penis using Nesbitt's operation (Fig. 7.9) or to insert permanent penile prostheses to give sufficient stiffness to allow intercourse.

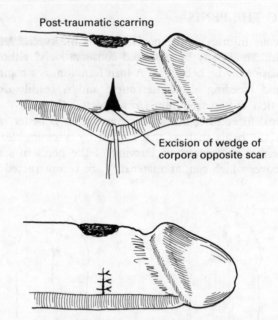

Post-traumatic scarring

Excision of wedge of
corpora opposite scar

**Fig. 7.9** Nesbitt's operation

In the long term some patients have permanent disability or deformity after penile injury but this can often be rectified by surgery. Some patients, however, inflict deliberate injury to their own genitalia and these patients, who require urgent psychiatric counselling, frequently remain disturbed.

## INJURIES TO THE SCROTUM AND TESTES

Direct blows to the scrotum are the usual cause of damage to the testes or scrotal skin. Avulsion of scrotal skin may require skin grafting or the exposed testes may need to be implanted into pockets of skin fashioned in the thighs, later being reconstructed into a neoscrotum.

Disruptive injuries to the testes are unusual, mainly because of their mobility within the scrotum. However, the presence of a large haematoma in the scrotum should alert the surgeon to the possibility of a haematocele or rupture of the testis. In this situation early surgical exploration is advisable to preserve testicular function if at all possible. Reconstruction of a ruptured testis can sometimes be accomplished, but often the testis is damaged beyond repair and requires removal. One should always be aware in this situation of a testicle which was abnormal in the first place and which was first noticed after trauma. The usual cause for this is a testicular tumour and, if this is suspected, the traumatised testis should be explored through an inguinal incision.

The scrotum and penis are especially prone to thermal burns from electric shocks since any electrical discharge, regardless of where it strikes, shows a propensity to exit from the genitalia. Such injuries usually produce significant skin loss which often heals by granulation but which may require skin grafting.

Any scrotal injury incurs the risk of developing Fournier's gangrene. If signs of infection with skin necrosis appear, aggressive treatment should be instituted with antibiotics and, if necessary, radical skin debridement (see Ch. 22).

# 8

# Urinary tract infection in adults

Infections of the urinary tract are common, affecting all ages and both sexes. Infection may be confined to one part of the urinary tract or there may be diffuse involvement; its effects vary widely, ranging from asymptomatic colonisation to severe disease complicated by renal damage or septicaemia (Fig. 8.1). In the male, infection of the genital tract (prostatitis, epididymitis) may also occur either separately or in conjunction with urinary infection.

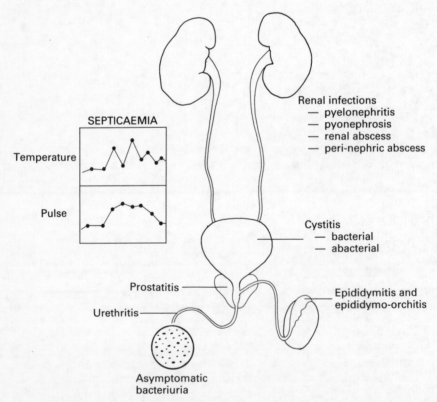

Fig. 8.1 Clinical syndromes associated with urinary tract infection

## AETIOLOGY AND PATHOGENESIS (Fig. 8.2)

The urinary tract is normally sterile above the distal urethra. The chief defence mechanisms are hydrokinetic and mucosal. Hydrokinetic defence is the more important, and is the dilution of bacteria by the flow of urine from the kidneys with periodic washout by voiding. The mucosal defences include secretion of immunoglobulin A (IgA) and the phagocytic capability of the urothelium itself. In the male, prostatic secretions also have antibacterial activity.

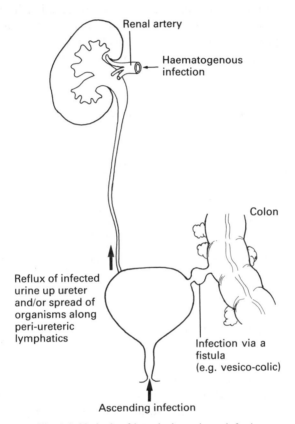

**Fig. 8.2** Methods of introducing urinary infection

### Factors predisposing to infection

Urinary tract infections are commoner in women than in men due to the shorter length of the female urethra; its site of opening at the vaginal vestibule is readily contaminated with faecal organisms. In many young women, infections are precipitated by sexual intercourse, bacteria-laden secretions from the perineum entering the urethra during sexual activity.

In either sex, infection may develop when the hydrokinetic clearance of organisms is impeded. Incomplete bladder emptying and the presence of residual urine due to outflow obstruction, bladder diverticula or neuropathic bladder leads to cystitis; upper tract stasis due to obstruction of the ureter, megaureter or stones predisposes to pyelonephritis. Vesicoureteric reflux interferes with both ureteric and bladder emptying and is commonly accompanied by infection.

Calculi, bladder tumours and foreign bodies (e.g. catheters) also predispose to infection, as may instrumentation of the urinary tract.

Factors that suppress the immune response are occasionally responsible for infection; these include diabetes mellitus and treatment with cytotoxic or immunosuppressive agents (e.g. after renal transplantation).

Common urinary pathogens are listed in Table 8.1.

**Table 8.1**   Urinary pathogens

| Ascending infection | Haematogenous infection |
| --- | --- |
| **Bacteria** | **Bacteria** |
| Gram-negative bacilli: | *Mycobacterium tuberculosis* |
|   *Escherichia coli* | *Salmonella* spp |
|   *Klebsiella* spp | *Staphylococcus aureus* |
|   *Proteus* spp | **Fungi** |
|   *Pseudomonas* spp | *Histoplasma duboisii* |
| Gram-positive cocci: | **Parasites** |
|   *Streptococcus faecalis* | *Schistosoma* spp |
|   *Staphylococcus aureus* | *Echinococcus* spp (hydatid disease) |
|   *Staphylococcus saprophyticus* | **Viruses** |
|   *Staphylococcus epidermidis* | Cytomegalovirus |
| **Fungi** | Adenovirus type II |
| *Candida* spp | |

## CLINICAL MANIFESTATIONS (Fig. 8.3)

### Symptoms

Patients with urinary tract infection (UTI) may have no symptoms, with infection being diagnosed on routine urine culture. When symptoms are present, they fall into two broad categories that reflect infection in either the lower or upper urinary tract.

In lower tract infection, voiding symptoms predominate with frequency and urgency of micturition accompanied by discomfort or a burning sensation (*dysuria*) and, occasionally, haematuria. There may be features related to an underlying cause (e.g. hesitancy and a poor stream in men with bladder outflow obstruction).

Upper tract infection is characterised by loin pain on the affected side and, unlike lower tract infection, is often associated with a systemic disturbance (fever, sweating and rigors). Some patients have lower tract symptoms as well.

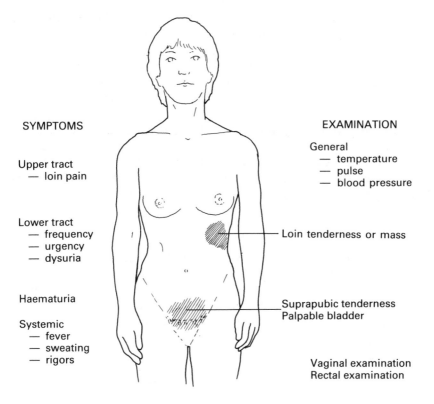

SYMPTOMS

Upper tract
 — loin pain

Lower tract
 — frequency
 — urgency
 — dysuria

Haematuria

Systemic
 — fever
 — sweating
 — rigors

EXAMINATION

General
 — temperature
 — pulse
 — blood pressure

Loin tenderness or mass

Suprapubic tenderness
Palpable bladder

Vaginal examination
Rectal examination

**Fig. 8.3** Clinical manifestations of UTI

## Physical signs

Physical signs are often scarce but there may be a fever or tachycardia and
hypertension is sometimes found in patients with significant renal damage.
Evidence of tenderness or a mass in the loin should be sought and the
suprapubic region examined for tenderness and bladder enlargement. A
vaginal examination must be performed in women to inspect the introitus
and external urethral meatus and to examine the pelvic organs. In men, the
epididymis may be inflamed and rectal examination may reveal enlargement
or tenderness of the seminal vesicles and prostate.

## DIAGNOSIS

The diagnosis of UTI depends on the presence of significant numbers of
organisms in a mid-stream specimen of urine (MSU); suprapubic needle
aspiration of the bladder can be used if collection is difficult (e.g. in children) or the urine is likely to be contaminated.

The presence of pus cells on microscopy suggests infection, although it is not diagnostic. A Gram stain may show bacteria, typically Gram-negative rods, and is often helpful diagnostically in the acute illness.

In addition to identifying the infecting organism on culture, a quantitative estimate of the number of bacteria present should be obtained; significant infection is present if there are more than 100 000 organisms per ml of urine. Lower counts suggest contamination but should be evaluated according to the clinical findings since significant infection can be present with 10 000–100 000 organisms/ml. All microbiology laboratories determine antibiotic sensitivities, using culture plates and antibiotic impregnated discs that inhibit the growth of susceptible organisms.

Specialised bacteriological techniques may be required in certain circumstances (tuberculosis, fungal infections, viral infections).

## FURTHER INVESTIGATIONS

Cystitis in young sexually-active women is rarely associated with underlying problems in the urinary tract, so immediate investigation is not required for a first attack unless it is accompanied by haematuria or loin pain. Investigation is, however, indicated in this group of women for recurrent infections and in older women with a recent onset of infection (Fig. 8.4).

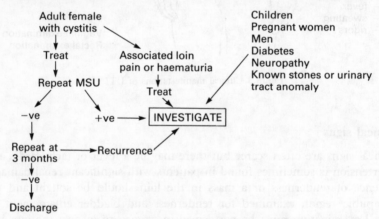

Fig. 8.4 Indications for investigation of UTI

As a routine, all patients with UTI should have a full blood count and measurement of the serum urea and creatinine.

An intravenous urogram (IVU) is the most widely used radiological investigation. Radio-opaque calculi may be seen on the plain film and other abnormalities predisposing to infection (e.g. hydronephrosis, bladder diverticula, residual urine) will be seen after contrast administration. A plain abdominal film and ultrasound of the urinary tract is normally used as a screening test instead of an IVU in patients with infection confined to the lower urinary tract.

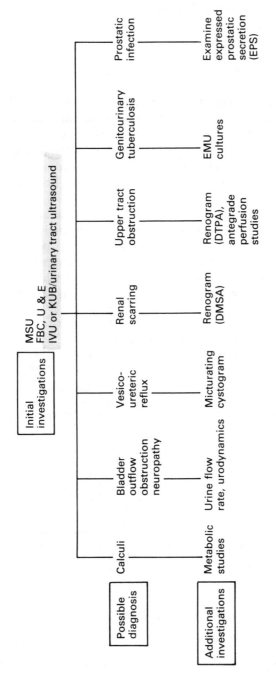

**Fig. 8.5** Investigation of UTI

Further investigations should be instituted on the basis of abnormalities detected by initial screening (Fig. 8.5).

## PRINCIPLES OF TREATMENT

Any predisposing factors found on investigation should be dealt with appropriately.

Simple measures to enhance the body's own defence mechanisms are useful; they include a high fluid intake and regular emptying of the bladder to promote hydrostatic clearance of bacteria. The patient should be instructed to empty the bladder twice on each occasion (*double micturition*) to ensure adequate bladder emptying. Attention should be paid to personal hygiene for women with recurrent cystitis and 'self-help' advice can be useful (Table 8.3).

The mainstay of treatment, however, is appropriate antibiotic therapy. The choice of agent is dictated by the results of bacteriological culture and sensitivity testing but treatment can be started on a 'best guess' policy, depending on the current pattern of infection and antibiotic resistance in the environment where the infection was acquired (Table 8.2).

In patients with collections of infected urine or pus (e.g. pyonephrosis, perinephric abscess), drainage is usually required.

**Table 8.2**   Antibiotics commonly used to treat UTI

| Agent | Oral/parenteral | Relevant antibacterial spectrum |
|---|---|---|
| Sulphonamides | O & P | Gram-negative bacilli except *Pseudomonas*. *Staphylococci*, some *Streptococci* |
| Co-trimoxazole & trimethoprim | O & P | Gram-negative bacilli except *Pseudomonas*. *Staphylococci*, *Streptococci* |
| Nitrofurantoin | O | Gram-negative bacilli except *Pseudomonas* and *Proteus*. *Staphylococci*, *Streptococci* |
| Nalidixic acid | O | Gram-negative bacilli except *Pseudomonas* |
| Ampicillin & amoxycillin | O & P | Gram-negative bacilli except *Pseudomonas* and *Klebsiella*. *Streptococci*, some *Staphylococci* |
| Cephradine | O & P | Gram-negative bacilli except *Pseudomonas*. *Staphylococci*, *Streptococci* |
| Gentamicin | P | Gram-negative bacilli including *Pseudomonas*. *Staphylococci*, some *Streptococci* |
| Ciprofloxacin | O & P | Gram-negative bacilli including *Pseudomonas*. *Staphylococci*, *Streptococci* |

## UPPER URINARY TRACT INFECTIONS

**Acute renal infections** (Fig. 8.6)

Most acute renal infections result from ascending infection (75% of patients have preceding lower tract symptoms), although some are the result of haematogenous spread.

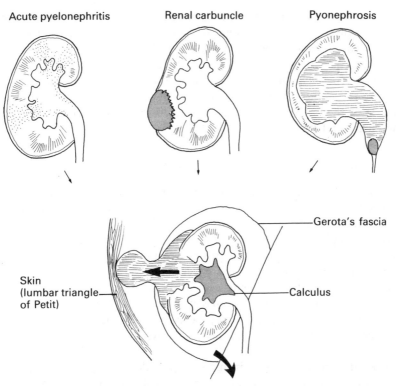

**Fig. 8.6** Acute renal infections

Several patterns of infection are seen, although the presenting features are very similar and the conditions tend to overlap. However, an important distinction must be made between infection alone and infection combined with upper tract obstruction; the latter combination may lead to rapid destruction of renal tissue unless prompt drainage of the obstructed kidney is established.

*Pathology*

*Acute pyelonephritis.* This is acute inflammation of the pelvic epithelium with bacteria entering the collecting ducts and fornices to produce inflammation of the renal parenchyma. Suppuration may ensue, producing pyonephrosis or perinephric abscess.

*Renal carbuncle.* This is an abscess in the renal parenchyma and is usually due to haematogenous spread of organisms. It typically follows a skin infection with *Staph. aureus* (from a boil or infected infusion site) or may occur in drug addicts from the use of contaminated needles. The abscess is usually confined to the renal cortex and does not communicate with the renal pelvis, so that bacteria are often absent from the urine.

*Pyonephrosis.* This is the result of infection within an obstructed kidney. The obstruction may be chronic or acute. There is rapid destruction of renal tissue if the obstruction is not relieved immediately.

*Perinephric abscess.* This can result from any of the above infective processes. Initially, the infection is confined by Gerota's fascia but may then rupture through this to reach the skin (in Petit's lumbar triangle), the psoas muscle or the bowel; it may even rupture through the diaphragm to reach the pleura and lungs.

### Clinical features

The classical symptoms of renal infection are loin pain and fever; there may also be rigors from accompanying bacteraemia and simultaneous lower tract symptoms are common.

In pyonephrosis, there may be a history of intermittent loin pain suggesting chronic obstruction. In renal carbuncle, a history of skin infection or intravenous drug abuse is often obtained.

Fever, tachycardia and tenderness in the loin are often found on examination. There may be scoliosis in severe cases, with its concavity towards the affected side and a mass may be palpable in the loin. Patients with septicaemia are occasionally shocked, with hypotension and poor peripheral perfusion.

The differential diagnosis includes intra-abdominal inflammatory lesions (e.g. diverticulitis, cholecystitis). Acute renal infections may also mimic pulmonary infection, with shallow and painful breathing on the affected side.

### Investigations

The urine should be examined for pus cells and bacteria. Urine culture is positive in most patients with ascending infection but may be negative in haematogenous infections confined to the renal cortex (e.g. renal carbuncle). Blood cultures should be taken from all patients with pyrexia or a clinical suspicion of septicaemia.

A plain abdominal X-ray may show a calculus and there may be a soft-tissue mass with absence of the psoas shadow on the affected side. Chest X-ray may show lower lobe collapse and a 'sympathetic' pleural effusion on the affected side.

An IVU will usually show enlargement of the infected kidney with poor concentration of contrast medium in acute pyelonephritis and, in renal carbuncle, a space-occupying lesion in the kidney; evidence of obstruction or non-function may be seen in pyonephrosis or perinephric abscess. In the acutely ill patient, ultrasound is of particular value in detecting pelvicalyceal dilatation from accompanying obstruction and it may also show the extent of any collections of pus.

A CT scan may help in the diagnosis of abscesses and allows guided percutaneous needle puncture to be performed to confirm the diagnosis and provide pus for culture. Renography using DMSA allows assessment of residual function on the affected side and diuresis (DTPA) renography may be used to evaluate obstruction.

## Management

In the severely ill and septicaemic patient, emergency resuscitation may be required to treat circulatory collapse. A central venous pressure line should be inserted to monitor the rapid intravenous fluid replacement that is necessary; intravenous hydrocortisone or methylprednisolone may be needed to restore an effective circulation. Parenteral antibiotics should be administered after blood cultures have been taken but subsequent management depends on the pattern of infection present.

*Acute pyelonephritis.* Antibiotic therapy is continued for 10–14 days, guided by the results of urine culture and sensitivity. The urine should then be monitored for infection over the next few weeks to detect recurrent or relapsing infection.

If not carried out in the acute phase, an IVU should subsequently be performed to evaluate the entire urinary tract and to detect any abnormality predisposing to infection. Any such predisposition should be treated as appropriate.

*Renal carbuncle.* Antibiotic therapy alone will not eradicate the infection once an abscess has become established. It may be possible to treat some patients by aspiration of the abscess under ultrasound or CT control followed by instillation of antibiotics. However, in a significant proportion of patients, formal surgical drainage is necessary.

*Pyonephrosis.* Prompt drainage under antibiotic cover is vital to prevent irreversible renal damage. This is best achieved by percutaneous nephrostomy performed under local anaesthetic. Sometimes the pus from the kidney is too thick to drain down the small cannulae that are inserted in this way so that formal surgical drainage and operative placement of a large nephrostomy tube may be necessary. Occasionally, the collecting system can be drained from below with a ureteric catheter passed retrogradely from the bladder at cystoscopy.

Once the patient's clinical condition has improved, the cause of the obstructive lesion should be investigated. An IVU may give useful information about how well the kidney works and a nephrostogram can be performed to identify the site and cause of the obstruction. DMSA renal scintigraphy will determine whether worthwhile function remains in an obstructed, infected kidney. If function is good, the obstruction should be dealt with appropriately; if poor, it is best to perform a nephrectomy.

*Perinephric abscess.* Surgical drainage under antibiotic cover is required. The precipitating cause should be dealt with in a kidney which functions well but, if function in the affected kidney is very poor, nephrectomy is the treatment of choice.

*Infection + Reflux in infancy*

## Chronic pyelonephritis (Fig. 8.7) — *Infection above an obstruction*

This is the term used to describe several different patterns of renal disease in which there is a combination of renal scarring and urinary infection. This may follow vesicoureteric reflux and infection in childhood or may develop in adult life as a result of persistent bacteriuria between repeated episodes of acute pyelonephritis. Its importance lies in the potential for serious renal damage. It has been estimated that chronic pyelonephritis accounts for 18% of adult cases of end-stage renal failure and 30% of childhood cases.

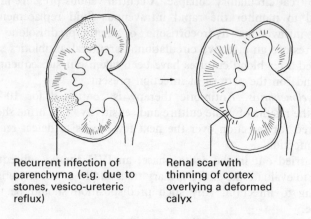

Recurrent infection of parenchyma (e.g. due to stones, vesico-ureteric reflux)

Renal scar with thinning of cortex overlying a deformed calyx

**Fig. 8.7** Chronic pyelonephritis

### Clinical features

Patients present either with recurrent symptomatic UTIs or the infection may be subclinical with bacteriuria detected only on routine urine screening; the latter is often detected during screening for hypertension or during pregnancy.

Occasionally, the disease presents at an advanced stage when chronic renal failure has occurred.

The diagnosis can be established by the finding of infection in the urine and cortical scarring which overlies a deformed calyx on the IVU.

### Management

Any predisposing cause for persistent infection should be dealt with as appropriate. Treatment is then directed towards eradicating infection and preventing further renal damage. Symptomatic infections should be treated with an appropriate antibiotic and long-term low-dose antibiotics should be considered in patients with asymptomatic bacteriuria or frequent symptomatic infections.

Nephrectomy may occasionally be required for a severely diseased kidney or for severe symptoms, provided the contralateral kidney is normal. If scarring and damage are confined to one pole of the kidney, a partial nephrectomy can be performed to preserve as many functioning nephrons as possible. The role of surgery in the treatment of vesicoureteric reflux associated with renal scarring is discussed in Chapter 9.

## Xanthogranulomatous pyelonephritis

This is the result of a granulomatous reaction within the kidney to chronic infection and is usually related to long-standing renal calculi. The resulting mass of chronically infected and poorly functioning renal tissue is often palpable and may resemble a tumour. Nephrectomy is the treatment of choice.

## LOWER URINARY TRACT INFECTIONS

The term 'cystitis' is used to indicate an inflammatory reaction within the bladder which gives rise to the typical symptoms of dysuria and frequency of micturition. Although bacterial infection is the commonest cause of cystitis, similar symptoms may occur in the absence of demonstrable infection (*abacterial cystitis*).

Primary infections of the urethra are discussed in Chapter 20.

## Acute bacterial cystitis

This is usually the result of ascending infection from the perineum. It is particularly common in women, even in the absence of any urinary tract abnormality, with up to 50% of women experiencing at least one attack during their lifetime. In men and children, infection is more likely to be associated with some abnormality of the urinary tract.

### Clinical features

Typically, there is frequency and urgency of micturition with dysuria. There may be suprapubic pain between voids and the urine often has a 'fishy' smell or may be bloodstained. In severe cases, there is a marked systemic upset with fever and even rigors from accompanying bacteraemia. Associated loin pain suggests spread of infection to the kidney (*acute pyelonephritis*).

It is important to enquire about previous infections and any predisposing factors (e.g. voiding difficulty in men, association with sexual intercourse in women).

Clinically, there is often little to find in uncomplicated cystitis, although the temperature may be elevated and there may be suprapubic tenderness. Occasionally, there are signs related to upper tract involvement or an underlying abnormality predisposing to the infection.

*Management*

It is essential that an MSU is obtained to confirm the diagnosis before treatment is commenced. However, symptoms are often severe enough to merit treatment before the MSU result is available. Simple measures that help include an increased fluid intake and alkalinising agents such as sodium bicarbonate or potassium citrate. A suitable antibiotic should be started immediately and given for a 5-day period; this can be changed, if necessary, on the basis of antibiotic sensitivity tests.

If the initial course of antibiotics produces resolution of symptoms, the MSU should be repeated at 2 weeks and again at 3 months to ensure that infection has been eradicated. The indications for further investigation following an episode of acute bacterial cystitis have been outlined earlier.

## Chronic and recurrent bacterial cystitis

In some patients, the urine may contain bacteria nearly all the time whilst, in others, recurrent bouts of infection occur with periods of sterile urine in between. Symptoms vary considerably, from minor frequency to recurrent episodes of severe acute cystitis.

Chronic inflammation in the bladder may lead to problems in the long term. Histologically, the chronically inflamed bladder may show cystic changes (*cystitis cystica*) and the development of *squamous metaplasia*. Squamous carcinoma may develop in areas of squamous metaplasia in long-standing inflammation.

*Management*

Investigation of the urinary tract with a plain film and ultrasound is useful to identify any underlying problems. An IVU is not necessary unless there are symptoms or signs of upper tract involvement. Any underlying problem should be dealt with as appropriate.

In women, 'self-help' advice may abort the full-blown symptoms of infection (Table 8.3). The empirical practice of cystoscopy and urethral dilatation helps a proportion of women and is still widely used; an alterna-

**Table 8.3**  Self-help advice for patients with cystitis

Increase fluid intake — approximately half a pint every 2 hours at the onset

Take potassium citrate or sodium bicarbonate to reduce urinary acidity

Pass urine every 2 hours by the clock once the symptoms are resolving, and try to empty the bladder twice each time ('double micturition')

Regular washing of the vulva and introitus. Avoid bubble baths, personal deodorants and talcum powder

Wipe from front to back after bowel actions

If the symptoms are precipitated by sex, empty the bladder after intercourse. The use of lubricant jelly may help

tive procedure is to irrigate the periurethral glands with saline to try and eradicate chronic infection within them.

If infection persists despite adequate treatment of any predisposing factors, the patient should be treated with long-term low-dose antibiotics to suppress multiplication of bacteria in the bladder; drugs which do not seriously affect the large bowel flora are best in this situation (e.g. trimethoprim 100 mg twice daily, nitrofurantoin 100 mg daily, co-trimoxazole one tablet twice daily). This regime should be continued for 6–12 months and, in many women, the infection does not recur after stopping treatment.

In women whose infections are precipitated by sexual intercourse, voiding and a single dose of antibiotic after intercourse may prevent infections developing.

## Abacterial cystitis

Cystitis may also be due to trauma, toxic drugs, chemicals, irradiation or viruses and related organisms such as *Chlamydia trachomatis*. In addition, interstitial cystitis is a well-recognised syndrome of unknown aetiology.

Although pus cells may be present in the urine, there are no organisms on standard culture. This clinical picture must be differentiated from that of genitourinary tuberculosis and other irritative lesions of the bladder such as calculi or tumours.

### Infective causes

Organisms such as *Chlamydia* can be isolated from the urine of some patients with abacterial cystitis if special culture techniques are used. Similarly, obligate anaerobes such as *Lactobacillus* and *Corynebacterium* may be found. These organisms are usually sensitive to the antibiotics normally used for cystitis; this explains why some patients with sterile urine seem to improve with antibiotic therapy.

Certain adenoviruses have been implicated in acute haemorrhagic cystitis and urinary symptoms sometimes accompany involvement of the sacral nerves by herpes zoster. It is possible that other cases of abacterial cystitis also have a viral origin.

### Irradiation and chemicals

Radiotherapy, given for tumours of the pelvic viscera, can give rise to florid cystitis with typical symptoms. Subsequent fibrosis may then lead to shrinkage of the bladder and persistent frequency of micturition.

Similarly, chemical cystitis can be induced by certain agents excreted in the urine. The best known example of this is *cyclophosphamide* during chemotherapy. Late fibrosis can occur from drug-induced cystitis and tumours may even develop in the long term.

Treatment of this condition is difficult. Hydrostatic bladder distension or cystoplasty may help in improving bladder capacity but urinary diversion is sometimes necessary for intractable symptoms.

### Interstitial cystitis

This unusual condition may be a form of autoimmune disease but, essentially, its cause is obscure. Symptoms, however, are often severe with frequency, nocturia, dysuria and suprapubic pain. There may be associated suprapubic tenderness on examination.

The typical finding on cystoscopy is generalised reddening of the bladder mucosa with bleeding when the bladder is emptied. Occasionally, a mucosal (*Hunner's*) ulcer can be seen, usually in the vault of the bladder. The diagnosis is made on bladder biopsy which shows an inflammatory infiltrate in the submucosa with numerous mast cells. In the long term, progressive fibrosis may lead to a small capacity bladder.

Treatment is not always effective. Systemic steroids, bladder instillations of steroids or dimethylsulphoxide (DMSO) and hydrostatic bladder distension have all been used with varying degrees of success. In some patients, symptoms are severe enough to merit excision of the bulk of the bladder and its replacement with intestine (ileum or caecum) or even urinary diversion.

## ASYMPTOMATIC BACTERIURIA

In screening studies, 1–2% of schoolgirls and 3–5% of adult women have asymptomatic bacteriuria. Males have a lower incidence, with 0.05% of schoolboys and 0.5% of adult males affected. By using ureteric and bladder sampling at cystoscopy, it has been shown that the infection originates in the upper tracts in 30–50% of patients.

To make the diagnosis of asymptomatic bacteriuria, it is important to pay meticulous attention to the collection of urine samples for culture; only when 'clean' samples are infected can it be assumed that genuine bacteriuria is present and the specimen is not simply contaminated.

### Management

In men, asymptomatic bacteriuria is usually associated with some abnormality of the urinary tract and full investigations should be instigated.

The situation is less clear in women but a distinction can be made between pregnant and non-pregnant women. If untreated, 30% of pregnant women with asymptomatic bacteriuria go on to develop acute pyelonephritis, perhaps because of the hormone-induced ureteric stasis that occurs during pregnancy. Treatment should, therefore, be given to clear the infection in pregnant women with follow-up urine cultures to confirm eradication. Investigation in pregnancy is limited to a plain abdominal film (after shielding the pelvis) and ultrasound of the urinary tract, although full radiological screening can be performed in the post-partum period.

In non-pregnant women, asymptomatic bacteriuria rarely causes long-term problems. Since the bacteriuria often recurs, the value of antibiotic treatment is doubtful. The simplest practical approach is to treat the initial finding of bacteriuria with an antibiotic and then perform post-treatment urine cultures; if infection recurs, an IVU should be performed to exclude underlying urinary tract abnormalities. If no such abnormalities are revealed on X-ray, further treatment for continued bacteriuria is probably unnecessary.

## INFECTIONS OF THE MALE GENITAL TRACT

Infections of the male genital tract may arise as a result of urinary tract infection or may occur in isolation. Infections of the epididymis and testis are discussed in Chapter 22.

### Prostatitis

The prostate may be subject to acute or chronic bacterial infection. In addition, prostatitis can occur in the absence of bacterial growth (*non-bacterial prostatitis*) and some patients present with typical symptoms but without objective evidence of inflammation or infection (*prostatodynia*).

Prostatic infection can be confirmed by examination of fractional urine specimens and expressed prostatic secretions (EPS) obtained after prostatic massage. Specimens of urine are taken from the initial part of the voided urine, from midstream and after prostatic massage. In prostatic infection, the EPS contains pus cells and bacteria whilst the post-massage urine has a higher cell and bacterial count than the MSU. In non-bacterial prostatitis, pus cells only are seen and the culture is sterile, whilst in prostatodynia, both the EPS and post-massage urine are normal.

The organisms implicated in bacterial prostatitis include *E. coli*, other faecal organisms and *Staph. albus*; in non-bacterial prostatitis, some patients have been shown to have infection with *Chlamydia trachomatis*.

#### Clinical features

Prostatitis is seen in adult men of all ages. Typically, it causes pain in the perineum, sacrum, suprapubic area and groins. There may be associated urinary symptoms with frequency, urgency of micturition and dysuria; some patients complain of ejaculation pain and haemospermia. In acute prostatitis, there is often a systemic disturbance with fever, sweating and rigors. Spread of infection down the vas deferens can lead to concurrent epididymitis.

Abdominal examination is usually normal. On rectal examination in acute prostatitis, the prostate feels enlarged and 'boggy' and is usually exquisitely tender. If suppuration has occurred, a fluctuant abscess may be palpable within the gland. In other types of prostatitis, the physical signs are less florid with variable enlargement and tenderness of the prostate; the prostate often feels firm and it can be difficult to exclude prostatic carcinoma.

### Investigation

At presentation, the diagnosis is established by culture of EPS and fractionated urine samples. In general, an IVU or ultrasound should be performed to identify any underlying abnormalities. Cystoscopy is helpful to exclude a urethral stricture as a cause of infective prostatitis and tumours of the bladder or prostate as causes of non-infective prostatic pain.

Transrectal ultrasound is a new technique of looking at the prostate which may prove useful in assessing prostatic disease.

In patients with recurrent prostatitis, it is helpful to assess the patient's sexual partner as a possible source of re-infection; swabs should be taken from the vagina and cervix and cultured for bacteria as well as for *Chlamydia*.

### Management

Treatment of bacterial prostatitis is with antibiotics. In general, antibiotics do not penetrate the prostatic stroma well but satisfactory levels can be achieved with trimethoprim, tetracyclines, ciprofloxacin and erythromycin; prolonged treatment (for 6–12 weeks) is often required to eradicate the infection completely.

In the event of abscess formation in acute prostatitis, the pus should be drained transurethrally by cystoscopic resection of the overlying prostatic tissue to 'de-roof' the abscess. Long-term antibiotic therapy may be required in chronic prostatitis and prostatectomy should be considered in older patients.

The treatment of non-bacterial prostatitis and prostatodynia is less satisfactory. Antibiotics do help some patients, possibly by eradicating undetected *Chlamydia*. Anti-inflammatory agents (e.g. flurbiprofen) or mild sedatives (e.g. diazepam) sometimes improve symptoms. A significant proportion of these men have an underlying anxiety about cancer or venereal disease and firm reassurance is necessary to allay these fears.

## GENITOURINARY TUBERCULOSIS

The genitourinary tract is involved in 3–5% of cases of tuberculosis. Although the condition is becoming less common in the UK, it remains an important disease to diagnose at an early stage to prevent extensive damage to the urinary tract.

## Pathology

The human variety of *Mycobacterium tuberculosis* is usually responsible, although infection with bovine strains still occurs. The organism reaches the urinary tract via the bloodstream from a primary focus elsewhere, usually in the lungs. However, genitourinary tuberculosis may manifest itself years after the primary infection so that only a small minority of patients have active pulmonary disease at the time of presentation. In men, infection may also spread to the genital tract (Fig. 8.8).

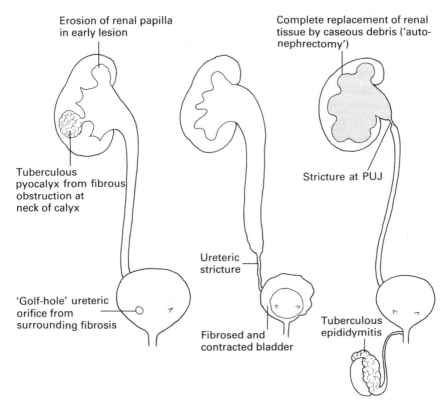

Erosion of renal papilla in early lesion

Complete replacement of renal tissue by caseous debris ('auto-nephrectomy')

Tuberculous pyocalyx from fibrous obstruction at neck of calyx

Stricture at PUJ

Ureteric stricture

'Golf-hole' ureteric orifice from surrounding fibrosis

Fibrosed and contracted bladder

Tuberculous epididymitis

**Fig. 8.8** Pathological changes in genitourinary tuberculosis

## Clinical features

The commonest presenting complaints are urinary frequency and dysuria. Other symptoms include loin pain (from upper tract obstruction), haematuria and symptoms from genital involvement. Non-specific symptoms such as lethargy, malaise and anorexia are common.

Occasionally, patients present with hypertension or end-stage renal failure. In some patients, there may also be symptoms from the primary focus (e.g. respiratory symptoms, haemoptysis).

In a proportion of patients, the disease is asymptomatic and is discovered only after finding sterile pyuria on a routine urine specimen or calcification in the urinary tract on plain X-ray.

Examination is often unhelpful. The blood pressure should always be measured and the chest examined carefully. A renal mass may occasionally be palpable and there may be signs of chronic genital infection in men.

### Investigation

The diagnosis can usually be made from culture of the urine. On a routine MSU there is sterile pyuria although secondary bacterial infection can occur. Since tubercle bacilli are scanty in the urine, they are best detected in the first early-morning specimen of urine (EMU); three such specimens should be taken on consecutive days. Acid-fast bacilli are occasionally seen on microscopy with Ziehl-Neelsen stain but confirmation of the diagnosis requires culture on Lowenstein-Jensen medium for 6 weeks. Guinea pig inoculation is rarely performed nowadays. The tuberculin skin test is usually positive in affected patients.

An IVU should be performed to assess the extent of the disease and a chest X-ray to exclude active pulmonary tuberculosis.

Cystoscopy in the acute stage of the disease reveals superficial granulations around the ureteric orifices and generalised bladder inflammation. Later, fibrosis reduces the bladder capacity and fibrosis around the ureteric orifices causes them to gape open ('golf-hole' orifices). Bladder biopsies may show histological changes of tuberculosis but should, in principle, be avoided in the acute stage because of the risk of disseminating organisms and precipitating tuberculous meningitis.

Additional investigations that may be useful include ultrasound and renography for assessment of obstruction and function.

### Management

Chemotherapy is the mainstay of treatment. Triple therapy should be commenced with isoniazid, rifampicin and pyrazinamide and continued for 2 months; pyrazinamide is then stopped and the other drugs continued for a further 2–4 months. Other agents may be needed if culture reveals resistance to first-line treatment. Careful long-term follow-up by regular urine culture is needed to confirm cure and detect any recurrence of the disease.

Chemotherapy can lead to accelerated fibrosis and this occasionally results in rapid stricturing of one or both ureters. Ureteric dilatation must be carefully monitored by urography (IVU), especially during the first few weeks of treatment. If there is any evidence of obstruction during treatment, steroids may prevent further progression but surgery is occasionally necessary to prevent renal damage.

Reconstructive surgery is required to treat obstruction of the ureter (pyeloplasty for obstruction at the pelviureteric junction, reimplantation for a lower ureteric stricture). Ablative surgery may be needed for a non-functioning kidney or for chronic epididymitis with sinus formation.

## PARASITIC INFECTIONS (Table 8.4)

A number of parasites may infect the urinary tract but all are rare in the UK. A diagnosis of parasitic infection must always be considered in patients originating from abroad or in those who have travelled abroad for business or recreation. Only schistosomiasis will be mentioned here; specialist texts should be consulted for details of other disorders.

**Table 8.4** Parasitic infections of the urinary tract

| Class of organism | Species | Clinical syndrome |
| --- | --- | --- |
| Cestode (tapeworm) | Echinococcus — granulosus — multilocularis | Hydatid disease |
| | Taenia — solium — saginata | Cysticercosis |
| Trematode (flukes) | Schistosoma — haematobium — mansoni — japonicum | Schistosomiasis (Bilharzia) |
| Nematode (roundworm) | Wuchereria bancrofti | Filariasis |

### Schistosomiasis (Fig. 8.9)

Schistosomiasis is also known as *bilharzia* after the German pathologist, Theodor Bilharz. It is endemic in Africa, the Middle East, the Far East and parts of South America. The disease is caused by a trematode fluke whose natural life cycle involves a larval stage in certain species of snail and an adult stage in man. Transmission between the two hosts is water borne. Three species cause disease in man (*Schistosoma haematobium, S. mansoni* and *S. japonicum*) but only *S. haematobium* commonly affects the urinary tract.

### Pathology

In man, the adult worms lie in pairs in the veins of the bladder; eggs are laid in the bladder submucosa and shed in the urine. The eggs cause an intense inflammatory reaction within the bladder wall. Calcification of the lesions then follows, together with marked fibrosis and shrinkage of the bladder.

Squamous metaplasia of the bladder mucosa is common and this may, eventually, progress to squamous carcinoma. The lower ends of the ureters, seminal vesicles and vasa may also be involved by calcification and fibrosis.

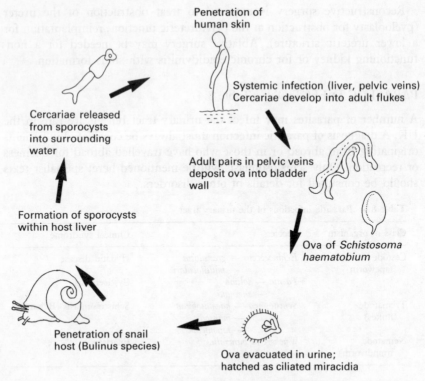

**Fig. 8.9** Life cycle of *Schistosoma haematobium*

## Clinical features

Symptoms include frequency and severe dysuria, often with accompanying haematuria. There may be painful ejaculation and haemospermia from involvement of the seminal vesicles. Later, fibrosis of the bladder wall leads to a small capacity bladder and ureteric obstruction can occur. Squamous carcinoma may be the presenting feature in some patients; in Egypt where schistosomiasis affects 35% of the population, 60% of patients with carcinoma of the bladder have schistosomal eggs in the bladder wall.

## Investigation

Diagnosis depends on the identification of schistosomal eggs in biopsies of the bladder wall or in the urine; eggs in the urine are most plentiful in the terminal part of a mid-morning specimen. A serological test (enzyme-linked immunosorbent assay, ELISA) is now available as a diagnostic aid.

There may be calcification in the bladder wall or seminal vesicles on the plain abdominal X-ray. An IVU allows evaluation of ureteric obstruction and bladder capacity and, in squamous carcinoma, a filling defect may be seen in the bladder.

*Management*

Treatment of the acute infestation with praziquantel or metrifonate is effective, although re-infection is frequent in endemic areas. Public health measures are required in endemic areas to kill the snails and break into the normal life cycle by providing clean water supplies and safe sewage disposal.

Surgery is reserved for complications of the disease. This includes augmentation cystoplasty for bladder contracture and reimplantation of the ureters for lower ureteric fibrosis. Ureteric reimplantation has a high failure rate because of the abnormal bladder into which the ureters must be implanted. Squamous carcinoma of the bladder has a poor prognosis, is often invasive at presentation and frequently requires total cystectomy with urinary diversion.

# 9

# Urinary tract infection in children

At first glance there would seem to be no difficulty in diagnosing and treating a child with urinary infection: two problems, however, can make diagnosis difficult. First, symptoms of urinary infection in small children may be non-specific (failure to thrive, vomiting, generalised abdominal pain or fever), and several systems may be investigated before the urinary tract is implicated. Second, the collection of urine, particularly in small girls, may be difficult and bacterial contamination of the urine may be misleading. If a urinary infection is suspected it should not be difficult to prove it by showing a pure bacterial growth of 100 000 organisms per ml and more than 50 pus cells per ml. A pure culture of 10 000–100 000 organisms per ml with symptoms justifies treatment. In boys, more than 10 pus cells per ml usually indicates an infection.

After being given a drink most chidren will be able to void into a plastic or foil container. Stick-on bags are useful in very small children but occasionally suprapubic puncture may be necessary.

The nature of the organisms may also be relevant. Persistent *Proteus* infection suggests a urinary anomaly or calculi; *Staph. epidermidis* and *Strep. faecalis* are usually contaminants. The purpose of investigating a child with suspected urinary infection is to categorise the child into one of three groups. In the first and most important group there are underlying anomalies, such as reflux or obstruction that can, under certain circumstances, lead to rapid deterioration in renal function. These may need urgent treatment with antibiotics or immediate operative management. In the second group, relatively harmless anomalies are identified such as duplications of the upper tract or a bladder diverticulum. Knowledge of these anomalies may be important in long-term management but they do not usually require urgent action.

Approximately 40% of children who present with a first urinary infection will fall into one or other of the above groups. The remainder will be found to have a normal urinary tract; it is just as important to know this so that child and parents can be reassured.

## PHYSICAL EXAMINATION

This is essential to look for a palpable bladder, enlarged kidneys or other abdominal masses, phimosis or fused labial folds. A fresh specimen of urine should be tested for evidence of infection. A dip slide is a simple culture medium stick that allows the specimen to be taken by the parents at home or by the general practitioner (Fig. 9.1).

## INVESTIGATION (Fig. 9.1)

### Intravenous urogram (IVU)

This test remains an important investigation but is now rarely the best initial test in small children. This is because neonatal kidneys do not handle urographic contrast medium well and the results may, therefore, be inconclusive. In this age group, other less invasive studies can give the same information and, in many cases, are *more* helpful than the IVU.

### Micturating cystourethrography (MCU)

This is a key investigation in neonates and other small children in whom it is important to diagnose reflux. In boys it also gives information about the outflow tract and is useful to exclude problems such as a posterior urethral valve. It is, however, an uncomfortable investigation and most children dislike it.

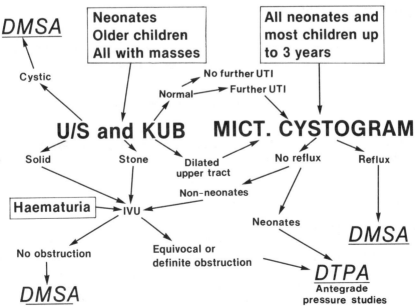

**Fig. 9.1** Flow chart of investigations. From Whitaker R H, Sherwood T 1987 Lancet i: 1266, with permission.

## Ultrasound

This procedure should always be accompanied by a *plain abdominal X-ray* to look for bony lesions and stones. Ultrasound is capable of detecting even minor degrees of pelvicalyceal dilatation consistent with obstruction, atonic dilatation or reflux. It can detect all but the most minor degrees of renal scarring as well as anomalies such as duplications and ectopic ureteroceles. Scanning of the full bladder may show ureteroceles, tumours, diverticula and abnormal thickening. A dilated ureter may be detected behind the full bladder, suggesting ureteric obstruction or vesicoureteric reflux.

Ultrasound is a harmless, painless and cheap investigation but the quality of the results is dependent on the skill of the operator.

## DTPA (diethylenetriamine penta-acetate) renal scintigraphy

Using a gamma camera and computerised calculations, this test can give an accurate assessment of the differential function of the two kidneys and the rate of accumulation by and excretion from the kidney. If necessary, a diuretic can be given to increase urine flow from the kidney. Kidneys with poor function, however, may not respond to a diuretic, resulting in an impression of obstruction when none exists: similarly, grossly dilated pelvicalyceal systems may not empty in response to diuretic and may seem obstructed when they are not. Neonates with immature kidneys may show a response to a diuretic that is difficult to interpret.

## DMSA (dimercaptosuccinate) renal scintigram

This allows the functioning parenchymal mass of each kidney to be mapped out and also gives an assessment of differential function. It is the most reliable method of showing renal scars in reflux nephropathy.

## Percutaneous antegrade pyelography and pressure flow studies

These are carried out under X-ray control and may be needed to display the anatomy in detail and to help in determining whether a dilated system is obstructed to a significant extent.

## INFLUENCE OF PRESENT AND PAST HISTORY

It is widely agreed that a child of any age who has had multiple urinary infections should be investigated fully with an IVU and micturating cystogram. It is more difficult to advise on the child who has had one infection and is now perfectly well. In a child under 2–3 years of age who has infection for the first time, and in whom it may still be possible to prevent the kidney from scarring, a micturating cystogram is essential to look for reflux. In conjunction with the cystogram an ultrasound should be performed to look for abnormal dilatation of the upper tract, since early detection of obstruction may prevent possible renal damage.

In older children (those over 5 years of age) new scarring from reflux is most unusual so the emphasis should be less on discovering reflux; ultrasound and plain abdominal X-ray can be the first investigations in these children. Other investigations may be indicated by the results of these simple studies.

A strong family history of urinary tract abnormalities, such as reflux or hydronephrosis, a poor response to adequate antibiotics for the initial infection or the presence of fever and loin pain amongst the initial symptoms are features which should encourage early investigation by cystography and urography.

In dilated non-refluxing systems, a DTPA scintigram and antegrade puncture are the best method of showing the anatomy and degree of obstruction. It should always be remembered that there are children with conditions such as the prune and pseudo prune belly syndromes in whom there is dilatation without obstruction and in whom an operation is not only unnecessary but can make the situation worse by causing obstruction.

## UNDERLYING PROBLEMS IN CHILDREN WITH URINARY INFECTIONS

Most of the conditions detailed in Chapters 5 and 6 can present with urinary infection and they represent a broad spectrum of anomalies that may be detected during the investigation of a child with a first or subsequent infection. The management of these conditions has already been discussed, but vesicoureteric reflux merits separate consideration.

### Vesicoureteric reflux

Reflux is the passage of urine from the bladder back into the ureter. It occurs when the ureter passes through the bladder wall directly with no submucosal tunnel, either as a form of immaturity of development of that area or perhaps secondary to another anomaly such as a paraureteric diverticulum. Reflux of urine occurs when the bladder pressure exceeds the lower ureteric pressure. This reflux is demonstrated by contrast medium passing up the ureter during micturating cystography (Fig. 9.2).

As the child grows and the base of the bladder and trigone mature, the submucosal tunnel may lengthen. Thus, there is a tendency for reflux to resolve spontaneously in 75% of refluxing ureters, and this is particularly likely with lesser grades. Children with reflux are liable to urinary infections because of stasis associated with inadequate clearance of urine. However, in only a proportion of affected kidneys is there scar formation.

It is now believed that scarring only occurs when infected urine enters the renal parenchyma via collecting ducts that open abnormally. Such ducts

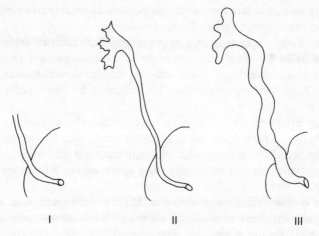

Fig. 9.2 Grading of reflux

open on to the concave part of a complex papilla. These abnormal papillae are found mostly in the upper and lower poles of kidneys and they may permit *intrarenal reflux* which can occasionally be seen during micturition cystography (Fig. 9.3). Scarring of the parenchyma drained by these abnormal collecting ducts occurs within days of the first infection and can only be modified or prevented by rapid commencement of effective treatment with antibiotics.

Thus, unless a child with intrarenal reflux is seen within a day or two of the first infection, there is little chance of preventing scarring. It is because of this risk to the kidney that the emphasis is now on the earliest possible diagnosis of reflux. Despite our efforts to detect reflux early, the fact remains that the vast majority of children who are seen with scarred kidneys already have the scarring at the initial presentation and, indeed, it is rare to see a child with a normal kidney subsequently developing a scar.

Because of this, it must be conceded that we probably have little influence over the natural history of renal damage associated with reflux. What is

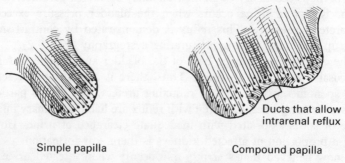

Ducts that allow intrarenal reflux

Simple papilla

Compound papilla

Fig. 9.3 Shape of papillae

needed is a test to diagnose reflux in the neonatal period before scarring has occurred but so far this test has eluded us.

Scarring of the kidney leads to a diminution in renal function in proportion to the degree of damage. It also leaves the patient more prone to the development of hypertension: 15–20% of patients with scarred kidneys develop raised blood pressure.

### Aims of treatment of reflux

It would be ideal if scarring could be prevented but achieving this is very difficult. As long as reflux is present, the patient is liable to repeated infections which can be a considerable source of morbidity; this can be a significant problem in women during pregnancy. Thus, in the lesser grades of reflux, where there is a good chance of spontaneous cessation, the treatment is directed to keeping the urine sterile with a long-term low-dose antibiotic such as trimethoprim, encouraging regular voiding and maintaining a high fluid intake. This antibiotic treatment may be needed for several years until the reflux is shown to have stopped. If a break-through infection occurs, an alternative antibiotic to which the bacteria are sensitive is given for a 2-week period and then the original suppressive antibiotic is recommenced. Cystography is needed at 2–3 year intervals to assess the reflux and either an IVU or DMSA scintigram at somewhat longer intervals to document renal growth and scarring.

In children who do not respond to this conservative management, and in some children who have more severe degrees of reflux, reimplantation of the refluxing ureters may be appropriate (Table 9.1).

Contraindications to reflux surgery include established hypertension, chronic renal failure and dysplastic ureters that lack effective peristalsis.

**Table 9.1**  Indications for surgery in vesicoureteric reflux

---

1. Poor response to antibiotics or break-through infections
2. Poor compliance to antibiotic treatment or difficulty in instituting adequate follow-up
3. Associated anomalies such as excessive ballooning of the pelvis on voiding, certain duplications of the ureter, paraureteral saccules in boys and gaping ureteric orifices (as seen cystoscopically)
4. Persistence of reflux into puberty

---

### Surgery for reflux

For lesser degrees of reflux, surgery offers a 95% cure rate without causing obstruction if one of the well-tried methods of reimplantation is used. The best known methods are the Cohen (Fig. 9.4) and Politano–Leadbetter operations, the former now being the more popular. A more recently adopted approach is to inject Teflon paste endoscopically under the ureteric orifice to prevent reflux; the early results of this procedure are encouraging.

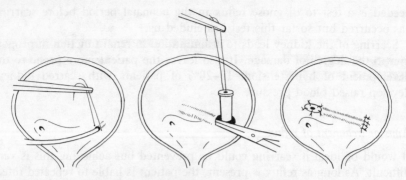

**Fig. 9.4** Cohen reimplantation of ureter

Trials comparing operative with conservative treatment in very severe reflux in infants have, so far, failed to show an advantage for either type of management.

# 10

# Urinary tract calculi

## INCIDENCE

The first records of urinary calculi are probably those of stones found among the bones of an Egyptian skeleton dating from 4800 BC and operations for stone are among the earliest surgical procedures described. There is little doubt that since the 19th century the true incidence of renal calculi has increased amongst developed nations whilst bladder calculi have become less common, except in endemic stone areas (Fig. 10.1).

Accurate figures on the prevalence of renal calculi are difficult to obtain but it has been estimated that 2–3% of the UK population have a stone in the upper urinary tract. The incidence of new stone formation shows a wide geographical variation and is between 45 and 80 per 100 000 of the population. Renal calculi are especially common in Europe, North America and Japan. The underlying reason for this is thought to be a relatively high intake of refined carbohydrate and animal protein with a low intake of crude fibre.

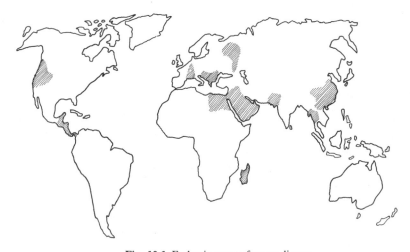

Fig. 10.1 Endemic areas of stone disease

This theory is borne out by several observations. In southern Africa, native Africans have a very low incidence of urinary calculi but white settlers, living under similar climatic and geographical conditions, have a high incidence of calculi. The number of patients presenting with stones also fell during the two world wars, times when refined food products were in short supply and crude fibre became increasingly used in the diet of the population.

Urinary calculi are more common in professional groups, particularly doctors, and less common in people with active physical occupations, provided they are not exposed to continuous high environmental temperatures. Most patients with renal calculi present in early adult life, with a peak incidence around 28 years. There is, however, a second peak at 55 years, almost exclusively as a result of infective stones in women. Overall, renal calculi are 4 times more common in men than women, although if one considers infective stones alone, they have a male/female ratio of 2:3.

## THE PATHOGENESIS OF RENAL CALCULI

The basic mechanism of stone formation remains unknown even after years of research. There are, however, a number of factors which have been recognised over the years as predisposing to stone formation (Table 10.1).

**Table 10.1**  Common identifiable causes of renal calculus formation

| | | |
|---|---|---|
| Idiopathic hypercalciuria | 65% | Some patients |
| Urinary infection | 20% | have more than |
| Cystinuria | 5% | one cause |
| Hyperparathyroidism | 4% | identified. |
| Medullary sponge kidney | 3% | |
| Hyperoxaluria | 2% | |
| Hyperuricosuria | 2% | |
| Urinary diversion (incl. ileostomy) | <1% | |
| Steroids/unknown | 5–10% | |

## Metabolic abnormalities

Most patients with a stone forming tendency have abnormal crystallisation in the urine. Stones form in the urine when solute concentrations reach supersaturation and this is especially likely to occur at low urine volumes, e.g. when a patient becomes markedly dehydrated. This tendency to crystallisation is exacerbated by diseases which result in excess urinary excretion of solutes such as calcium, oxalate, amino acids (e.g. cystine) or urate. In addition, there are naturally occurring inhibitors of crystallisation in the urine (citrate, pyrophosphate and magnesium) which may be deficient in stone formers.

The nucleus of many renal calculi is made up of microcrystals of precipitated solute embedded in a substance known as matrix, which is a mucoprotein/protein complex, probably secreted by renal tubular cells. Eighty-five per cent of stone forming patients have matrix substance A in their urine and this substance has calcium binding properties very similar to those of plasma calcium-binding proteins. Since substance A is not found in the urine of patients free from renal disease it is possible that matrix deposition may be the precursor of stone formation.

## Anatomical abnormalities

Where gross anatomical abnormalities of the kidney or ureter are not responsible for stone formation, abnormalities of microanatomy have been proposed. One theory is that the kidneys of patients who form stones possess areas of subepithelial papillary calcification (Randall's plaques) on which solutes crystallise to form microcalculi: these plaques then slough off into the collecting system to form the nucleus of a larger stone. Intrarenal micro-concretions (Carr's concretions) have also been identified in some patients: these are said to form as a result of damage or obstruction to the intrarenal lymphatics and are thought to ulcerate into the collecting tubules whence they are discharged into the urine.

## Urinary infection

Typically, infective stones are large 'staghorn' calculi made of struvite (calcium magnesium ammonium phosphate; 'triple' phosphate). These are formed by the action of Enterobacteria, usually *Proteus*, which produce an enzyme, urease, that splits urinary urea to form ammonium ions, resulting in a rise in urinary pH. Urea splitting organisms are frequently found in the interstices of infective stones and are difficult to eradicate, even with prolonged courses of antibiotics.

## Idiopathic stone formation

In 5–10% of all stone formers, no abnormality can be found to account for the stone forming tendency. Most of these patients have calcium oxalate calculi and a tendency to excrete an alkaline urine. This group presents a major challenge to the metabolic physician as well as the surgeon, since these patients often continue to form stones over a period of years.

## ASSESSMENT OF THE STONE FORMING PATIENT

### History

It is important to obtain a detailed history from all such patients and special attention should be paid to the number of urinary infections, calcium and fluid intake, occupation, symptoms of hypercalcaemia, hypertension or renal failure and periods of residence in the tropics. In addition, there may be a strong family history of stone disease in patients with conditions such as cystinuria and hyperoxaluria.

## Clinical examination

A full examination is essential which must include taking the temperature and a careful abdominal examination to detect subcostal and loin tenderness or enlargement of the kidneys. In women, it may be possible to feel a stone in the lower ureter per vaginam in the lateral fornix.

## Laboratory investigations

Urine microscopy reveals microscopic haematuria in 80% of patients with upper tract calculi. Pyuria is also common in the presence of stones and large crystal aggregates of calcium oxalate or urate may be seen. The presence of cystine crystals in the urine is diagnostic of cystinuria. A mid-stream specimen of urine should be cultured for bacteria and the urinary pH measured.

Calcium and phosphate concentrations should be measured in more than one 24-hour urine collection and this collection should, if possible, be performed with the patient at home on a normal diet to provide representative levels. If indicated, urine can also be assayed for urate, cystine and oxalate, although cystine can now be simply detected in urine on a single 'spot' sample (Table 10.2).

## Stone analysis (Table 10.3)

Stones which have been passed by the patient or removed by the surgeon can be analysed by simple biochemical testing, X-ray crystallography or

Table 10.2   Recommended blood investigations in stone disease

| | |
|---|---|
| Full blood picture & ESR | Urea & electrolytes |
| Creatinine | Calcium & phosphorus |
| Alkaline phosphatase | Urate |
| Total protein | Protein electrophoresis |
| Albumin | Globulin |
| Parathormone (if hyperparathyroidism is suspected) | |

Table 10.3   Relative incidence of stone types

| | |
|---|---|
| Pure calcium oxalate | 45% |
| Calcium oxalate + phosphate | 25% |
| 'Triple' phosphate (infective) | 20% |
| Calcium phosphate | 3% |
| Uric acid | 5% |
| Cystine | 3% |

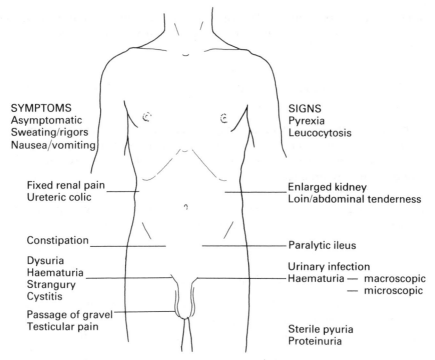

SYMPTOMS
Asymptomatic
Sweating/rigors
Nausea/vomiting

Fixed renal pain
Ureteric colic

Constipation

Dysuria
Haematuria
Strangury
Cystitis

Passage of gravel
Testicular pain

SIGNS
Pyrexia
Leucocytosis

Enlarged kidney
Loin/abdominal tenderness

Paralytic ileus

Urinary infection
Haematuria — macroscopic
— microscopic

Sterile pyuria
Proteinuria

**Fig. 10.2** Symptoms and signs in upper urinary tract calculi

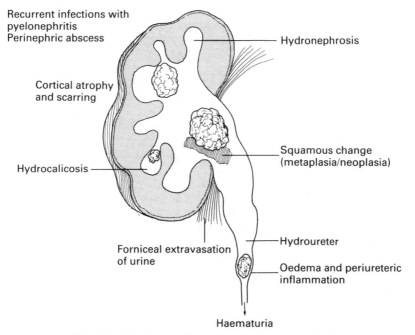

Recurrent infections with
pyelonephritis
Perinephric abscess

Cortical atrophy
and scarring

Hydrocalicosis

Forniceal extravasation
of urine

Hydronephrosis

Squamous change
(metaplasia/neoplasia)

Hydroureter

Oedema and periureteric
inflammation

Haematuria

**Fig. 10.3** Pathological effects of renal and ureteric calculi

infra-red spectrophotometry. Whilst this gives only limited information to the clinician, it may detect unsuspected stone constituents such as cystine, urate or xanthine.

## CLINICAL FEATURES OF UPPER URINARY TRACT CALCULI
(Figs 10.2, 10.3)

Stones in the kidney and ureter may produce problems ranging from no symptoms at all to severe pain radiating from loin to groin. Typically, this pain renders the patient nauseated, sweaty and pale, causes extreme restlessness and may produce hypotension.

In elderly patients with apparent left renal colic, it is important to be aware of the possibility of a leaking abdominal aortic aneurysm producing similar symptoms; such patients may even have microscopic haematuria, producing further diagnostic confusion.

## INVESTIGATIONS IN THE ACUTE PHASE

It is useful to measure the haemoglobin and white cell count together with non-specific measurements of renal function (urea, electrolytes and creatinine). The more specific investigations aimed at determining the underlying

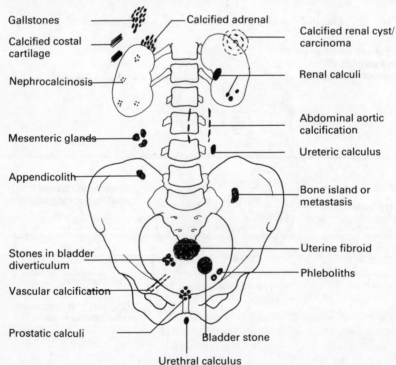

Fig. 10.4 Common calcific lesions on the abdominal film confused with stones

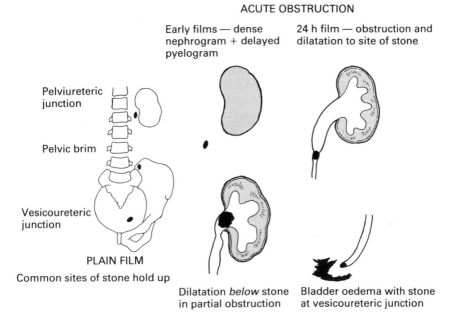

ACUTE OBSTRUCTION

Early films — dense nephrogram + delayed pyelogram

24 h film — obstruction and dilatation to site of stone

Pelviureteric junction

Pelvic brim

Vesicoureteric junction

PLAIN FILM

Common sites of stone hold up

Dilatation *below* stone in partial obstruction

Bladder oedema with stone at vesicoureteric junction

**Fig. 10.5** Urographic findings in patients with urinary calculi

cause of the stone formation can usually be performed at leisure after the acute episode has been dealt with.

A plain abdominal film will reveal 90% of all urinary calculi (Fig. 10.4). This is because nine out of ten stones contain either calcium or cystine, both of which are radio-opaque, cystine because of its sulphur content. A plain film is usually performed as a prelude to an intravenous urogram (IVU) which should be carried out as soon as possible after admission in any patient with suspected renal or ureteric colic (Fig. 10.5).

It may be difficult to determine from a simple IVU whether a stone is causing significant obstruction to urine outflow from the kidney. The simplest way to determine this is to perform a renogram (a simple probe renogram is adequate) which will give an accurate indication of whether the stone is causing significant obstruction and to what degree there is functional impairment.

## MANAGEMENT OF THE ACUTE EPISODE

This is essentially conservative in most cases. Pain should be relieved by adequate regular doses of analgesia. The drugs recommended are pethidine, buprenorphine and prostaglandin synthetase inhibitors such as indomethacin, ketoprofen or diclofenac. The latter group of drugs may be given by mouth, by suppository or by intravenous infusion. Antispasmodic drugs have little effect on pain and are not now used routinely. Anti-emetic drugs are often necessary to combat the nausea of the disease itself or that induced by pethidine.

The patient should be encouraged to remain as mobile as possible within the constraints of pain and it has become traditional to maintain a high fluid intake. All urine passed should be strained in an attempt to retrieve the stone if it is passed in hospital.

On this conservative regime, 60% of all stones pass spontaneously (half of these within 48 hours). The majority of stones that are passed spontaneously do so within 1 week of the onset of symptoms. However, 30% of stones do require surgical removal, whilst the remaining 10% may be followed expectantly.

Surgery is indicated for large stones (> 5 mm), infection with severe obstruction, failure of conservative measures and to correct anatomical abnormalities.

## SURGERY FOR RENAL CALCULI (Fig. 10.6)

Stones in the kidney may be removed by one of three methods: first, conventional open surgery via an incision in the loin, second, percutaneous puncture of the kidney or, third, extracorporeal shockwave lithotripsy.

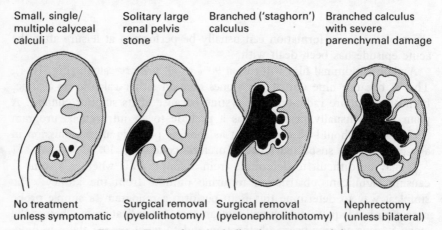

| Small, single/ multiple calyceal calculi | Solitary large renal pelvis stone | Branched ('staghorn') calculus | Branched calculus with severe parenchymal damage |

| No treatment unless symptomatic | Surgical removal (pyelolithotomy) | Surgical removal (pyelonephrolithotomy) | Nephrectomy (unless bilateral) |

Fig. 10.6 Types of renal calculi and treatment needed

## Conventional open surgery

Classically, this is carried out with the patient in the lateral position and the affected kidney uppermost. The kidney may then be exposed and the stone(s) removed via the renal pelvis (pyelolithotomy).

A similar exposure of the kidney can be obtained using a longitudinal incision parallel to the lateral border of the erector spinae muscle deepened through the underlying muscle of the abdominal wall (vertical lumbotomy).

For a 'staghorn' calculus, it may not be possible to remove all the stone fragments via the renal pelvis. In this situation, it is necessary to incise into the calyces directly through the renal substance to pick out the calyceal fragments (nephrolithotomy) after first detaching the pelvic component of the stone and removing it by pyelolithotomy. Incisions into the renal parenchyma bleed profusely so the renal artery must be dissected out and clamped to achieve haemostasis.

The kidney can tolerate the ischaemia of renal artery occlusion only for 15 minutes. If more prolonged arterial clamping is needed to remove multiple intra-renal stone fragments, the metabolic requirements of the kidney must be reduced dramatically. This can be accomplished by cooling the kidney to 15°C or by giving intravenous inosine before arterial clamping (both act as renal preserving agents). At the end of such a procedure, contact X-rays of the kidney should be taken on the operating table to ensure complete clearance of stones.

## Percutaneous nephrolithotomy (Fig. 10.7)

The morbidity associated with loin incisions has prompted a search for safer methods of removing renal calculi without incisions. This has resulted in the development of percutaneous methods of stone removal. In essence, the kidney is punctured under X-ray or ultrasound control with a needle — this can be carried out under local anaesthesia. A tract is then dilated into the kidney to gain access to the stone using graduated dilators, up to a diameter

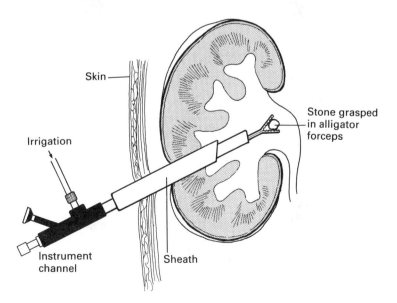

**Fig. 10.7** Percutaneous stone removal

of approximately 1 cm (30 French gauge; 30 FG). The stone can then be
removed down this tract immediately or the tract can be drained with a
nephrostomy tube and the stone removed after a delay of 48 hours.

Stone removal is accomplished under direct vision within the kidney
using special nephroscopes and a variety of grasping instruments. Stones
that are larger than the tract (> 1 cm) need to be broken into smaller pieces
before they can be removed. This can be accomplished using an ultrasound
probe which 'scales' the stone, reducing it to a fine powder, and aspirates
the powder down the centre of the probe. Alternatively, an electrohydraulic
probe may be used. This produces a shock wave within the irrigating fluid
in the kidney which breaks the stone into multiple fragments.

*or laser*

This technique has the obvious advantage that the stone can be dealt with
under direct vision without a formal incision in the loin. In addition, it is
time-saving for the patient who spends less time in hospital (often only 48
hours), it has a low complication rate and convalescence is short.

### Extracorporeal shockwave lithotripsy (Fig. 10.8)

This technique avoids the use of any sort of surgical intervention. The
procedure involves aiming shockwaves from a spark generator or piezo-

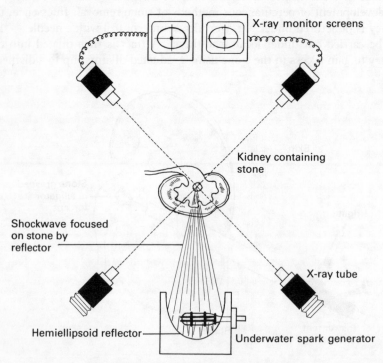

**Fig. 10.8** Extracorporeal shockwave lithotripsy

electric dish directly onto the stone under X-ray or ultrasound control. The shockwaves pass through the skin into the kidney and disintegrate the stone in situ. The patient must then pass the powdered stone fragments down the ureter over the next days and weeks.

A small proportion of patients develop ureteric colic due to passage of fragments and some require further operative intervention to remove these. Although most stones could be dealt with by this method, the initial capital outlay for equipment is substantial, and certain stones (particularly those which are radiolucent and cystine stones) are difficult to disintegrate using this method.

Contraindications :

## Post-operative follow-up

After any surgery for renal stones, long-term follow-up is important since stone recurrence is frequent. In the early stages after surgery, renography gives good information about renal function and the presence of residual obstruction and is generally performed after 6–8 weeks. At 3 months, a follow-up IVU is useful to assess renal anatomy.

## The poorly-functioning kidney containing stones

In some patients, long-standing stones in the kidney may have damaged renal function so much that the kidney is not worth preserving. A DMSA renal scintigram is a useful method of determining renal function in this situation. If the other kidney is functioning well and the kidney containing the stone contributes less than 10% of overall renal function, it is better, in this situation, to remove the entire kidney with its stones rather than attempt to remove the stones alone. However, renography whilst the kidney is acutely obstructed may underestimate the function of the kidney, so results should be interpreted with caution.

If both kidneys are affected by stones, then the best policy is to operate first on the kidney whose function is worse, delaying the second operation on the better kidney for at least 8 weeks.

Patients who present with acute obstruction and proximal infection resulting in pyonephrosis should also be assessed by renal scintigraphy. In most of these patients, the combination of infection and obstruction destroys the kidney and there is rarely much to be gained by removing the stone alone: it is usually necessary to remove the kidney.

In the past, stones in the lower pole of the kidney have been dealt with by lower pole partial nephrectomy. This, however, does not reduce the overall stone recurrence rate, since calculi form again in the new 'lower pole' of the kidney. If the lower pole of the kidney is severely thinned and excavated, then lower pole partial nephrectomy may be performed although the indications for this nowadays are rare.

## SURGERY FOR URETERIC CALCULI

Ureteric calculi may be removed by open operation (ureterolithotomy) or by endoscopic means. The indications for surgical intervention have already been discussed. In open operations, the ureter is approached extraperitoneally and incised longitudinally to remove the stone. The ureteric incision is sutured and the wound closed with drainage of the peri-ureteric area.

Stones in the lowest 5 cm of the ureter may be removed endoscopically, provided they are less than 5 mm diameter. At cystoscopy, a stone basket (Dormia, Pfister–Schwarz) is inserted into the ureteric orifice and passed up above the stone. The basket is opened within the ureter and then pulled back to engage the stone. If the stone is 'snared' it can be extracted from the ureteric orifice and washed out of the bladder (Fig. 10.9). If the stone cannot be retrieved, diathermy incision of the ureteric orifice (ureteric meatotomy) may encourage the stone to pass spontaneously over the ensuing days.

There is, however, a danger of damage to the ureter (avulsion, mucosal stripping, perforation) with this technique. To lessen this risk, rigid ureteroscopes have been developed which can be passed under direct vision into the ureteric orifice (which first requires dilatation with bougies). The ureteric calculus can then be seen directly, snared in a stone basket and removed more safely than by blind basketry. Large ureteric calculi may be disintegrated in situ and the fragments retrieved individually.

This technique may be used for stones in the upper ureter, but success

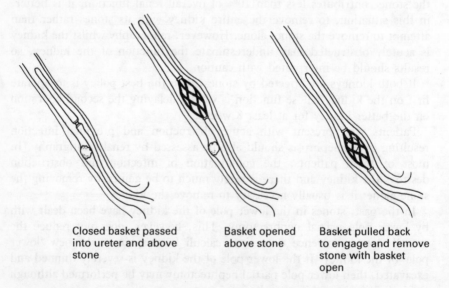

Closed basket passed into ureter and above stone

Basket opened above stone

Basket pulled back to engage and remove stone with basket open

**Fig. 10.9** Basketry for stones in the lower ureter

rates are best for stones in the lower half. Ureteric damage, however, is still a possibility even with optical instruments. If ureteroscopic manipulation fails, it may be possible to push the stone back into the kidney, whence it can be removed by one of the methods outlined above.

Occasionally, a ureteric calculus may be snared in a stone basket but the basket becomes impacted in the ureteric orifice. If this occurs, the ureteric orifice should be incised with a 'cold' knife to release the basket and stone.

## RECURRENT UPPER TRACT CALCULI

Recurrence of stones is a common occurrence in many patients. Although a recurrent stone should be treated on its own merits according to the guidelines above, there are some specific measures which have been shown to help in such patients (Table 10.4).

Stone recurrence rates in patients with idiopathic hypercalciuria may be reduced by as much as 90% by controlling the hypercalciuria using thiazide diuretics or vegetable bran. Patients with hypercalcaemia should be investigated further for hyperparathyroidism and offered parathyroidectomy if there is strong evidence of a parathyroid tumour. Cystine stones may be dissolved in situ simply by increasing the patient's fluid intake, alkalinising the urine and, sometimes, giving D-penicillamine.

Some ingenious surgical approaches have also been described but are rarely used. The replacement of the ureter by an isolated segment of ileum between the pelvis of the kidney and the bladder may allow stones forming in the kidney to pass rapidly into the bladder without causing problems. This technique, however, does result in reflux, infections and metabolic disturbances due to reabsorption of urine from the ileal segment. A better alternative may be to autotransplant the kidney into the iliac fossa and join the renal pelvis directly on to the bladder. This, too, allows stones to pass rapidly out of the kidney and, if they do not, allows cystoscopic visualis-

**Table 10.4** Medical treatment of stone disease

| | |
|---|---|
| *Hypercalciuria* | *Cystine stones* |
| low calcium diet | high fluid intake (water) |
| phytates/bran | urinary alkalinisation |
| orthophosphates | D-penicillamine |
| thiazide diuretics | |
| sodium cellulose phosphate | *Infective (struvite) stones* |
| allopurinol | urinary acidification |
| | urease inhibitors |
| *Uric acid stones* | |
| urinary alkalinisation | *Stone dissolution* |
| allopurinol | heparin |
| | citrate compounds |
| *Renal tubular acidosis* | saline |
| urinary alkalinisation | (relatively ineffective) |

ation of the kidney at which the stone may be retrieved easily from the kidney using grasping instruments.

## BLADDER CALCULI

Bladder calculi may be the result of stones passed down the ureter which have lodged and enlarged in the bladder but, more usually, bladder stones form de novo in the bladder. The usual reason for this is *bladder outflow obstruction*, although stones may form in diverticula or on foreign bodies (including catheters) in the bladder. Fifteen to twenty per cent of patients with bladder calculi do, however, have co-existing upper tract calculi.

The classical picture is one of sudden cessation of the urinary stream during voiding with severe penile or perineal pain and, often, the passage of a small amount of blood (Fig. 10.10). The pain is relieved when the patient lies down, as the stone falls back away from the trigone. Urinary infection is common when stones and outflow obstruction co-exist.

A common cause of bladder stones is a long-term indwelling catheter. Stones tend to form around the balloon of the catheter, typically taking on a crescentic shape. Stone formation may be inhibited by regular bladder washouts (usually containing citrate) and by keeping the urine acidic.

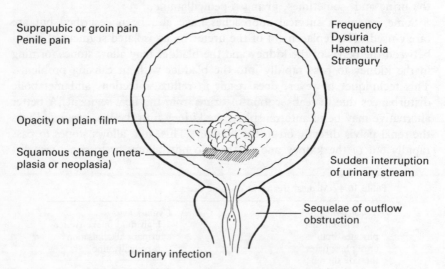

Suprapubic or groin pain
Penile pain

Frequency
Dysuria
Haematuria
Strangury

Opacity on plain film

Squamous change (meta-plasia or neoplasia)

Sudden interruption of urinary stream

Sequelae of outflow obstruction

Urinary infection

**Fig. 10.10** Symptoms and signs of bladder calculi

## Surgery for bladder calculi

Surgery involves the removal of stones and relief of the underlying cause for the stone formation (usually bladder outflow obstruction). Bladder calculi may be removed endoscopically or may require open surgical removal.

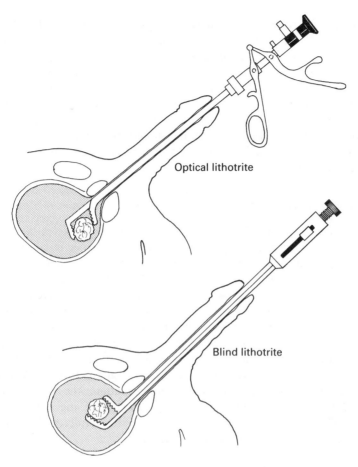

Optical lithotrite

Blind lithotrite

**Fig. 10.11** Litholapaxy for bladder calculi

Endoscopically, small stones may simply be washed out of the bladder via a cystoscope. Larger stones, however, need to be broken into fragments before removal. This can be accomplished using ultrasound or electro-hydraulic lithotripsy under direct vision. The time-honoured method, however, is *litholapaxy* (Fig. 10.11). The crushing instrument (*lithotrite*) is introduced into the bladder via the urethra and rotated with its jaws open until the stone can be gripped in the jaws. Once gripped, the stone is crushed into pieces small enough to be washed out of the bladder via a cystoscope. The traditional 'blind' lithotrite has now been replaced by optical versions which allow the stone to be seen through the instrument and crushed under vision without the risk of damaging the bladder wall.

For stones which cannot be crushed safely, open removal is indicated. This involves a suprapubic incision, opening of the bladder vault and direct removal of the stone (*cystolithotomy*).

If outflow obstruction is the cause of stone formation in the bladder, this should be dealt with appropriately. Open stone removal may be combined with retropubic or transvesical prostatectomy, although it is often safer to resect the prostate transurethrally first and then open the bladder simply to remove the stone. If the bladder is opened for stone removal, it should be drained by catheterisation for a minimum of 7 days to allow healing.

If a long-standing stone has resulted in the development of squamous carcinoma of the bladder, the stone should be removed, any outflow obstruction dealt with and the tumour managed as appropriate for its stage, grade and histology.

## URETHRAL CALCULI

Urethral stones rarely form de novo in the urethra (except in urethral diverticula) but are usually stones of bladder, ureteric or renal origin that have been passed into the urethra. Most small stones (less than 1 cm diameter) pass spontaneously down the urethra, albeit with some pain, but larger stones may impact, causing pain, bleeding and even acute retention.

In women, the stone can often be seen in the urethra and can be either removed directly or pushed back into the bladder and evacuated. Stones in the male urethra can usually be pushed back into the bladder under vision with a cystoscope and evacuated. However, impaction of the stone in the urethra can occasionally be severe enough to thwart attempts to return the stone to the bladder. In this situation, the stone must be retrieved by direct incision through the ventrum of the penis into the urethra. The urethral incision should be closed carefully and the patient subsequently catheterised for a minimum of 7 days.

## PROSTATIC CALCULI

Stones within the prostate are common and can often be seen on a plain abdominal radiograph in men with outflow obstruction. They usually form between the adenoma of benign prostatic hypertrophy and the compressed rim of prostatic tissue encircling it (the *prostatic capsule*). They are therefore not free to migrate into the urethra and are usually only released at the time of prostatectomy. It is important during prostatectomy to evacuate all these calculi since, if they remain, they may be passed subsequently and impact in the urethra.

Submucosal calculi are occasionally seen in the prostatic urethra. They may cause bleeding but rarely ulcerate through the mucosa to migrate down the urethra.

# 11

## Upper urinary tract obstruction

Whatever the cause, prolonged or severe obstruction of the upper urinary tract results in functional impairment of the obstructed kidney. It is important to recognise obstruction and to treat it promptly to avoid irreversible damage to the kidney. Obstruction which is relieved promptly may result in a return to normal renal function.

### PATHOPHYSIOLOGY

When a ureter is obstructed, continuing urine production results in distension above the site of the obstruction. This, in turn, causes a rise in intra-ureteric pressure. This pressure is transmitted via the papillae of the kidney to the nephrons and negates the filtration gradient in the glomeruli. If this situation persisted, all obstructed kidneys would cease functioning completely within a short time. Studies in chronically obstructed kidneys, however, have shown that glomerular filtration is restored even in kidneys with unrelieved obstruction. This restoration of glomerular filtration is brought about by a number of inter-connected mechanisms.

#### Ureteric dilatation

This occurs progressively with chronic obstruction of the upper tract: the ureteric muscle becomes at first hypertrophic and then, later, floppy and atonic. To some extent, this dissipates the pressure rise within the ureter caused by obstruction. Dilatation, however, is a long-term event and cannot explain why glomerular filtration continues in the short term.

#### Alternative routes for urine removal

In the early stages of obstruction, urine is redirected into renal lymphatics and collecting ducts. As obstruction continues, urine is predominantly re-absorbed into the renal veins by back-diffusion through the vasa recta. These mechanisms result in a lowering of pressure within the nephrons and restoration of a filtration gradient in the glomeruli.

155

## Papillary shutdown

This occurs when intra-ureteric pressures exceed 80 mmHg and is particularly important during episodes of acute obstruction.

## Intra-renal vascular changes

These changes are important in maintaining nephron function when the kidney is obstructed. In the first few hours after obstruction, filtration is restored by an increase in renal blood flow due to preglomerular vasodilatation; this effect is mediated by intra-renal prostaglandin E2 ($PGE_2$), a potent vasodilator, and there is some evidence that the renin–angiotensin system is also involved. As the obstruction becomes more chronic, renal blood flow begins to fall due to increased post-glomerular venous resistance and superimposed preglomerular vasoconstriction; this is mediated by the potent vasoconstrictor, thromboxane A2 ($TXA_2$). The exact mechanism of these vascular changes is poorly understood but the precipitating factor is always *raised pressure in the collecting system*. If the obstruction continues unrelieved, blood flow through the kidney does continue but at a much reduced rate.

## THE EFFECTS OF OBSTRUCTION ON RENAL FUNCTION

Glomerular filtration rate and renal blood flow are reduced in both acute and chronic obstruction, although renal blood flow rises in the early stages after obstruction. If it is accepted that raised pressure in the collecting system is the main factor in 'switching on' hormonal changes within the kidney, one would expect the most distal part of the nephron to be affected first by obstruction. Indeed, distal and collecting tubule function is impaired first, with concentrating ability in particular being reduced at an early stage. This impairment is brought about by enzymatic and metabolic changes within the tubular cells which result in altered reabsorptive capability of the distal nephron for sodium and water.

## CLINICAL FEATURES

Typically, acute obstruction of the upper urinary tract produces loin pain. This is usually localised to the loin but can radiate into the groin (cf ureteric colic). It may be associated with haematuria (microscopic or macroscopic) and with pyrexia if the urine proximal to the obstruction is infected. In addition, symptoms specific to the underlying cause of obstruction may be present.

Chronic obstruction may be totally silent. However, most patients have occasional episodes of loin pain, whilst children often describe ill-defined central abdominal pain. Any agent which produces a diuresis (e.g. alcohol) stimulates urine output by the obstructed kidney and may exacerbate the pain. This symptom pattern is especially common in patients with pelvi-ureteric junction obstruction.

Physical signs in acute obstruction are few, but the symptom of loin pain with the findings of tachycardia, pyrexia and loin tenderness are usually sufficient to suggest the possibility. In chronic obstruction, there may be little to find apart from slight tenderness in the loin although an enlarged obstructed kidney may be palpable. Bilateral upper tract obstruction is usually due to disease within or below the bladder, so it is important to feel for an enlarged bladder and to perform rectal examination for any suggestion of prostatic malignancy.

## DIAGNOSIS

In acute upper tract obstruction, diagnosis can usually be made on the characteristic history and physical findings combined with intravenous urography. The typical urographic appearances of a dense nephrogram, delayed pyelogram and dilatation of the ureter down to the site of obstruction have already been described in Chapter 10.

In chronic obstruction, the diagnosis may also be clear on an IVU. The usual appearances are of an enlarged kidney with thin renal cortex and grossly dilated calyces, often filled with layered contrast medium. When long-standing obstruction has produced gross calyceal dilatation, a *negative pyelogram* may be seen because a nephrogram develops but the calyces do not fill with contrast.

One problem area is the patient who has genuine intermittent obstruction of the kidney. Between attacks of obstruction, the IVU in a patient may appear almost normal. However, one common feature that suggests intermittent obstruction is the presence of a flat medial edge to the renal pelvis where it lies on the psoas muscle, suggesting that the pelvis has an unfulfilled capacity for distension (Fig. 11.1).

If this sign is seen during the course of an IVU, a diuretic (e.g. frusemide) should be given intravenously. This may result in further distension of the renal pelvis, making obstruction more obvious. If the use of diuretic does not clarify the situation, then an IVU performed during an attack of pain (*acute urography*) may reveal the obstruction.

Not all ureters and kidneys which are dilated on urography are obstructed. Non-obstructive dilatation, which is usually due to atony or congenital dysplasia of the ureter, does not normally cause functional impairment of the kidneys and is not an indication for surgical intervention. It is crucial, therefore, to differentiate between obstructive and non-obstructive dilatation.

If this distinction cannot be made by urography alone, radionuclide renography or antegrade perfusion studies may help. Renography, using

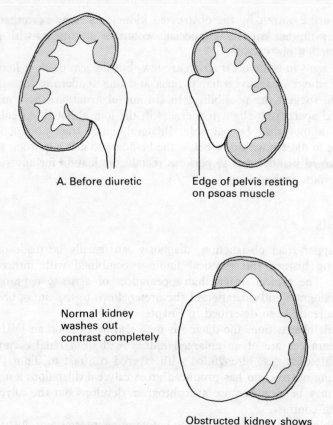

A. Before diuretic

Edge of pelvis resting
on psoas muscle

Normal kidney
washes out
contrast completely

B. After diuretic

Obstructed kidney shows
typical PUJ obstruction

Fig. 11.1 Flat medial edge in underdistended pelvis

gamma camera analysis, can be supplemented by a diuretic stimulus and
the rate of isotope transit through the renal parenchyma can be measured
to determine whether obstruction is present (obstruction causes prolonged
isotope transit) (Fig. 11.2). Renography has the advantage over an IVU that
it can also give an accurate reflection of individual renal function.

Perfusion studies involve puncturing the dilated kidney under local
anaesthesia with a small cannula and perfusing contrast medium down the
ureter under X-ray control at a constant rate (10 ml/min). The pressure
drop between kidney and bladder in response to this perfusion is measured.
A high pressure gradient (>22 cm of water) suggests obstruction, whilst a
low gradient (<15 cm of water) is regarded as normal. In difficult cases,
both renography and perfusion studies should be performed to obtain the
maximum information about anatomy and function.

Once the presence of obstruction has been confirmed and its effect on
renal function measured, it is necessary to determine the site and cause of

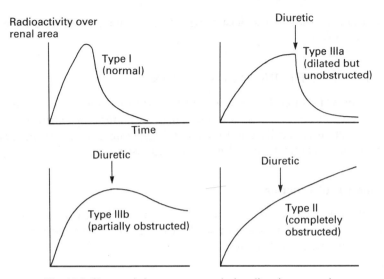

**Fig. 11.2** Characteristic patterns seen during diuretic renography

the obstruction. The site and nature of the obstruction may be obvious on the IVU but, if not, may be clarified by retrograde or antegrade uretero-pyelography, CT scanning or ultrasound.

If function is significantly impaired or symptoms are severe, then urgent relief of the obstruction is indicated. In the past, this involved operative insertion of a nephrostomy tube or retrograde cystoscopic insertion of a ureteric catheter. Nowadays, it is better to use double-J ureteric stents or radiological percutaneous nephrostomy, performed under X-ray, ultrasound or CT control (Fig. 11.3). These techniques allow the obstruction to be

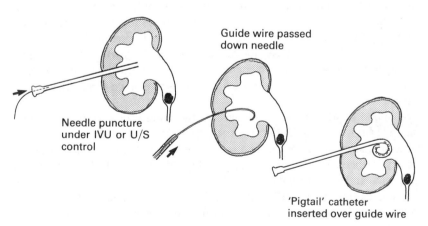

**Fig. 11.3** Percutaneous nephrostomy

relieved and investigated at leisure whilst renal function recovers from its obstructive insult.

## CAUSES OF URETERIC OBSTRUCTION

In common with all occlusive lesions of hollow tubes, the causes of ureteric obstruction can be classified as intraluminal, intramural or extrinsic. Bilateral obstruction is usually due to bladder outflow obstruction or malignant lesions of the bladder base and is considered elsewhere.

### Intraluminal obstruction

The commonest obstructive lesion seen within the lumen of the ureter is a ureteric calculus. The diagnosis and treatment of calculi obstructing the ureter are discussed in Chapter 10.

#### Renal papillary necrosis

Necrosis of renal papillae usually occurs as a result of analgesic abuse, sickle cell disease or diabetes mellitus although it can itself be the result of ureteric obstruction and infection.

The underlying cause of papillary necrosis seems to be vascular occlusion in the vasa recta causing ischaemia: as a result, the devascularised papillae are sloughed into the collecting system. The papillae are usually radiolucent, although they may calcify peripherally.

The majority of patients with renal papillary necrosis are abusers of analgesics. The typical clinical picture is of a woman with a long history of back pain and analgesic consumption who is found to have sterile pyuria, haematuria and functional impairment of the kidneys.

Intravenous urography shows 'holes' in the medulla where the sloughed papillae have been lost. In some patients, papillae which have not yet sloughed may be seen on IVU surrounded by contrast medium, giving a 'halo' appearance. A degree of renal parenchymal scarring is not unusual. Sloughed papillae may pass down the ureter and obstruct it. If calcified, a sloughed papilla is easily recognised but, if not, histology of the lesion passed by the patient or removed by the surgeon confirms that it is a papilla.

Sloughed papillae may be removed in the same way as ureteric or pelvic calculi. Endoscopic extraction is usually possible and open removal is rarely necessary, since the papillae themselves are soft and easily pulled out of the ureteric orifice from below. Subsequently, patients should be told to avoid analgesics and non-steroidal anti-inflammatory agents.

A small proportion of patients with kidneys badly damaged by analgesic abuse develop chronic renal failure and require dialysis and/or transplantation.

## Intramural obstruction

### Idiopathic pelviureteric junction obstruction

Obstruction at the pelviureteric junction (PUJ obstruction) is usually congenital. Although a number of possible causes have been postulated, the aetiology remains obscure.

It is a popular misconception that lower pole renal vessels are the cause of obstruction in most cases. Such vessels are often present and run across the pelviureteric junction, but they are truly the prime cause of obstruction in less than 5% of patients affected.

Histologically, the pelvis and pelviureteric junction show an increase in collagen and elastin with increased endoplasmic reticulum and Golgi bodies; whether these changes are primary or secondary to the obstruction is not known.

Idiopathic PUJ obstruction is commoner in males and is seen slightly more often in the left kidney. Ten to fifteen per cent of patients affected have bilateral disease. In children, obstruction may also be caused by polyps, papillomas or mucosal folds and can, occasionally, be precipitated by reflux of bladder urine into the renal pelvis (*reflux-induced PUJ obstruction*).

The basic defect at the PUJ results in ineffective peristalsis from pelvis to ureter. The result of this is that the pelvis dilates, intra-pelvic pressure rises and renal function may be progressively impaired, especially during episodes of high urine flow.

The typical clinical picture is of a child or young adult with loin pain, often precipitated by a fluid load. PUJ obstruction is occasionally asymptomatic and may be picked up only during urography or ultrasound for another problem. Some patients have microscopic or macroscopic haematuria and, if the condition is bilateral, the patient may present with hypertension or chronic renal failure.

The diagnosis is usually clear from a standard IVU. In cases where the clinical picture is less clear, renography and perfusion studies may be needed to clarify the situation. Renography should be performed in all patients to assess the contribution to overall function of the obstructed kidney. It should be noted, however, that renography may underestimate the potential function if performed whilst the kidney is still obstructed.

Treatment is by *pyeloplasty* (Fig. 11.4). In many cases, the obstruction means that the ureter below the PUJ cannot be seen on an IVU. If this is the case, a retrograde ureterogram should be performed before pyeloplasty to ensure that the ureter is normal. After pyeloplasty, the anastomosis should be temporarily splinted, by either a long-tailed nephrostomy tube or a ureteric stent.

If function in the obstructed kidney is less than 10% of overall renal function on renography, there is little point in reconstructing the PUJ, except in infants in whom the kidney has a greater potential for recovery. Other-

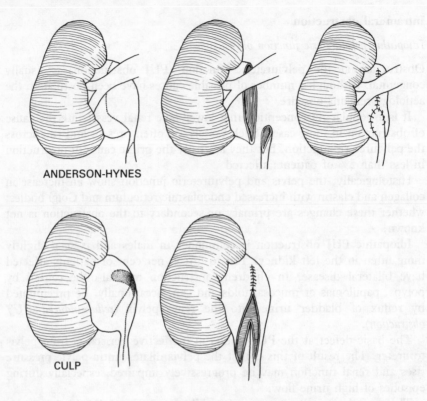

ANDERSON-HYNES

CULP

**Fig. 11.4** Pyeloplasty

wise, it is best to perform a nephrectomy, provided the contralateral kidney is functioning normally. In bilateral disease, provided overall renal function is reasonable, the poorer of the kidneys should be operated upon first, followed 3 months later by the other kidney.

Follow-up is by renography 6 weeks after surgery and by IVU 3–6 months postoperatively. Renal function in kidneys subject to PUJ obstruction improves in only one third of patients after surgery but drainage function improves in 90%. Dilatation of the calyces often persists after surgery but, provided drainage function has been improved, persistent dilatation does not mean surgical failure.

*Ureteric folds and polyps*

These can occur in adults and cause ureteric obstruction, but are more common in infants and children. The clinical picture is indistinguishable from idiopathic PUJ obstruction but the IVU shows an obvious obstructing lesion at the PUJ. Although the obstructing lesion can simply be removed, pyeloplasty is usually the best treatment.

### Ureteric strictures

The commonest causes of ureteric strictures are iatrogenic trauma (usually after pelvic or ureteric surgery) and radiation for carcinoma of the cervix, prostate or bladder. A small proportion of ureteric strictures are idiopathic and probably congenital. Local resection is appropriate for short strictures, although ureteric reimplantation is best for strictures close to the bladder.

Post-irradiation strictures, which occur in 1.5% of patients after radiotherapy for carcinoma of the cervix, present a difficult problem. Irradiated tissue heals poorly after reconstructive surgery and the presence of recurrent malignant disease must be excluded before undertaking surgical repair or urinary diversion.

### Ureteric tumours

The treatment of transitional cell tumours of the ureter is described in Chapter 16.

### Chronic inflammatory conditions

Chronic inflammatory conditions such as tuberculosis and schistosomiasis typically affect the lower ureter. Specific treatment for the underlying condition may result in an improvement in the obstruction, which should be followed carefully using serial renography. In tuberculosis, rapid progressive stricturing of the ureter can occur during treatment and should be treated by ureteric stenting.

Reimplantation of the chronically inflamed lower ureter may involve constructing a Boari bladder flap, since many strictured segments are long, fibrotic and relatively ischaemic.

### Congenital anomalies of the ureter

Orthotopic or ectopic ureteroceles may also produce ureteric obstruction. The diagnosis and treatment are discussed in Chapter 5.

### Intravesical obstruction

The lower ureter may be obstructed within the bladder by intravesical disease. The commonest causes for this are gross bladder distension by chronic retention of urine, carcinoma of the bladder and carcinoma of the prostate invading under the trigone. Treatment is directed specifically towards the underlying aetiological factor, although proximal diversion may be required temporarily to relieve the obstruction.

## Extrinsic obstruction

### Vascular lesions

Iliac or aortic aneurysms may obstruct the ureter, either by direct compression or by peri-aneurysmal fibrosis. The aneurysm should be treated as appropriate. The ureter may be freed from the obstruction (*ureterolysis*) or simply intubated until the inflammation around the aneurysm site has settled.

The right ureter is often dilated in women, especially in those who have had children. The right ovarian vein at $S_1$ level very occasionally produces genuine ureteric obstruction which can be relieved simply by resection and ligation of the vein.

Retrocaval ureter always occurs on the right side. It is due to persistence of the ventral subcardinal vein which remains as the infrarenal segment of the inferior vena cava. The ureter loops behind the inferior vena cava and may be obstructed by it. Relief of the obstruction is obtained by dismembered (*Anderson–Hynes*) pyeloplasty, although nephrectomy may be necessary if function is severely impaired.

### Benign disorders of the female reproductive system

Pregnancy commonly results in dilatation of the ureters. This is partly due to hormonal changes resulting in atony, but the enlarged uterus may compress the ureters and cause genuine obstruction. If this is the case, a ureteric stent should be inserted to relieve the obstruction which normally resolves after completion of the pregnancy.

Third degree uterine prolapse (*complete procidentia*) may obstruct the ureter by pressure on the cardinal ligaments of Mackenrodt or against the edges of the levator ani muscles. Reduction and fixation of the prolapse is usually curative.

Endometriosis occurs in 15% of pre-menopausal women. Of those women affected, 20% have urinary tract involvement, although the ureters are rarely involved. Surgical oophorectomy or danazol may relieve the obstruction. A radiation menopause should not be used, since the radiation itself may damage the ureter. If this fails, ureterolysis or reimplantation of the ureter into the bladder may be needed.

### Gastrointestinal disease

Any inflammatory condition of the gastrointestinal tract (appendicitis,

Crohn's disease, diverticular disease) may obstruct a ureter that lies in close proximity to the inflamed bowel. Ureteric obstruction usually resolves with treatment of the primary condition, although ureterolysis may be necessary.

Gastrointestinal tumours may also obstruct the ureter by direct invasion. Ureteric reimplantation, resection and ureteroureterostomy or nephrectomy may be necessary during resection of the bowel tumour.

### Retroperitoneal tumours

Although benign tumours of the retroperitoneal space may obstruct the ureters, most retroperitoneal tumours are malignant. Seventy per cent of all such tumours obstructing the ureter arise from cervix, prostate, bladder, breast, colon, ovary or uterus. Ureteric splinting is rarely helpful in such malignant conditions. Ureterolysis, reimplantation, urinary diversion or nephrectomy are usually necessary. If such procedures are contemplated, their benefit must be balanced against the problem of leaving untreatable malignancy in the pelvis and condemning the patient to a painful and unpleasant death.

### Retroperitoneal disease

The commonest retroperitoneal disease producing ureteric obstruction is *retroperitoneal fibrosis* (RPF). One third of cases are secondary to malignancy, irradiation or drugs (e.g methysergide, beta-blockers) whilst the remainder are idiopathic. There is convincing evidence that idiopathic RPF may be due to a fibrotic retroperitoneal reaction to the leakage of insoluble lipids from atheromatous plaques in the abdominal aorta.

Whatever the cause, the ureters become involved in a fibrotic plaque of tissue which pulls them towards the midline and obstructs them (Fig. 11.5). The process may also produce obstruction of the blood vessels to the lower limbs and pelvis.

Men are affected twice as commonly as women by idiopathic RPF. Typically, the clinical picture is of a man 40–60 years old with backache, a vague systemic illness and signs of renal functional impairment. There are few physical signs other than those associated with hypertension, chronic renal failure or venous occlusion.

IVU shows the typical indrawing of the ureters and this can be confirmed by retrograde ureteropyelography if necessary. Renography is useful to determine the degree of functional impairment of each kidney. Abdominal CT scanning shows the typical appearance of a peri-aortic plaque of fibrosis involving the ureters. If there is any question of malignant RPF, CT guided needle aspiration biopsy may be performed.

There is often a normochromic normocytic anaemia with raised levels of urea and creatinine and the ESR is often markedly raised. The initial treat-

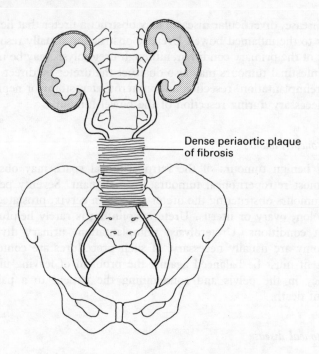

Dense periaortic plaque
of fibrosis

**Fig. 11.5** Site of the plaque in retroperitoneal fibrosis

ment is to improve renal function by ureteric stents or percutaneous nephrostomy. Once renal function has returned to stable levels, definitive treatment should be instituted.

Treatment with systemic steroids and ureteric stents has gained popularity in recent years. This technique is particularly useful when the ESR is raised: the dose of steroid can be titrated against the ESR to keep the disease under optimum control. If necessary, ureteric stents can be left in place indefinitely, especially in elderly patients.

In younger patients, the risks of long-term steroid treatment are significant and definitive surgery is preferred. This involves a laparotomy and complete freeing of both ureters from renal pelvis to bladder from the fibrotic process (*ureterolysis*) (Fig. 11.6). To prevent recurrent obstruction, the ureters are then wrapped in omentum and remain intraperitoneal. Temporary ureteric stenting and/or nephrostomy tube drainage are used in the postoperative period.

The main causes of death in idiopathic RPF are hypertension and venous thromboembolic disease. A proportion of patients with irreversible functional damage to the kidneys develop chronic renal failure requiring specific treatment.

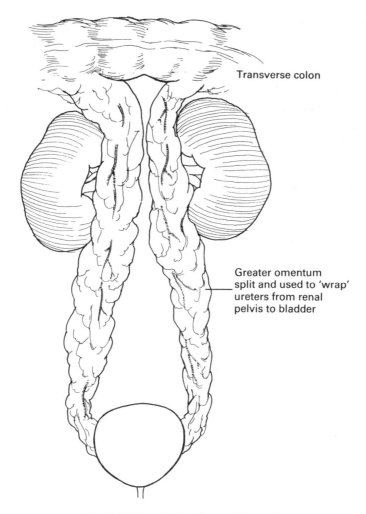

Transverse colon

Greater omentum
split and used to 'wrap'
ureters from renal
pelvis to bladder

**Fig. 11.6** Ureterolysis and omental wrapping

## Special types of ureteric obstruction

### Obstruction after renal transplantation

The transplant ureter may be obstructed after kidney transplantation by narrowing at the site of its reimplantation into the bladder. This type of obstruction can be relieved temporarily by nephrostomy drainage but eventually requires further reimplantation of the ureter.

The transplant ureter may also be obstructed by a collection of lymph in the pelvis (*lymphocele*). Small lymphoceles can be aspirated but larger ones usually require drainage by marsupialisation into the peritoneal cavity.

*Urinary diversion*

There are many problems for the patient with a long-term urinary diversion. One of these is obstruction of the ureter as it enters the organ into which it has been diverted: this causes ureteric dilatation, stasis, functional deterioration in the kidneys and, sometimes, stone formation.

Obstruction is usually due to fibrosis of the ureteric anastomosis or kinking of the ureter, but may be caused by local infiltration of recurrent malignancy in patients diverted for malignant pelvic tumours. Most obstructed ureters above urinary diversions require reconstruction, although there is increasing experience now with balloon dilatation of obstructive narrowing. The best treatment, however, is prevention, with meticulous attention to technique in the construction of the original anastomosis.

# 12

# Renal failure, dialysis and transplantation

## ACUTE RENAL FAILURE

Acute renal failure (ARF) is an abrupt decline in renal function resulting in a fall in urine output and retention of hydrogen ions, potassium ions and nitrogenous waste products. A daily urine output of less than 500 ml in an adult is termed *oliguria*, whilst the absence of urine formation is known as *anuria*.

The underlying cause of ARF is a persistent fall in renal blood flow (RBF) to levels 30–40% of normal with glomerular filtration (GFR) being reduced as a result to less than 5 ml/min. This is thought to occur as a result of tubular damage and intratubular obstruction, although such histological changes are seen only in a patchy distribution throughout the kidney.

### Aetiology

There are many possible causes of ARF which can be divided broadly into three categories: pre-renal, renal and post-renal (Fig. 12.1).

Pre-renal ARF is usually due to *hypovolaemia*. Typically, it follows a circulatory catastrophe (e.g. trauma, blood loss, surgery, septicaemia) although it may follow other causes of fluid loss such as burns or severe diarrhoea; these conditions are usually associated with acute tubular necrosis (ATN).

Renal ARF may be caused by vascular, glomerular, interstitial or tubular lesions and is often associated with ATN.

It is important to recognise post-renal causes for ARF because they are related to *obstruction*. Such obstruction may occur as a result of blockage of the collecting tubules, ureteric occlusion (e.g. by stones, tumour) or bladder outflow obstruction (e.g. by prostatic hypertrophy or carcinoma). Immediate relief of such obstructive lesions by the appropriate means may result in rapid resolution of the ARF.

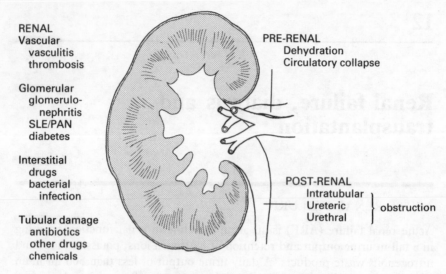

RENAL
Vascular
   vasculitis
   thrombosis

Glomerular
   glomerulo-
      nephritis
   SLE/PAN
   diabetes

Interstitial
   drugs
   bacterial
      infection

Tubular damage
   antibiotics
   other drugs
   chemicals

PRE-RENAL
Dehydration
Circulatory collapse

POST-RENAL
Intratubular
Ureteric      } obstruction
Urethral

**Fig. 12.1** Principal causes of acute renal failure

## Acute tubular necrosis (ATN)

This is a specific morphological feature of ARF but is not, in itself, synonymous with ARF. It is seen histologically in 75% of patients with ARF and, typically, microscopy shows no intratubular obstruction and no glomerular or interstitial lesions.

Pathological examination of affected kidneys shows them to be swollen with a yellowish cortex and an engorged, purple-red medulla. The urine in the renal pelvis is usually blood-stained. Microscopically, there is dilatation of the proximal tubules with necrosis and flattening of the tubular epithelium. Milder changes are seen in the distal tubules, often with casts in the tubular lumen. The interstitium of the kidney is usually oedematous with infiltration of polymorphonuclear leucocytes. Electron microscopy in ATN shows disruption of mitochondria, abnormalities of the nuclei and shedding of the brush borders of tubular cells.

The most important practical point, however, is to distinguish between the physiological oliguria not infrequently seen with hypovolaemia and the more sinister oliguria of established ARF. Early treatment of the former by volume replacement may prevent the development of the latter.

## Diagnosis

The diagnosis is usually clear from the history, the finding of oliguria or anuria and the biochemical features of uraemia, acidosis, hyperkalaemia and raised serum creatinine levels. The biochemical parameters described above will help to determine whether the situation is potentially reversible or

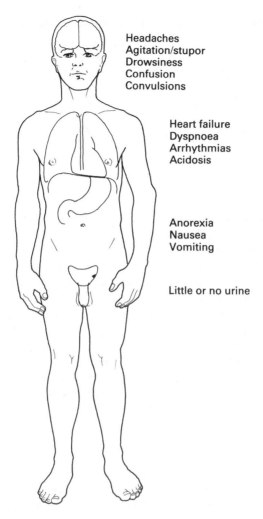

Headaches
Agitation/stupor
Drowsiness
Confusion
Convulsions

Heart failure
Dyspnoea
Arrhythmias
Acidosis

Anorexia
Nausea
Vomiting

Little or no urine

**Fig. 12.2** Symptoms of acute renal failure

established (Table 12.1). In most patients the cause will be clinically obvious, although in some it may be necessary to perform a renal biopsy to obtain more accurate information which is useful both in terms of treatment and prognosis.

The standard intravenous urogram (IVU) has now largely been replaced as the prime investigation in an oliguric/anuric patient by ultrasound of the kidneys and bladder. A plain abdominal film is still essential to exclude calculi in the urinary tract. Ultrasound can detect dilatation of the ureter and kidneys which might suggest a treatable obstructive lesion and abdominal CT scanning, antegrade or retrograde pyelography may help in assessing the nature and site of the obstruction. A skilled radiologist can

**Table 12.1**   Biochemical recognition of established acute renal failure

|  | Physiological oliguria | Established ARF |
|---|---|---|
| Urine volume | Low (?high) | Low |
| Urine specific gravity | > 1020 | 1010 |
| Urinary osmolality (mosm/kg) | > 500 | 250–300 |
| Urinary sodium (mmol/l) | < 15 | > 60 |
| Urinary urea (mmol/l) | > 250 | < 160 |
| Urine/plasma osmolality | > 1.3 | <= 1.1 |
| Urine/plasma urea | > 10 | <10 |
| Response to fluid load | Always | Occasional |

now insert fine nephrostomy tubes into the kidneys to relieve ureteric obstruction. Bladder outflow obstruction is best dealt with by urethral or suprapubic catheterisation.

Radionuclide investigation (renal scintigraphy) is useful in determining arterial patency to the kidneys and gives information about excretion and differential function between the two kidneys. Radionuclide studies are also useful in follow-up as a method of charting progress without the risk of excessive radiation exposure.

An IVU may be useful, particularly in the early stages after contrast injection (the 'nephrogram' phase). A persistent nephrogram is seen in glomerulonephritis and ATN, whilst a dense nephrogram progressing to a negative pyelogram is very suggestive of obstruction. Polycystic kidneys may also be seen at this stage, although they are best seen on ultrasound.

### Treatment

The general aim of treatment is to keep the patient alive whilst assessing the cause of the ARF and instituting treatment appropriate to that cause. A catheter may be useful in the early stages to monitor urine output but is not essential. Fluid intake is best restricted to 500 ml every 24 hours plus the daily urine volume, giving further fluid supplements to make up any other losses. Fluids are best given orally but may need to be administered intravenously if the patient's condition demands this. Improved urine output may be obtained by infusing dopamine ($2–5$ $\mu$g/kg/min) and frusemide ($10–15$ mg/kg/h) and there is good evidence that this may be useful in improving renal blood flow by reversing renal vasoconstriction. Higher doses of frusemide should not be used. Such a regime may not shorten the duration of ARF or decrease the mortality but can convert the patient from an oliguric state to a non-oliguric one.

These measures are intended to prevent renal ischaemia from progressing to ATN and renal cortical necrosis. Overexpansion of the plasma volume, either intravenously or by high oral intake, should be avoided since this may result in water intoxication. Accurate fluid balance is, therefore, essential and daily weighing of the patient is a useful method of assessing this.

Sodium intake should be restricted to 20–30 mmol per day but the main problem is hyperkalaemia and its risk to the heart. Serum potassium levels can be lowered in an emergency by intravenous infusion of glucose (50 g) and insulin (10 units) and maintained at safe levels by ion exchange resins (e.g. calcium resonium) administered orally or rectally. There is little point in trying to correct acidosis by infusion of sodium bicarbonate, since this is usually ineffective and may constitute an excessive sodium load.

Maintenance of nutritional status can be very difficult and may require the help of a clinical nutrition team. Ideally, patients should receive 100 g of carbohydrate and 3000–3500 kilocalories daily, with 60–80 g of nitrogen.

ARF impairs both cellular and humoral immunity so that infection is a common problem, accounting for up to 50% of deaths. There is probably no place for prophylactic antibiotics but all proven infections should be treated vigorously and potential foreign bodies (e.g. catheters, intravenous cannulae) should be avoided if possible.

H2-receptor antagonists and antacids are very useful in patients with ARF, since upper gastrointestinal haemorrhage is a major contributory factor in the death of these patients.

When prescribing antibiotics or any other drug in renal failure, it is important to be aware of potential problems with toxicity due to impaired renal excretion. Most drug formularies now give advice on prescribing for patients with impaired renal function.

Dialysis may be indicated if conservative measures fail to control the situation (Table 12.2). Peritoneal dialysis is the simplest form of treatment, although haemodialysis may be necessary.

**Table 12.2**  Indications for dialysis in acute renal failure

| Clinical | Biochemical |
|---|---|
| Fluid overload | Potassium > 7.0 mmol/l |
| Pulmonary oedema | Urea > 35 mmol/l |
| Poor clinical condition | Bicarbonate < 12 mmol/l |
| Pericarditis | (arterial pH < 7.15) |
| Before surgery | Urea rising by > 16 mmol/l/day |

One of the main dangers of ARF is the development of persistent anuria. This usually implies bilateral renal infarction at renal artery or arteriolar level and eventually progresses to renal cortical necrosis. Persistent anuria may be an indication for renal biopsy to exclude vascular occlusion which, if present, has a very poor prognosis and is normally irreversible.

## Clinical course

This can be highly variable but can usefully be divided into oliguric, diuretic and post-diuretic phases. The oliguric phase normally starts early, although it may be delayed for a week or so and may last for up to 60 days. The development of a diuresis can be quite abrupt and is usually a sign that recovery is taking place. Great care is needed during this stage with fluid and electrolyte intake, since the kidneys are unable to deal with a solute load. Some patients may need dialysis when they develop a diuresis and 50% of deaths occur during this phase.

After this, renal function gradually improves over 3–12 months but GFR only returns to normal levels in younger patients. Distal tubular function remains permanently impaired, although this impairment is often clinically undetectable. There is no reliable evidence that ARF leads to the development of hypertension in later life. If function does not recover as expected, this raises the possibility of obstruction, acute nephritis/vasculitis or acute pyelonephritis, all of which are potentially reversible conditions.

## Prognosis

The mortality of ARF is high (50%) and is normally a reflection of the precipitating cause. Mortality has not changed much in the last 25 years, probably because of patient selection rather than any lack of progress in treatment. The worst outlook is seen in patients with gastrointestinal haemorrhage, ATN after trauma, peritonitis or jaundice and in the elderly. Twenty per cent of all deaths are due to infection alone and infection contributes significantly to 50% of deaths from ARF. The best prognosis is seen in obstetric patients (10% mortality) who often manage to maintain reasonable urine volumes despite ARF.

## CHRONIC RENAL FAILURE

Approximately 60 patients per million of the UK population present in end-stage renal failure each year. Half of these patients have either chronic glomerulonephritis or pyelonephritis.

Some causative factors are reversible and their treatment may produce an improvement, to a greater or lesser extent, in renal function (Table 12.3). This is true, however, in only a minority of cases.

When no reversible factor can be found causing chronic renal failure (CRF), the aim of assessment is to differentiate the condition from ARF, to define the cause if possible and to determine the severity of the disease so that treatment can be planned and an accurate prognosis given.

Clinical examination may reveal signs associated with the symptoms (Fig. 12.3) but the kidneys are rarely palpable unless they are grossly enlarged as a result of obstruction or polycystic disease. Rectal examination should

**Table 12.3**  Principal causes of chronic renal failure

| | |
|---|---|
| Chronic glomerulonephritis | 38% |
| Chronic pyelonephritis | 18% |
| Other identified rare disease | 8% |
| Renovascular disease (including hypertension) | 8% |
| Aetiology uncertain | 8% |
| Cystic renal disease | 5% |
| Hereditary/congenital | 4% |
| Analgesic abuse | 4% |
| Others | 7% |

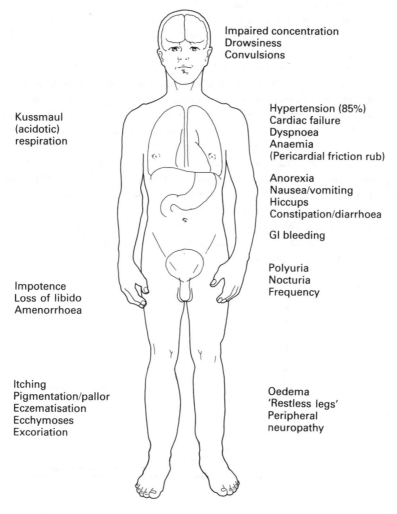

Impaired concentration
Drowsiness
Convulsions

Kussmaul
(acidotic)
respiration

Hypertension (85%)
Cardiac failure
Dyspnoea
Anaemia
(Pericardial friction rub)

Anorexia
Nausea/vomiting
Hiccups
Constipation/diarrhoea

GI bleeding

Polyuria
Nocturia
Frequency

Impotence
Loss of libido
Amenorrhoea

Itching
Pigmentation/pallor
Eczematisation
Ecchymoses
Excoriation

Oedema
'Restless legs'
Peripheral
neuropathy

**Fig. 12.3**  Clinical features of chronic renal failure

always be performed to exclude treatable prostatic disease as a cause of CRF.

### Biochemical features

Patients with CRF usually have polyuria due to a loss of normal concentrating ability. Nocturia is often an early sign that all is not well. The urine often contains protein together with granular casts and white blood cells. A characteristic but rare finding in the urine is the presence of 'broad' casts which are probably dilated nephrons shed in the urine.

Sodium is gradually retained in CRF, although the serum sodium is a poor reflection of this. Potassium levels are affected less frequently, although they may rise in end-stage CRF. Acidosis is inevitable due to decreased ammonium ion excretion and decreased excretion of buffer phosphate; the urine pH is usually less than 5.

Calcium levels may be low or normal and secondary hyperparathyroidism or osteomalacia is common. Calcium excretion is reduced and there is little or no absorption of calcium due to decreased levels of 1,25-dihydroxycholecalciferol, whose synthesis is dependent on the presence of intact renal mitochondria. The osteomalacia is sometimes vitamin D resistant.

Magnesium levels in serum are usually unchanged but absorption is impaired, as is the ability to excrete a magnesium load. Magnesium based purgatives, therefore, should be avoided. The decreased glomerular filtration results in a fall in tubular reabsorption of phosphate. Phosphate levels do not normally rise until the GFR falls below 10 ml/min and can usually be maintained at stable levels by restriction of protein intake.

Urea and uric acid levels rise in chronic renal failure. Urea itself causes little in the way of symptoms but hyperuricaemia may cause gout. Creati-

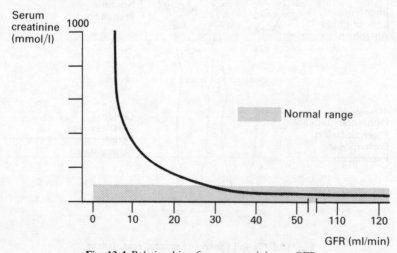

**Fig. 12.4** Relationship of serum creatinine to GFR

nine levels rise in proportion to the GFR but creatinine itself causes no specific symptoms (Fig. 12.4). Chromogens in the urine do increase with poor renal function, resulting in yellow coloration of the skin and the effect of a 'good suntan'. Many symptoms of CRF are thought to be due to increased levels of unidentified 'toxins': many substances (e.g. parathyroid hormone) have been suggested but none has yet been definitely implicated.

Anaemia is common: it is usually normochromic and normocytic and is probably due to marrow suppression combined with decreased red cell survival, although some patients have evidence of occult or overt gastrointestinal blood loss.

## Conservative treatment

The aim of conservative treatment is to delay the progressive deterioration in renal function and to prevent its consequences. More aggressive measures (i.e dialysis or transplantation) are used when conservative treatment fails.

Fluid intake should be tailored to produce a urine output of approximately 1 litre per 24 hours, unless the patient is grossly oedematous when more stringent restriction is necessary.

Sodium supplements may be used if there is evidence of a negative sodium balance (i.e hypotension or clinical evidence of dehydration). The acidosis of CRF does not usually respond to treatment with sodium bicarbonate, although bicarbonate may delay the development of bone changes. Ideally, the aim is to prevent metastatic calcification developing. This can be achieved by keeping the calcium–phosphate product constant by administering aluminium hydroxide gel (50–100 ml per day) or by giving calcium carbonate. Care must be exercised, however, to avoid aluminium toxicity resulting in dementia and osteomalacia. Vitamin D in high doses may be used for established osteomalacia.

Blood pressure can usually be controlled by antihypertensive drugs and by reducing sodium intake. Cardiac failure is treated by the standard measures. Infections should be treated with the appropriate antibiotics, if indicated. Hiccups often respond to treatment with chlorpromazine or antihistamines but are a late sign and respond best to dialysis.

The anaemia of CRF only responds to transfusion. This is not normally indicated unless there are obvious signs of bleeding or symptoms which can be directly attributed to the anaemia. 'Good' dialysis can increase circulating levels of erythropoietin and synthetic erythropoietin is now available. Transfusion runs the risk of further impairing renal function, of transmitting hepatitis B or AIDS and of sensitising some patients to develop antibodies which make them untransplantable.

Nausea and vomiting can normally be helped by decreasing protein intake (to 20–40 g per 24 hours) and are also relieved by dialysis. The aim of any protein restriction is to try to produce a decreased concentration of nitrogenous waste products without producing a prolonged negative nitrogen balance. There is, nowadays, a move to restrict protein intake at an early stage (before the plasma urea is greater than 25 mmol/litre).

## DIALYSIS

Dialysis allows patients with CRF to relax their dietary restrictions and is generally considered once the serum creatinine has risen above 1000 $\mu$mol/l with a creatinine clearance of less than 5 ml/min. Maintenance dialysis should be started before the patient is moribund. The rate-limiting factor, however, is the availability of resources and facilities for dialysis. There is good evidence that those patients who have suffered long periods of protein restriction, peripheral neuropathy or pericarditis do badly on dialysis.

The options for dialysis are between haemodialysis and peritoneal dialysis.

### Haemodialysis

The principle of haemodialysis is to allow selective diffusion of molecules below a certain size from the peripheral blood through a semi-permeable membrane to a dialysis fluid. Most dialysis machines use a disposable membrane within a hollow-fibre or flat plate and have a special mechanism to remove calcium and aluminium from the incoming water supply before mixing the water with electrolytes to produce the dialysis fluid. The hyperosmolar dialysis fluid removes water by osmosis and, by applying a relative positive pressure to the blood, it is possible to produce ultrafiltration.

In the UK, 65% of patients on haemodialysis are treated in their own homes, compared with only 19% in Europe as a whole. Home dialysis allows the patient greater freedom, greater independence, a decreased risk of blood-borne disease and improved survival, although the latter may simply be a selection phenomenon.

Access to the patient's circulation is necessary for haemodialysis (Fig. 12.5). This can be obtained in the short term by direct cannulation of large vessels (e.g. subclavian or femoral veins) with single or double lumen tubes or by external (Quinton–Scribner) shunts. In the long term vascular access is best achieved by arterialisation of a peripheral vein which then expands and can be cannulated repeatedly (Cimino–Brescia fistula).

Most patients require dialysis 2 or 3 times per week for 4–8 hours each time, although there is now a move towards more frequent, shorter dialysis periods. However, shorter dialysis periods seem to be associated with an increased risk of cardiovascular mortality.

One recently developed form of dialysis that is gaining increasing respectability is *haemofiltration*. In this technique, a high ultrafiltration capacity membrane is used which allows large volumes of plasma to be filtered in a short time with appropriate replacement of fluid and electrolytes. This

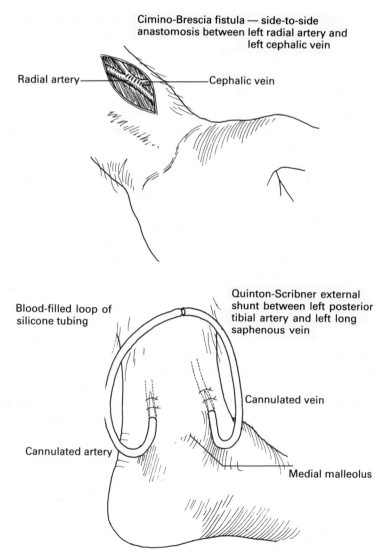

**Fig. 12.5** Common methods of vascular access

technique provides better control of blood pressure than conventional dialysis, with more efficient removal of medium-sized molecules and less risk of hyperlipidaemia. The technique, however, is expensive and has not yet gained widespread acceptance except in West Germany, where its use is widespread.

Patient survival after 2 years is 88% on home dialysis and 75% on hospital dialysis, which compares with 88% for renal transplantation. Ten-year survival on haemodialysis is approximately 50%. Survival is worst in the elderly and those with multisystem disease (e.g. SLE, amyloid, diabetes) and best in those with polycystic kidneys. Death is usually due to vascular disease, infection or hyperkalaemia.

### Peritoneal dialysis (Fig. 12.6)

Peritoneal dialysis is a less efficient means of dialysis than haemodialysis but is very useful in emergency situations. A trocar cannula can be inserted into the abdominal cavity percutaneously under local anaesthetic to allow immediate fluid exchange and dialysis.

In the chronic situation, a custom-built cannula (Tenckhoff, Oreopoulos) is inserted through a small puncture hole in the abdominal wall, just below the umbilicus in the midline. This must be inserted under aseptic conditions and the bladder should be emptied first to avoid its accidental penetration. The catheter may be inserted under general or local anaesthesia, but the tip of the cannula must be positioned in the recto-vesical pouch.

Dialysis fluid is run into the peritoneal cavity and then drained off again. Adequate control requires three treatment sessions per week, each session lasting up to 12 hours. Most dialysis units now have automatic cycling systems which instil and drain the dialysis fluid automatically.

There are mechanical, infective and intestinal problems associated with this technique. These often limit its use to the short term and have led many dialysis units to prefer haemodialysis.

Chronic ambulatory peritoneal dialysis (CAPD) is a more recent development which has found favour in many centres. This employs rather more frequent changes of dialysate (4 cycles per day, 7 days per week). Each fluid

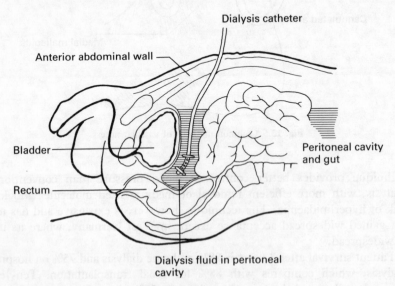

Fig. 12.6 Peritoneal dialysis

installation is left in situ for 6–8 hours before draining but, being performed by the patient at home, such exchanges can be carried out at times convenient to the patient (i.e. meal times, before bedtime). CAPD has the advantages of preserving nutritional status and minimising the risk of anaemia, and it may protect the patient in the long term from bone disease. The technique is rapidly and easily learnt. In addition, it is considerably cheaper than haemodialysis. The main problem, however, is one of infection.

## RENAL TRANSPLANTATION

Organs can only be exchanged without the risk of rejection between identical twins: transplants between unrelated individuals will inevitably be rejected and the main problem of renal transplantation has been developing safe methods of suppressing this rejection process.

The potential for rejection is assessed by looking at the antigenic match between donor and recipient. The major histocompatibility antigens that

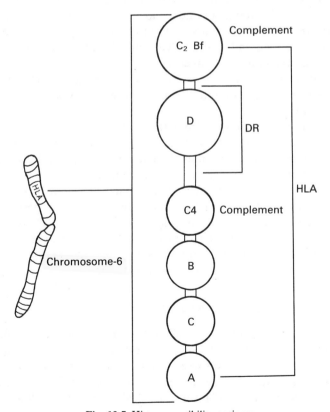

**Fig. 12.7** Histocompatibility antigens

are routinely assessed in preparation for renal transplantation are the ABO (blood group) antigens and the human leucocyte antigens (HLA) (Fig. 12.7). HLA is determined by genes on chromosome 6. There are four broad sub-groups of HLA (A–D), of which the most strongly antigenic are A and B. Compatibility between donor and recipient is now assessed by an 'identical' match of ABO antigens and HLA-A/HLA-B. More recently, it has been realised that other antigen matches, in particular DR typing of B-lymphocytes, have an important influence on the outcome of a renal transplant.

## Donor selection

The majority of donated kidneys come from cadavers, although a small proportion of transplants are taken from live-related donors. If a good antigenic match can be obtained from a live-related donor, that donor should undergo intravenous urography and renal angiography to assess the potential kidney for donation. Measurement of creatinine clearance or radionuclide divided studies for each kidney are also useful in determining whether the kidney is suitable for transplantation. If the kidney proves suitable, it is removed through a standard loin approach, with great care taken to preserve the renal artery and vein and to avoid devascularising the ureter. The kidney is cooled and transplanted immediately, usually in an adjacent operating theatre, into the recipient.

Cadaveric donors are usually patients with irreversible brain stem damage who are dependent upon artificial ventilation but who have no evidence of malignant disease.

Both kidneys are removed from the donor via an anterior abdominal approach, usually removing the kidneys en bloc with a patch of aorta and inferior vena cava. Great care must be taken not to devascularise the upper ureter by stripping it of adventitial tissue. The kidneys are then perfused via the renal artery with cold hypertonic citrate solution and packed in ice. Ideally, kidneys for transplantation should have a minimal period of warm ischaemia (detachment from blood supply within the donor) and no longer than 24 hours cold ischaemia (packed in ice). A better method of preservation may be to institute continuous hypothermic perfusion at 10°C, although this has not gained widespread acceptance.

## Recipient assessment (Table 12.4)

Patients should be admitted for full reassessment prior to transplantation and should also receive a urological assessment of bladder and bladder outflow function to identify those patients whose lower urinary tracts do not work well. Some of these patients, if considered for renal transplantation, may require a transplant into an ileal or colonic conduit.

**Table 12.4**  Contraindications to renal transplantation

| Relative | Absolute |
| --- | --- |
| Age > 65 years | Severe diabetes with large vessel disease |
| Very young children | Active tuberculosis or other systemic |
| Hyperoxaluria with oxalosis | infection |
| Some types of glomerulonephritis (focal glomerular sclerosis, mesangiocapillary) | Active malignant disease |
| Bladder/bladder outflow problems | |

The question of whether the recipient's native kidneys should be removed prior to transplantation is still a vexed one. Patients with grossly dilated or refluxing ureters should probably have their kidneys and ureters removed, because of the risk of developing a potential sump of infected urine which may cause problems when immunosuppressive treatment is commenced. Nephrectomy may be necessary in recipients with persistent hypertension, in those with recurrent urinary infections and in those with polycystic disease (if the kidneys are large or infected). If left in the recipient, the native kidneys do fulfil a useful function after transplantation by producing erythropoietin and vitamin D metabolites, although the transplanted kidney will also do this.

The techniques used in renal transplantation are summarised in Figure 12.8.

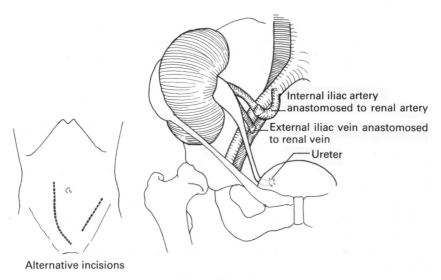

Internal iliac artery anastomosed to renal artery

External iliac vein anastomosed to renal vein

Ureter

Alternative incisions

**Fig. 12.8** Renal transplantation

*Immunosuppression*

In the postoperative period, it is, of course, necessary to give the patient immunosuppressive drugs to prevent rejection of the transplanted kidney. Traditionally, this has been achieved using steroids (100 mg prednisone per day reducing to 10 mg per day maintenance) and azathioprine (2.5–3 mg/kg body weight). These drugs are associated with significant side-effects, including bone marrow toxicity. More recently the antifungal agent cyclosporine A (Cy-A) has been developed as an immunosuppressive drug. In some transplant units, Cy-A is now the sole form of immuno-suppression, given initially in doses of 4 mg/kg body weight intravenously until bowel function is normal and then orally in doses of 10–12 mg/kg body weight. Therapeutic levels can be monitored in the peripheral blood to minimise toxicity (particularly to the transplanted kidney itself).

Most transplant units use combinations of Cy-A, prednisolone and azathioprine in low doses to minimise the side-effects of immunosuppression.

**Prognosis** (Table 12.5)

Survival after transplantation, both for patient and graft, has been improved dramatically by the use of Cy-A.

**Table 12.5** Graft and patient survival after renal transplantation

| Donor | Graft survival (%) | | | Patient survival (%) | | |
|---|---|---|---|---|---|---|
| | 1 yr | 3 yr | 5 yr | 1 yr | 3 yr | 5 yr |
| Sibling | 80 | 70 | 60 | 85 | 80 | 70 |
| Parent | 70 | 60 | 45 | 80 | 70 | 65 |
| Cadaver | 55 | 40 | 35 | 65 | 50 | 45 |

(Related to HLA matching, ABO matching, presensitisation of the recipient, previous blood transfusions, age and time spent on dialysis)

Rejection remains a major problem after transplantation. Hyperacute rejection normally means that the kidney needs to be removed urgently. In accelerated rejection, the patient becomes systemically unwell with graft tenderness, and graft biopsy shows cellular infiltration with arteriolar necrosis. The treatment is high-dose steroids (methylprednisolone 1 g intra-venously) but the graft failure rate is high (67%). Acute rejection presents with similar symptoms but is usually reversible with a short period of high-dose steroid therapy. Chronic rejection is associated with recurrent hyper-tension and fluid retention and is treated with high-dose steroids or azathioprine.

Much importance has been attached to the relative costs of the various forms of treatment for chronic renal failure. Home dialysis is an expensive prospect, costing approximately £9000 per year after an initial installation cost of £7–10 000. Hospital dialysis is, naturally, more expensive. Transplantation costs much the same as home dialysis for the first year after a successful graft, but thereafter is much cheaper.

# 13

# Renal and adrenal hypertension

Ninety-four per cent of all hypertensive patients have no readily identifiable cause for their high blood pressure (*essential hypertension*). In the remainder, the hypertension is secondary to an underlying problem which is usually adrenal or renal in origin. Only 1–2% of hypertensive patients have a surgically remediable cause for their high blood pressure (Table 13.1).

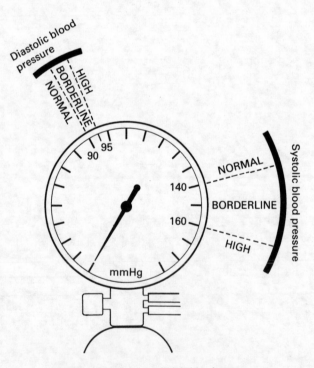

**Fig. 13.1** A definition of high blood pressure

**Table 13.1**  Causes of hypertension

| | |
|---|---|
| Essential hypertension | 92–94% |
| Renal hypertension | |
| *Parenchymal* | 2–3% |
| connective tissue disease | |
| glomerulonephritis | |
| pyelonephritis | |
| polycystic disease | |
| analgesic nephropathy | |
| hydronephrosis | |
| *Renovascular* | 1–2% |
| Endocrine hypertension | |
| *Conn's syndrome* | 0.3% |
| *Cushing's syndrome* | <0.1% |
| *Phaeochromocytoma* | <0.1% |
| *Oral contraceptives* | 2–4% |
| *Adrenogenital syndrome* | <0.1% |
| 17α hydroxylase deficiency | |
| 11β hydroxylase deficiency | |
| Miscellaneous causes | 0.2% |

# DETECTION OF SECONDARY HYPERTENSION

The clinical history may give a clue to the cause of high blood pressure. Hypertension in children, adolescents and young adults (less than 50 years old) should be suspected as being secondary to an underlying cause. A history of oral contraceptive intake, analgesic abuse, urinary infection in childhood or pregnancy and symptoms referable to the kidneys may all suggest an underlying precipitating cause. A family history may be present in patients with polycystic kidneys, vesicoureteric reflux or hydronephrosis. In addition, patients who do not respond satisfactorily to appropriate anti-hypertensive therapy should be suspected of having a secondary cause for high blood pressure.

Some symptoms are specific to certain diseases. For example, episodic headaches, sweating and hypertension are characteristic of phaeochromocytoma whilst muscle weakness is often seen in Conn's syndrome. Other endocrine disease such as myxoedema or acromegaly may also cause hypertension, but the clinical features of the disease itself usually precede the development of hypertension in affected patients.

The finding of an abdominal bruit on examination of the patient may suggest the possibility of renal artery stenosis: 30–60% of affected patients have a bruit over the partially occluded renal artery, compared with 10% of patients suffering from essential hypertension.

Specific investigations should be instituted if any of the above factors suggest the possibility of secondary hypertension. The finding of proteinuria, haematuria and casts in the urine may be indicative of underlying renal disease. Infection in the urine and glycosuria should also prompt further investigation. If there is clinical suspicion of renal artery stenosis, an IVU and radionuclide renogram may confirm the diagnosis.

Biochemical tests on the blood may also be helpful; simple measurement of plasma electrolytes may show abnormalities such as the hypokalaemia, alkalosis and raised sodium levels seen in patients with Conn's syndrome.

## HYPERTENSION DUE TO RENAL PARENCHYMAL DISEASE

Most of the disease entities which cause renal parenchymal hypertension have been dealt with elsewhere in this volume. In many cases, the underlying disease is untreatable and therapy is simply directed towards alleviating the effects of renal failure. For details on the management of hypertension in patients with renal disease, the reader is referred to a specialist text on this subject.

The only clinical problem that regularly confronts the urologist is whether to remove a hydronephrotic kidney in a hypertensive patient. Although the response of blood pressure to nephrectomy cannot be accurately predicted, it is, as a general rule, poor in patients with established hypertensive changes in the contralateral normal kidney and relatively good in those patients with high renin levels from the hydronephrotic kidney.

## RENOVASCULAR HYPERTENSION

Seventy per cent of patients with renovascular (renin-dependent) hypertension are elderly males with generalised atherosclerosis of which renal artery stenosis is only a part. The remaining 30% are less than 50 years old and often female. The majority of these young patients have medial fibromuscular hyperplasia of the renal artery, although a small proportion have intimal or periarterial fibroplasia.

The possibility of renal artery stenosis should be suspected in the presence of accelerated hypertension, severe hypertensive retinopathy, hypertension refractory to conventional treatment and a progressive deterioration in renal function despite adequate blood pressure control.

The only specific sign is an arterial bruit in the abdomen or loin. Intravenous urography detects 85% of patients with extra-renal arterial stenosis. The typical findings are of a small kidney, a delayed nephrogram progressing to a dense pyelogram and ureteric notching by collateral vessels around the upper ureter. Radionuclide renography (Fig. 13.2), however, is probably the most reliable method of establishing the diagnosis.

Aortography and renal arteriography usually confirm the diagnosis by showing either atheroma in the aorta and renal artery or the typical 'beaded' appearance of the renal artery in fibromuscular hyperplasia, often with post-stenotic dilatation. In addition, it may also be possible to collect blood from the renal veins for renin levels. A renal vein renin ratio (abnormal/contralateral

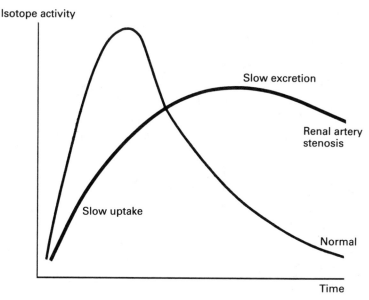

**Fig. 13.2** Radionuclide renography in renal artery stenosis

renal vein level) of 1.5 or greater is strongly suggestive of arterial stenosis which will respond to surgery. The mere presence of an angiographic stenosis, however, does not necessarily mean that this is the cause of the hypertension.

Angiotensin converting enzyme (ACE) inhibitors have been used to treat renin-dependent hypertension but are often ineffective. Operative intervention is indicated if blood pressure control is poor on ACE inhibitors or if there is a specific need for preservation or improvement of renal function. Nowadays, *percutaneous transluminal angioplasty* is widely used to dilate stenotic areas in renal arteries. It is especially indicated for localised atherosclerotic lesions, short fibromuscular dysplastic lesions and patients with deteriorating renal function. In the short term, the results of angioplasty are as good as those of surgery (Fig. 13.3).

After reconstructive surgery, 60% of patients become normotensive, 30% have their blood pressure lowered (but not to normal levels) and the remainder are unchanged; there is a mortality rate of 1–2% associated with surgery. Success rates for reconstructive surgery are diminished in elderly patients, patients with generalised atherosclerosis, patients with bilateral arterial stenosis and those with marked impairment of renal function. Nowadays, surgery is rarely recommended for patients older than 45 years.

The blood pressure after surgery does not always fall immediately but may take several months. Untreated, 50% of patients with hypertension due to renal artery stenosis progress to malignant hypertension.

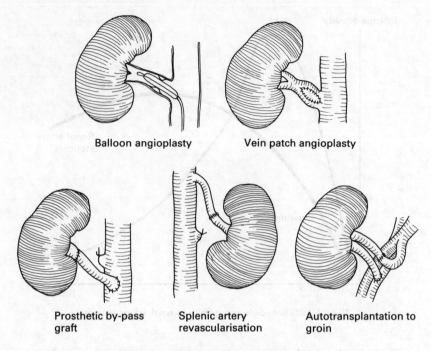

Balloon angioplasty        Vein patch angioplasty

Prosthetic by-pass    Splenic artery        Autotransplantation to
graft                revascularisation     groin

**Fig. 13.3** Surgery for renal artery stenosis

## PRIMARY HYPERALDOSTERONISM

Seventy per cent of patients with hypertension due to primary hyperaldos-teronism have an aldosterone-producing adrenal adenoma arising from the zona glomerulosa (*Conn's syndrome*) (see Fig. 13.4). The remaining 30% have idiopathic, bilateral adrenal hyperplasia. The hypertension is due to raised circulating levels of aldosterone which produce sodium retention by the kidney, an increase in exchangeable body sodium, hypokalaemia and an increase in extracellular fluid volume.

Conn's syndrome should be suspected in young to middle-aged women with severe hypertension. Weakness, tetany, nocturia and constipation are also occasionally seen in this condition.

The standard imaging technique for Conn's syndrome has traditionally been *adrenal venography*. This also permits venous sampling for measure-ment of aldosterone levels in the adrenal veins. Adrenal venography, however, may miss small adrenal adenomas and has been replaced by abdominal CT scanning. Radionuclide scanning with [131]I-iodocholesterol has also been used and is 60–90% accurate in localising aldosterone-producing tumours if CT is inconclusive.

The differentiation between adenoma and hyperplasia is made on the response of plasma aldosterone levels to changes in posture: aldosterone

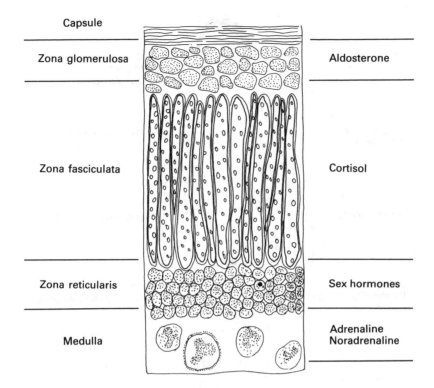

| Capsule | |
| Zona glomerulosa | Aldosterone |
| Zona fasciculata | Cortisol |
| Zona reticularis | Sex hormones |
| Medulla | Adrenaline Noradrenaline |

**Fig. 13.4** Structure and function of the adrenal gland

levels fall in the erect position in the presence of an adenoma and rise with hyperplasia of the adrenal.

In Conn's syndrome, surgical removal of the adenoma cures the hypertension in 60% of affected patients. Twenty per cent have their blood pressure improved and 20% are unchanged. Surgical removal is normally performed via a conventional extraperitoneal loin approach to the adrenal gland. In bilateral hyperplasia, surgery is curative in only 30%. In those patients who fail to respond to surgery, treatment with spironolactone (100–400 mg/day) is indicated. In the event of side-effects from spironolactone (nausea, rashes, gynaecomastia, impotence and amenorrhoea), amiloride (10–40 mg/day) may be used as an alternative.

## CUSHING'S SYNDROME (Fig. 13.5)

The commonest cause of Cushing's syndrome is the administration of steroids (prednisolone, prednisone) to treat other diseases. Of the remainder, 80% have a basophil or chromophobe adenoma of the pituitary (*Cushing's disease*) whilst 20% have either ectopic ACTH production or an adrenal tumour.

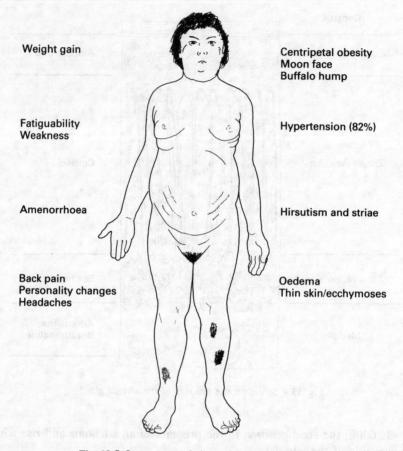

Weight gain

Centripetal obesity
Moon face
Buffalo hump

Fatiguability
Weakness

Hypertension (82%)

Amenorrhoea

Hirsutism and striae

Back pain
Personality changes
Headaches

Oedema
Thin skin/ecchymoses

**Fig. 13.5** Symptoms and signs of Cushing's syndrome

When not caused by steroids, the disease is commonest in the third and fourth decades and is seen four times more often in women than in men. The hypertension is due to the mineralocorticoid activity of cortisol, a glucocorticoid-induced increase in vascular reactivity of vasopressor agents and inappropriate renin-angiotensin activity as a result of increased renin substrate levels.

The diagnosis of Cushing's syndrome is made on the typical clinical features, together with laboratory investigations. Plasma cortisol levels are raised, with loss of the normal circadian rhythm. Urinary excretion of free cortisol, 17-oxogenic steroids and 17-oxosteroids is raised. The normal rise in cortisol levels in response to insulin hypoglycaemia is blunted in Cushing's syndrome and plasma ACTH levels may be abnormal.

To establish the cause of the disease requires more sophisticated investigations. Skull X-ray shows an enlarged pituitary fossa in 20% of patients with Cushing's syndrome. Chest X-ray may show a bronchial neoplasm responsible for ectopic ACTH production. Localisation of tumours in the adrenal glands can be performed by adrenal angiography but abdominal CT scanning has now taken over as the imaging technique of choice. Adrenal scintigraphy with $^{131}$I-labelled cholesterol may be useful to demonstrate an adrenal adenoma.

Further biochemical tests may be needed to confirm the underlying cause and, for details of these specific tests, the reader is referred to a specialist endocrinological text.

Cushing's disease due to a pituitary tumour is best treated by hypophysectomy. This can be performed by irradiation (external beam or interstitial) or by surgical ablation. If no pituitary tumour can be identified but the adrenals are both hyperplastic, bilateral adrenalectomy is usually preferred to 'blind' hypophysectomy. This may be performed through bilateral loin incisions or transabdominally. After bilateral adrenalectomy, the patient requires glucocorticoid and mineralocorticoid supplements for life and has a 10–20% risk of developing a pituitary tumour over the next 10 years (*Nelson's syndrome*). In those patients considered unfit or unsuitable for surgical adrenalectomy, medical adrenalectomy can be accomplished using metyrapone and aminoglutethimide.

Adrenal tumours causing Cushing's syndrome should be removed surgically. It must be remembered, however, that non-functioning adrenal adenomas are seen in 10–15% of the population, so the presence of an adrenal tumour is not always associated with Cushing's syndrome. Two-thirds of adrenal tumours causing Cushing's syndrome are benign adenomas and can be removed with the adrenal gland through a loin incision. Replacement therapy is usually necessary after surgery, since the contralateral adrenal is suppressed by high circulating levels of ACTH. Malignant adrenal tumours causing Cushing's syndrome have a poor prognosis, with death usually occurring from metastatic disease within 3 years.

## PHAEOCHROMOCYTOMA

Phaeochromocytoma is a tumour of the adrenal medulla which produces pressor agents (adrenaline, noradrenaline). It has often been called the *ten per cent tumour*; 10% of phaeochromocytomas are extra-adrenal (Fig. 13.6), 10% are malignant, 10% are bilateral and 10% are multiple. It may also be associated with multiple endocrine adenomatosis.

The tumour usually occurs in the third, fourth or fifth decades and is equally common in men and women. Hypertension is the usual presenting feature and, in 35% of patients affected, the hypertension is intermittent with periods of normotension intervening (Fig. 13.7).

The diagnosis is confirmed by the finding of raised levels of catecholamines (adrenaline, noradrenaline) and their metabolites (e.g. vanillylmandelic acid) in at least three 24-hour urine collections. Prior to urine collection, the patient should avoid ingestion of any substances which contain

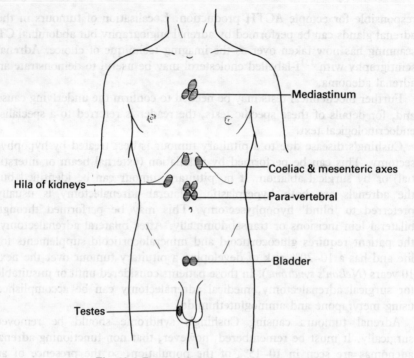

**Fig. 13.6** Extra-adrenal sites of chromaffin tissue

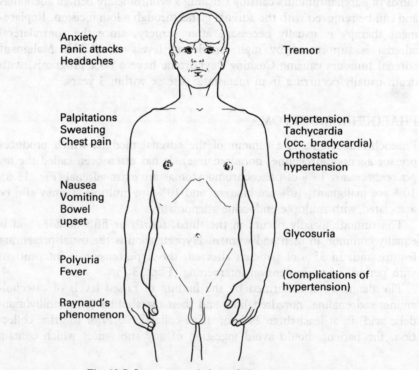

**Fig. 13.7** Symptoms and signs of phaeochromocytoma

phenols (coffee, bananas, vanilla flavourings), methyldopa or any drugs which interfere centrally or peripherally with sympathetic function.

Once the diagnosis has been confirmed, it is usually possible to localise the adrenal tumour using adrenal angiography or abdominal CT scanning. If this does not demonstrate the tumour, $^{131}$I-metaiodobenzylguanidine scintigraphy is useful to localise a biochemically proven phaeochromocytoma.

Treatment is surgical removal of the tumour, which usually lies in the adrenal gland. Surgery can be hazardous in patients with phaeochromocytoma, since handling of the tumour peroperatively may release large quantities of catecholamine into the circulation resulting in severe, acute hypertension. For this reason, all patients should receive alpha- and beta-blockers for at least 72 hours before surgery; the drugs used to accomplish this are phenoxybenzamine (20–40 mg/day) and propranolol (120–240 mg/day). During surgery, intravenous alpha- and beta-blockers should be used in the event of sudden hypertension and vasodilator agents such as sodium nitroprusside may also be used to lower the blood pressure. Pressor agents and intravenous fluid replacement are important in the event of 'rebound' hypotension.

Removal of the tumour (or tumours, if multiple) is always effective in curing the hypertension.

Other adrenal tumours are described in Table 13.2.

**Table 13.2** Other adrenal tumours

| Adrenal cortex | Adrenal medulla |
|---|---|
| Adenoma | Ganglioneuroma |
| Carcinoma | Neuroblastoma |
| | |
| Cysts | Hamartomas |
| Parasitic | Lipoma/myelolipoma |
| Epithelial | Fibroma/neurofibroma |
| Endothelial | Myoma |
| Pseudocysts | Haemangioma |
| | Lymphangioma |

*Metastases*
Reported in 10% of all malignancies.
Especially common in breast, gastric, colonic,
   bronchial, biliary and renal tumours

# 14

# Haematuria

The presence of blood in the urine is an important finding in the urological patient. This may vary from frank bleeding to the microscopic detection of red cells. There is, however, a poor correlation between the degree of haematuria and the severity of the underlying disorder. All patients with blood in the urine should, therefore, be fully investigated to establish a cause (Table 14.1).

Haematuria may occur in a wide variety of disorders but a careful history and examination often provide important clues to the source of the bleeding and help determine the nature and extent of investigations required.

**Table 14.1**  Causes of haematuria

| Congenital disorders | Hydronephrosis, renal cysts, polycystic disease |
| Trauma | Blunt or penetrating injuries |
| Infections | Bacterial (including TB), parasitic (e.g. bilharzia) |
| Calculi | Renal, ureteric or bladder |
| Tumours | Renal parenchyma, urothelium, prostate |
| 'Medical' causes | Glomerulonephritis, renal emboli, renal vein thrombosis |
| Bleeding diatheses | Haemophilia, thrombocytopenia, sickle cell disease |
| Drugs | Anticoagulants, cyclophosphamide, penicillamine |
| 'Benign' causes | Exercise, prostatic 'varices' |

## HISTORY

It is helpful to know whether blood is present throughout the stream or not; blood seen only at the beginning or end of micturition suggests bleeding from the bladder neck, prostate or urethra. A history of injury to the loin, pelvis or perineum is important because congenital abnormalities of the urinary tract are prone to bleed even after seemingly minor trauma.

In many patients, the underlying disorder may be suspected from a detailed enquiry about associated urinary symptoms. Unilateral loin pain suggests bleeding from that kidney due, for example, to calculi, tumours, hydronephrosis or cystic disease. A ureteric calculus should be suspected if the pain radiates in a colicky fashion to the groin, although blood clots may cause similar pain as they pass down the ureter (*clot colic*). An accompanying fever with these symptoms is strongly suggestive of renal infection.

Disturbances of micturition suggest a lower urinary tract cause for the bleeding. Frequency and urgency accompanied by dysuria are typical of cystitis and lower tract infection is a common cause of haematuria in children and young women. In men, such infections are usually secondary to bladder outflow obstruction and are associated with additional symptoms such as hesitancy, a reduced urinary stream and dribbling. Pain and bleeding occurring at the end of the urinary stream are typical of a bladder stone.

Painless haematuria throughout the urinary stream should raise the suspicion of a neoplasm in the urinary tract. Bladder tumours commonly present in this way and tumours of the kidney, ureter or prostate may also present with haematuria as the only symptom. In view of the established links between certain carcinogens and urinary tract tumours, all patients should be asked about smoking habits and about any previous occupations in which exposure to carcinogens might have occurred.

In addition to enquiring about other urinary symptoms, a full general history is essential. A recent sore throat or upper respiratory tract infection followed by oedema or joint pains raises the suspicion of glomerulonephritis, whilst a history of atrial fibrillation may be relevant as a possible source of renal emboli.

A history of inherited coagulation disorders (e.g. haemophilia, von Willebrand's disease) or of other genetic disorders that give rise to bleeding (e.g. sickle cell disease) may occasionally be obtained. A recent purpuric rash may be reported by patients with bleeding secondary to idiopathic thrombocytopenic purpura or Henoch–Schonlein disease.

All medications should be recorded. Anticoagulants may cause haematuria but should not be assumed solely responsible until appropriate investigations have ruled out other possible causes. Other drugs known to be associated with urinary tract bleeding include cyclophosphamide and D-penicillamine. The ingestion of beetroot causes red urine but stick testing and microscopy reveal that this is not due to haemoglobin or red cells in the urine.

Less common causes of haematuria may be suspected from the history, such as the occurrence of bleeding after vigorous exercise in some individuals (*jogger's haematuria*). Finally, a family history should be taken, noting particularly any inherited renal disorders such as polycystic disease or Alport's nephritis.

## EXAMINATION (Fig. 14.1)

General assessment of the patient should include examination for signs of anaemia or a bleeding tendency (e.g. bruising, purpura). The patient's

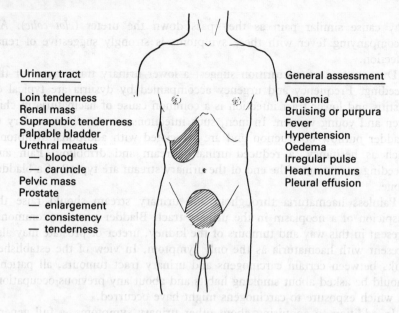

**Urinary tract**

Loin tenderness
Renal mass
Suprapubic tenderness
Palpable bladder
Urethral meatus
— blood
— caruncle
Pelvic mass
Prostate
— enlargement
— consistency
— tenderness

**General assessment**

Anaemia
Bruising or purpura
Fever
Hypertension
Oedema
Irregular pulse
Heart murmurs
Pleural effusion

**Fig. 14.1** Physical examination of the patient with haematuria

temperature may be elevated in infections, whilst hypertension and oedema may be present in glomerulonephritis. The rhythm of the heart and the presence of murmurs should be assessed to exclude emboli to the kidney. The chest should also be examined for the presence of a pleural effusion which may occur with renal or perinephric infections.

Local examination of the urinary tract should include abdominal palpation to look for tenderness in the costovertebral angle and to feel for a palpable, enlarged kidney. Renal enlargement may be due to a renal tumour or be the result of non-malignant disorders such as polycystic disease or hydronephrosis. The suprapubic region should be palpated to detect any tenderness or bladder enlargement; the latter is usually due to chronic retention of urine, although advanced tumours of the prostate or bladder can occasionally be palpable suprapubically.

Additional abdominal findings may include an enlarged, irregular liver if metastases have occurred from a urinary tract tumour and enlarged para-aortic nodes from lymphatic spread of tumour. An enlarged spleen suggests the possibility of a haematological disorder with impaired clotting.

In women, a vaginal examination should be carried out to detect pelvic masses arising either from the bladder or from the adjacent gynaecological organs. The urethral meatus should be inspected to exclude the presence of a urethral prolapse or caruncle. In the male, the prostate should be examined rectally to detect benign or malignant enlargement, or tenderness from prostatic infection. If the prostate feels malignant, the spine should be examined for any vertebral tenderness caused by metastases.

# INVESTIGATIONS

## Urine tests

Dipstix testing of the urine is a very sensitive method of detecting haemoglobin in the urine but the presence of red cells must always be confirmed on microscopy. Microscopy may reveal other features such as casts (in glomerulonephritis), crystals (in stone formers) and ova (in patients with schistosomiasis). Culture of the urine should be performed to exclude bacterial infection; if tuberculosis is suspected, three early-morning urines should be cultured for tubercle bacilli. Cytological examination of the urine is very helpful and may reveal malignant cells in the urine.

## Blood tests

General evaluation should include a full blood count, ESR and measurement of urea and creatinine. If glomerulonephritis is suspected, antistreptolysin-O (ASO) titres and serum complement levels should be measured; a nephrological opinion should then be sought regarding the need for renal biopsy. Additional haematological investigations (e.g. prothrombin time, bleeding time, haemoglobin electrophoresis) are needed if a bleeding disorder is suspected.

## Radiological investigations (Fig. 14.2)

The mainstay of investigation in patients with haematuria is the intravenous urogram (IVU). This is indicated in all patients who have blood in the urine unless there is a history of severe asthma or iodine allergy; when an IVU is contraindicated, a plain film and ultrasound of the urinary tract will usually suffice.

Urinary calculi may be visible on the preliminary plain film. After injection of contrast medium, a full sequence of films with nephrotomograms is taken to visualise the kidneys, ureters and bladder completely.

Subsequent radiological investigations depend on the IVU findings. A space-occupying lesion in the kidney requires further evaluation with ultrasound to determine whether it is cystic or solid. Aspiration of a cystic space-occupying lesion may be used to confirm that the lesion is a simple cyst, although improved ultrasound techniques now mean that cyst aspiration is rarely required.

## Other investigations (Fig. 14.3)

In all patients, regardless of the IVU findings, cystoscopy should be performed to look for a bladder tumour or other causes of bleeding in the lower urinary tract. This can be performed immediately before definitive

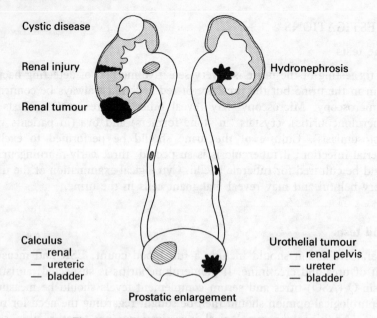

**Fig. 14.2** IVU findings in patients with haematuria

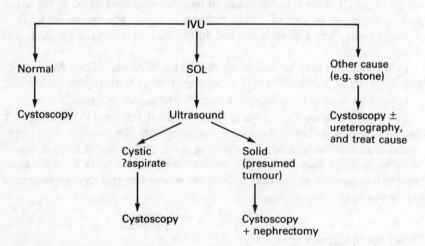

SOL = space occupying lesion

**Fig. 14.3** Investigation of haematuria

treatment of an already identified abnormality (e.g. prior to nephrectomy for a renal tumour). Cystoscopy should never be omitted because of the possibility of two independent causes of bleeding coexisting. An ascending ureterogram can be performed at the same time if a filling defect in the ureter or renal pelvis has been demonstrated by the IVU.

## THE PATIENT IN WHOM NO ABNORMALITY IS FOUND

If no cause for the haematuria is found as a result of the above investigations, the patient should not be discharged but kept under review for 3 months. At that time, the urine should be tested again and, if blood is still present, the entire investigative sequence repeated. In many patients, the bleeding does not recur in the long term.

Unfortunately, a small group of patients are seen in whom bleeding continues but in whom no cause can be found. This is especially likely to occur in patients with asymptomatic microscopic haematuria. In children with persistent haematuria, the possibility of glomerulonephritis should be considered. In young adults, the chance of a significant lesion in the urinary tract when bleeding persists is low (less than 2%) but such patients should probably be kept under regular review for at least 3 years. In older patients, 25% of those with haematuria are subsequently discovered to have a significant urological lesion and, of these, half are malignant. It is therefore important to maintain follow-up in elderly patients because of their tendency to develop a significant urological lesion over the ensuing years.

# 15

# Renal tumours

A variety of tumours may arise in the kidney either from the renal parenchyma or from the urothelial lining of the collecting system. Tumours of the kidney account for 3% of all malignancies. The most important parenchymal tumours are adenocarcinoma of the kidney (80% of all renal tumours) and Wilms' tumours (nephroblastoma) (Table 15.1). Transitional cell carcinomas account for the majority of tumours of the urothelium and are discussed separately in Chapter 16.

**Table 15.1** Types of renal tumour

| Parenchymal tumours | Tumours of the renal pelvis |
|---|---|
| *Benign* | *Benign* |
| adenoma | papilloma |
| haemangioma | *Malignant* |
| angiomyolipoma | transitional cell carcinoma |
| mesoblastic nephroma | squamous cell carcinoma |
| *Malignant* | adenocarcinoma |
| renal adenocarcinoma | |
| Wilms' tumour (nephroblastoma) | |
| sarcoma | |
| secondary tumours | |

## RENAL ADENOCARCINOMA

This tumour is of special interest because of its diversity of presenting symptoms. As a result, it may present initially to clinicians other than urologists and an awareness of the unusual syndromes associated with renal adenocarcinoma is essential in making the correct diagnosis.

The tumour arises from tubular epithelial cells and not from ectopic adrenal tissue as Grawitz originally proposed. The term renal adenocarcinoma reflects this origin and is preferred to other descriptive names such as hypernephroma, Grawitz tumour, renal cell carcinoma or clear cell carcinoma.

### Incidence and aetiology

The incidence increases steadily above the age of 40, reaching a peak at 65–75 years. It is almost twice as common in men as in women and bilateral tumours occur synchronously or asynchronously in 3% of patients. Benign adenomas, viruses, oestrogens, certain carcinogens and familial diseases (e.g. von Hippel–Lindau, tuberous sclerosis) have all been implicated in causing renal adenocarcinoma.

### Pathology

These tumours characteristically produce a discrete mass within the kidney that has a homogeneous yellowish appearance on cut section, although areas of haemorrhage and necrosis are often visible. Satellite nodules may be found adjacent to the primary tumour or, in poorly-differentiated tumours, there may be diffuse infiltration throughout the renal parenchyma.

On microscopy, the tumours have a solid or tubular pattern composed of cells with clear cytoplasm although some tumours contain cells with a granular eosinophilic cytoplasm. The histological appearances range from well-differentiated to anaplastic.

Figure 15.1 shows the spread of renal adenocarcinoma, while staging is depicted in Table 15.2.

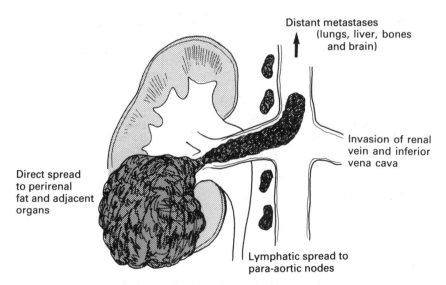

**Fig. 15.1** Spread of renal adenocarcinoma

**Table 15.2**   TNM staging for renal tumours

| | |
|---|---|
| Primary tumour: | T1 Small tumour not enlarging kidney |
| | T2 Large tumour distorting the kidney but confined within renal capsule |
| | T3 Spread through capsule to perinephric tissues |
| | T4 Invasion of abdominal wall or adjacent organs |
| Lymph nodes: | N0 Regional nodes not involved |
| | N1 Tumour in single regional node |
| | N2 Multiple regional nodes involved |
| | N3 Regional nodes fixed |
| | N4 Lymphatic involvement beyond regional nodes |
| Metastases: | M0 No distant metastases |
| | M1 Distant metastases present |

## Clinical features (Fig. 15.2)

Clinical examination may reveal a mass in the loin, signs of anaemia and, occasionally, enlarged nodes in the left supraclavicular fossa (*Troisier's nodes*).

Some patients present with symptoms due to metastases. Bone secondaries can lead to bone pain or pathological fractures, pulmonary deposits may produce respiratory symptoms or be detected on chest X-ray and metastases in the brain may produce neurological symptoms and signs. Tumour extension into the left renal vein may result in a varicocele and

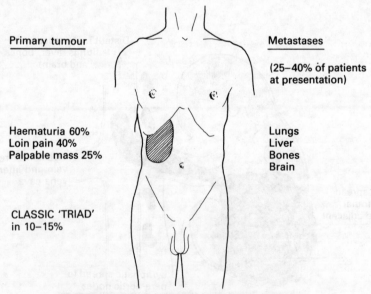

Primary tumour

Haematuria 60%
Loin pain 40%
Palpable mass 25%

CLASSIC 'TRIAD'
in 10–15%

Metastases

(25–40% of patients
at presentation)

Lungs
Liver
Bones
Brain

A left varicocele occurs in 1–2% of patients as a
result of renal vein invasion

**Fig. 15.2** Clinical features of renal adenocarcinoma

**Table 15.3** Paraneoplastic syndromes associated with renal adenocarcinoma

| Clinical effect | Incidence | Cause |
|---|---|---|
| Weight loss and fatigue | 48% | ? Tumour metabolites |
| Anaemia | 43% | Unknown |
| Raised ESR | 53% | Unknown |
| Abnormal LFTs | 15% | Unknown |
| Fever | 15% | ? Tumour associated pyrogens |
| Hypertension | 15% | Renin secretion |
| Erythrocytosis | 4% | Erythropoietin secretion |
| Hypercalcaemia | 4% | Ectopic parathyroid hormone production |
| Neuromyopathy | 3% | Unknown |
| Amyloidosis | 3% | Unknown |

extension into the inferior vena cava (IVC) may produce signs of IVC obstruction (bilateral leg oedema and collateral venous circulation).

In addition, renal carcinoma may give rise to a number of 'paraneoplastic' syndromes (Table 15.3). Systemic symptoms include fatigue, anorexia and weight loss which may be the result of toxic substances produced by the tumour. Many patients are anaemic to a greater degree than can be accounted for by haematuria, with circulating red cells that are normocytic but hypochromic.

Some tumours are diagnosed incidentally on an IVU or ultrasound performed for another reason.

### Investigations

Microscopy or dipstix testing of the urine is positive for blood in 67% of patients. Blood tests may reveal anaemia or polycythaemia, an elevated ESR and abnormal liver function tests but renal function is usually normal provided the other kidney is not diseased.

An IVU is the screening investigation of choice for a suspected renal tumour and typically reveals a space-occupying lesion within the kidney which causes distortion of the renal outline or calyceal pattern (Fig. 15.3). The main differential diagnosis is between a solid tumour and a benign cyst. Ultrasound scanning is normally used to distinguish between these two and, if a solid lesion is confirmed, the renal vein and inferior vena cava can be scanned for evidence of tumour extension (Fig. 15.4).

CT scanning is helpful to evaluate complex lesions not diagnosed with certainty by IVU and ultrasound alone. It also provides accurate pre-operative staging by detecting spread through the renal capsule, regional node enlargement and tumour in the renal vein or IVC.

Other diagnostic techniques may be indicated in certain circumstances. Arteriography was used routinely before the introduction of ultrasound and CT scanning to demonstrate the abnormal circulation associated with a tumour (as distinct from the avascular pattern of a cyst) and is still helpful

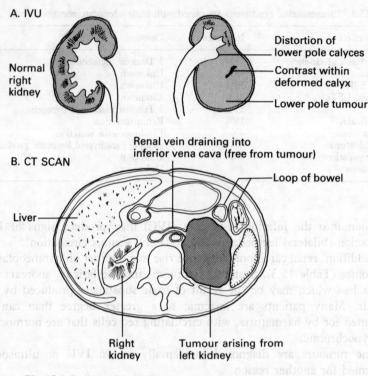

A. IVU

Normal right kidney

Distortion of lower pole calyces

Contrast within deformed calyx

Lower pole tumour

B. CT SCAN

Renal vein draining into inferior vena cava (free from tumour)

Loop of bowel

Liver

Right kidney

Tumour arising from left kidney

**Fig. 15.3** Radiographic findings in a patient with renal adenocarcinoma

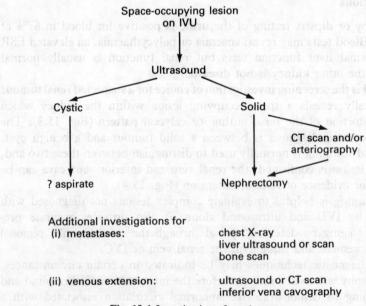

Space-occupying lesion on IVU

Ultrasound

Cystic

Solid

? aspirate

Nephrectomy

CT scan and/or arteriography

Additional investigations for
(i) metastases:        chest X-ray
                       liver ultrasound or scan
                       bone scan

(ii) venous extension: ultrasound or CT scan
                       inferior vena cavography

**Fig. 15.4** Investigation of renal tumours

where these scanning facilities are not readily available. Needle biopsy of the tumour is occasionally used to confirm the histological diagnosis, although it is not normally recommended because of the risk of tumour dissemination along the needle track.

Metastases in the lungs can be detected by simple chest X-ray, although CT scanning is a better method of demonstrating metastases in the mediastinum and lung fields. Bone scintigraphy may be helpful to detect asymptomatic spread to the skeleton. Venography via the femoral vein can be performed to show the extent of tumour spread within the IVC; this is helpful for planning the operative approach to such tumours.

## Treatment

In the absence of distant metastases, the treatment of choice for renal adenocarcinoma is *radical nephrectomy*. This involves removal of the kidney, adrenal gland and surrounding perinephric fat within Gerota's fascia, together with the upper ureter and any enlarged para-aortic nodes. A transperitoneal approach is preferred so that the renal vessels can be ligated before mobilising the kidney: this reduces the operative blood loss and prevents tumour thrombus being dislodged from the renal vein. Pre-operative occlusion of the renal artery by radiological embolisation is used by some surgeons but has not found widespread favour. Tumour extending into the inferior vena cava should be removed if possible after first controlling the contralateral renal vein and the IVC above and below the tumour.

Postoperative radiotherapy to the renal bed is preferred if there is evidence of invasion into perinephric fat or involvement of para-aortic lymph nodes.

### Tumour in a solitary kidney

In patients with a tumour in a solitary kidney, partial nephrectomy should be attempted. This may require extracorporeal 'bench surgery' which involves removal of the kidney, enucleation of the tumour and autotransplantation of the kidney remnant into the iliac fossa. If such conservative resection is not possible in a solitary kidney, nephrectomy followed by dialysis should be considered with the possibility of a renal transplant at a later date if the patient remains tumour free. In patients with bilateral tumours, the more affected kidney should be removed and conservative resection considered in the less severely affected kidney.

### Tumour in the presence of metastatic disease

The role of surgery in the presence of metastatic disease is controversial. If the metastasis is truly solitary (1–3% of patients), nephrectomy combined with removal of the metastasis (e.g by lobectomy for a pulmonary secondary) can sometimes be curative. More commonly, there are multiple metastases at the time of presentation.

Although there are reports of regression of metastases after removal of the primary tumour, this is very rare and probably occurs in less than 0.5% of patients with multiple metastases. Spontaneous regression of metastases undoubtedly occurs in untreated patients and many of the 'miraculous cures' achieved in the past can be attributed to this.

In patients with metastatic disease, the possible benefits of nephrectomy must be weighed against the morbidity and mortality of the operation. Surgery is best reserved for patients with intractable symptoms such as bleeding or pain. Nowadays, palliative radiotherapy or radiological embolisation may be equally effective in relieving local symptoms without resort to surgery; embolisation has the added advantage that it may stimulate an immune response to the tumour.

*Metastatic disease*

The treatment of metastatic disease is very unsatisfactory. Palliative radiotherapy may help in controlling symptoms from isolated deposits but systemic chemotherapy has proved very disappointing. Many chemotherapeutic agents have been tried, both singly and in combination, with response rates of 10% or less. Some tumours do respond to treatment with progestogens (e.g. medroxyprogesterone acetate 100 mg three times daily), although overall response rates are poor (10–20%).

The spontaneous regression occasionally seen in renal adenocarcinoma is thought to have an immunological basis. Immunotherapy has therefore been tried, using either BCG vaccine or interferon. Both agents produce measurable regression of metastatic disease in selected patients and are currently under evaluation in clinical trials.

**Prognosis** (Table 15.4)

The overall 5-year survival rate is 30–50% but metastases can develop many years after nephrectomy. The prognosis in individual patients is less

**Table 5.4**   Prognosis of renal adenocarcinoma

| Extent of spread | 5-year survival |
|---|---|
| Confined to kidney | 75% |
| Invading perirenal fat | 50% |
| Regional lymph nodes and/or tumour in renal vein or vena cava | 35% |
| Distant metastases | < 5% |

predictable and depends on tumour stage and grade at presentation. There is a markedly worse prognosis with capsular penetration by tumour or with lymphatic invasion and most patients with these features die from recurrent disease within 3 years. Involvement of the IVC is not necessarily an adverse prognostic sign provided the tumour thrombus can be removed.

## WILMS' TUMOUR (NEPHROBLASTOMA)

This tumour was first described by Wilms in 1899 and is found predominantly in children. It was formerly associated with a very poor prognosis but major advances in treatment in recent years have transformed the outlook for this condition.

### Incidence and aetiology

Wilms' tumour accounts for approximately 10% of all childhood malignancies. Eighty per cent occur before the age of 5, with a peak incidence at 2–3 years, although sporadic cases do occur in adults. In 5% of patients, there are bilateral tumours at the time of presentation.

The histogenesis of the tumour is unknown but it may arise in nests of embryonic blastema cells which are frequently found in areas of the kidney adjacent to the tumour. Genetic factors may also be important, since 15% of patients have associated congenital disorders including genitourinary tract anomalies, hemihypertrophy of the body and aniridia.

### Pathology

These tumours can reach a considerable size, causing distortion and compression of the remaining renal tissue. The tumour is usually soft and pale on cut section and may contain cysts or areas of haemorrhage. Microscopically, the tumour contains both epithelial and mesenchymal elements with connective tissue components such as muscle, fat, fibrous tissue and cartilage. The degree of differentiation varies from well differentiated (favourable histology) to anaplastic or spindle-cell lesions (unfavourable histology).

Staging of Wilms' tumour is shown in Table 15.5.

**Table 15.5**   Staging of Wilms' tumour

| | |
|---|---|
| Stage 1 | Tumour confined to kidney and completely excised |
| Stage 2 | Tumour extends beyond kidney but completely excised |
| Stage 3 | Residual non-haematogenous tumour confined to abdomen |
| Stage 4 | Deposits beyond stage 3 (lung, liver, bone or brain) |
| Stage 5 | Bilateral renal involvement at diagnosis |

## Clinical features (Fig. 15.5)

A palpable abdominal mass is present in 80% of patients. This may be the presenting symptom (often detected by the parents) or may simply be found at the time of initial examination. The mass is sometimes large enough to be visible on simple inspection of the abdomen.

Approximately 30% of children complain of abdominal pain which may be vague and ill-defined rather than specifically located in the loin. In contrast with renal adenocarcinoma in adults, haematuria occurs in only 25% of patients with Wilms' tumour and can often only be detected on dipstix testing or urine microscopy.

Non-specific symptoms such as anorexia, weight loss, anaemia or fever are common. Other systemic syndromes of the type seen with renal adeno-carcinoma are less common, although erythrocytosis and hypertension are occasionally encountered. Some children have signs of associated congenital anomalies.

Symptoms may also arise from metastases which are present in 20% of patients at presentation. These affect predominantly lungs and liver, although bone-metastasising tumours are occasionally seen (and are associated with a poor prognosis).

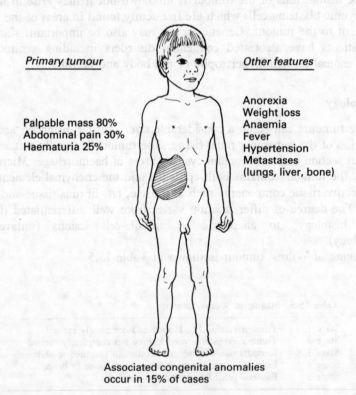

*Primary tumour*

Palpable mass 80%
Abdominal pain 30%
Haematuria 25%

*Other features*

Anorexia
Weight loss
Anaemia
Fever
Hypertension
Metastases
(lungs, liver, bone)

Associated congenital anomalies
occur in 15% of cases

**Fig. 15.5** Clinical features of Wilms' tumour

## Differential diagnosis

Other causes of an enlarged kidney in children include benign conditions such as hydronephrosis and multicystic or polycystic kidney disease. Wilms' tumour must also be differentiated from the rarer childhood renal tumours such as mesoblastic nephroma or sarcoma and from retroperitoneal tumours such as lymphoma and neuroblastoma.

## Investigations

The urine should be tested for blood and a 24-hour urine sample assayed for catecholamine production to help differentiate Wilms' tumour from neuroblastoma.

The IVU typically shows gross distortion of the calyceal pattern by an intrarenal mass. Ultrasound can be used to confirm this as solid rather than cystic, thus excluding benign cystic disease and hydronephrosis. CT scanning can help in difficult cases and is particularly useful in providing pre-operative staging of the disease. CT scanning has now largely replaced arteriography in pre-operative assessment.

Needle biopsy is occasionally necessary to establish the diagnosis, especially in patients with extensive disease in whom pre-operative chemotherapy is planned. Investigation for metastatic disease includes chest X-ray and CT scan, ultrasound or CT scanning of the liver and bone scintigraphy.

## Treatment

Treatment involves a combination of surgery, radiotherapy and chemotherapy. Treatment regimes have been formulated in large multicentre studies in Britain and the USA; they follow a carefully planned sequence according to the stage and histology of the tumour.

Nephrectomy is the initial procedure (except in 'inoperable' cases) and, at laparotomy, the other kidney should be examined to exclude bilateral tumour. If tumour is present in both kidneys, the more severely affected kidney should be removed; the other kidney should be treated by partial nephrectomy if possible, or (if partial nephrectomy cannot be performed) its margins marked with radio-opaque clips to aid post-operative radiotherapy. Occasionally, it may be necessary to undertake bilateral total nephrectomy and resort to haemodialysis in the postoperative period.

Postoperative radiotherapy was originally given to all patients to encompass the full area involved by the tumour, including the para-aortic area. Nowadays, with modern chemotherapy it has been shown that radiotherapy confers no additional benefit to surgery in children with either stage 1 or stage 2 favourable histology disease.

Chemotherapy has revolutionised the approach to Wilms' tumours, both as an adjuvant treatment in early disease and for the treatment of metastases. Actinomycin D was the first agent used successfully, although vincristine, adriamycin and cyclophosphamide are now also used. By using these drugs either singly or in combination, prolonged survival has been achieved even in advanced disease, with tumour response rates of 70%. Clinical trials currently in progress are aimed at refining this chemotherapy and minimising its toxicity without reducing its effectiveness.

In advanced cases considered 'inoperable' at presentation, the histological diagnosis should be confirmed by needle biopsy and treatment with chemotherapy commenced. If this produces sufficient regression, nephrectomy can be performed at a later date.

**Prognosis**

The overall 5-year survival rate with current cytotoxic regimes is 80% and the majority of patients with early disease can be cured. This figure seems likely to improve as the identification of poor prognostic factors (i.e. unfavourable histology, bone-metastasising tumours) enables such patients to be selected for more intensive chemotherapeutic regimes.

## OTHER MALIGNANT TUMOURS

**Sarcoma of the kidney**

Sarcomas are rare, accounting for less than 3% of all renal malignancies. Histologically, the tumour may be identifiable as a fibrosarcoma, leiomyosarcoma or liposarcoma, although it may be composed of unidentifiable undifferentiated tissue. Symptoms include haematuria, loin pain and a renal mass; investigation by IVU and ultrasound usually shows a solid lesion within the kidney and such tumours are often indistinguishable from renal adenocarcinomas before surgery. Treatment is by radical nephrectomy where possible, but these tumours are highly malignant and the prognosis is very poor.

**Secondary renal tumours**

These occur as a result of blood-borne emboli and are often multiple. The commonest primary sites are carcinoma of the bronchus or breast, malignant melanoma and lymphoreticular tumours. Occasionally, a tumour from one kidney metastasises to the other by retrograde spread along the renal vein. Renal metastases may cause loin pain and haematuria, although symptoms from the primary tumour usually predominate. Prognosis is very poor but palliation of symptoms can be obtained either by nephrectomy or by non-operative means (radiotherapy, radiological embolisation).

**Renal oncocytoma**

This is a tumour which is derived from proximal tubular cells and has a typical histological appearance. The tumour is composed of well-differentiated granular eosinophilic cells (*oncocytes*) arranged in a tubular, alveolar or papillary pattern. At presentation, oncocytoma is often large and difficult to distinguish from renal adenocarcinoma. Although it has a very good prognosis compared with other forms of renal tumour, metastases occasionally occur so that it cannot be regarded as totally benign. Treatment is by nephrectomy.

## BENIGN TUMOURS OF THE KIDNEY

### Adenoma

Adenomas are often seen in the kidney at autopsy and may also be encountered during operations on the kidney. They are well-demarcated lesions of varying size up to 3 cm and are composed of small cuboidal or columnar cells forming tubules. They rarely cause symptoms but a small proportion may undergo malignant change to adenocarcinomas.

### Haemangioma

This is a benign vascular tumour. Haemangioma is a rare cause of haematuria but the bleeding can be recurrent and profuse. The IVU is often normal but blood seen issuing from one ureteric orifice at cystoscopy may help to localise the side of the tumour. Arteriography is usually required to demonstrate the abnormal vessels and may allow therapeutic embolisation. Conservative resection is possible but, in most patients affected, the diagnosis is only made after nephrectomy for significant haemorrhage.

### Angiomyolipoma

This is a tumour composed of fat, blood vessels and smooth muscle which is often seen in patients with tuberous sclerosis. The tumour may be so large that an abdominal mass is the presenting symptom but, in most patients, haematuria is the mode of presentation. Pre-operative diagnosis is often possible from CT scanning because these tumours contain fat which has a characteristic tissue density. If removal of the tumour is needed for pain or bleeding, partial nephrectomy should be performed where possible since the tumour may be bilateral.

### Mesoblastic nephroma

This is a rare benign tumour which is usually found in neonates and infants, in whom it must be distinguished from a Wilms' tumour. It is composed of mesenchymal tissue with occasional epithelial structures within it. Nephrectomy is usually performed for the presence of the renal mass but no additional treatment is required after this.

# 16

# Urothelial tumours

The urinary tract is lined by specialised waterproof (transitional) epithelium. This extends from the tips of the renal papillae to the navicular fossa in men, and halfway along the urethra in women. Transitional cell tumours may occur at any site in this epithelium and are often multifocal. In patients with transitional cell tumours, the entire lining of the urinary tract is potentially unstable. Seventy per cent of urothelial tumours are superficial at presentation but, of these, two-thirds will subsequently recur locally or elsewhere in the urinary tract and, in 10–15%, the recurrence will be invasive.

## INCIDENCE

Bladder tumours are found in 20 per 100 000 of the population. Eight thousand new cases of urothelial cancer present in the UK each year. There is a wide geographical variation in incidence, with tumours common in the industrialised world but less common in undeveloped countries (except those in bilharzial areas). The peak incidence occurs at 65 years.

## AETIOLOGY

Rehn (1894) was the first to recognise the association between industrial carcinogens and bladder cancer. Many factors are now recognised as contributing to the development of urothelial tumours, but occupational exposure is nowadays a factor in only 10% of patients. Most carcinogens have a latent period of 15–20 years between exposure and the development of tumours: this means that occupational exposure could result in tumour formation at an earlier age than in those patients not exposed to industrial carcinogens.

In the majority of patients, no single causative factor can be identified (Table 16.1). In such patients, it must be presumed that endogenous carcinogens are the cause of tumour development. There is some evidence that tryptophane metabolism may be abnormal in these patients, that the

**Table 16.1**  Factors implicated in the development of urothelial cancer

*Occupational exposure*
  2-naphthylamine
  4-aminodiphenyl
  benzidine
  auramine and magenta dyes
  *o*-dianisidine
  *o*-tolidine
  chrysoidine/rhodamine

*Cigarette smoking* (× 2 risk)

*Drugs*
  phenacetin/aspirin
  cyclophosphamide

*Associated diseases*
  schistosomiasis
  Balkan nephropathy (× 200 risk)
  exstrophy (ectopia vesicae)
  leukoplakia
  urachal remnants
  pelvic irradiation

*Endogenous carcinogens*
  nitrosamines
  tryptophane metabolites (aminophenols)

*Chronic inflammation*
  bladder outflow obstruction
    + infection
    + stones/diverticulum

effects of this may be reduced by pyridoxine and that patients who smoke are more likely to suffer the effects of these endogenous carcinogens.

## PATHOLOGY (Table 16.2)

Very few premalignant conditions have been identified. Cystitis cystica or cystitis glandularis in an otherwise normal bladder are not premalignant conditions; squamous metaplasia of the trigone as seen in women with

**Table 16.2**  Histological types of urothelial tumour

*Benign*
  papilloma (0.5% of all tumours)
  fibroepithelial polyp

*Malignant*
  transitional cell carcinoma (90%)
  squamous carcinoma (5–8%)
  adenocarcinoma (1–2%)
  undifferentiated carcinoma
  sarcoma

trigonitis is not premalignant but the metaplasia seen in exstrophy, chronic bladder inflammation and schistosomiasis undoubtedly is. Bladder leuko-plakia is a premalignant condition, especially when associated with chronic infection.

The vast majority of urothelial tumours are malignant transitional cell carcinomas. There is still a tendency to refer to these tumours as 'papil-lomas' which, strictly, they are not. A true diagnosis of papilloma requires histological evidence of no increase in the number of cell layers in the tumour (usually < 7), a uniform cellular structure and little or no abnormal mitotic activity.

Squamous carcinomas usually develop in bladders which have been subject either to long-standing inflammation or to infestation by schisto-somiasis. Adenocarcinomas occasionally occur de novo anywhere in the bladder but more usually arise from urachal remnants in the vault of the bladder (Fig. 16.1).

The histological appearance of tumours arising in the upper urinary tracts is identical to that of bladder tumours. However, presentation of these tumours is often late so that a higher proportion of them are more advanced at the time of diagnosis (Fig.16.2).

The degree of histological differentiation of malignant urothelial tumours is an important factor in determining treatment and prognosis. Several methods of histological grading are used but it is most useful to regard tumours as well differentiated (G1), moderately differentiated (G2) or poorly differentiated (G3).

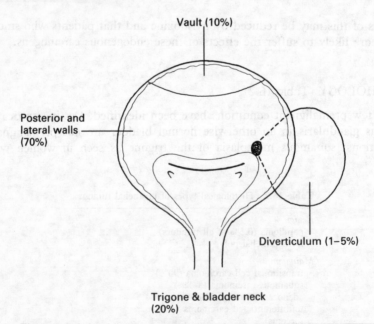

Vault (10%)

Posterior and lateral walls (70%)

Diverticulum (1–5%)

Trigone & bladder neck (20%)

**Fig. 16.1** Relative frequency of tumour development at sites in the bladder

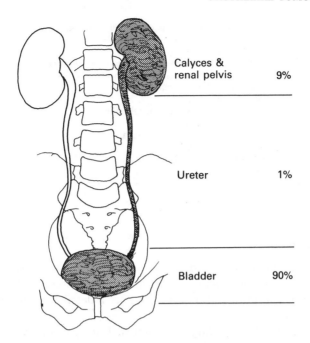

Calyces &
renal pelvis         9%

Ureter               1%

Bladder              90%

**Fig. 16.2** Relative frequency of tumours throughout the urinary tract

A special form of tumour that may occur anywhere in the urinary tract is *carcinoma in situ*. This is analogous with carcinoma in situ in other sites and is characterised by malignant change in the surface epithelial lining confined entirely to the mucosa of the bladder or upper urinary tract. Carcinoma in situ in the bladder, however, sometimes behaves in a very aggressive manner with early invasion or spread and this presents special problems to the urologist.

## SYMPTOMS (Table 16.3)

The classical presenting symptom of a urothelial tumour is *painless total haematuria*.

Twenty per cent of patients with haematuria are subsequently found to have a urinary tract tumour whilst 10% of patients with microscopic haematuria over the age of 45 years have a tumour as the cause of the bleeding. A bladder tumour may be an incidental finding at cystoscopy for another problem, and this accounts for approximately 10% of all tumours.

Some patients with carcinoma in situ of the bladder present with frequency, dysuria, urgency and perineal or groin pain. There may be no blood in the urine and the symptoms are often ascribed to infection or prostatitis. This symptom complex has been referred to as *malignant cystitis*.

**Table 16.3**   Symptoms of urothelial tumours

Painless haematuria (in 70–90%)
Cystitis — 40% have a proven urinary infection
       — 15% present with symptoms of cystitis
Bladder outflow obstruction
Ureteric obstruction
      — renal pain or renal failure
Non-specific symptoms
      — weight loss, anaemia, PUO
Metastatic disease
Incidental finding (10%)
Microscopic haematuria

## INVESTIGATIONS

The three cardinal investigations in patients with haematuria are urine culture/microscopy, intravenous urography and cystoscopy. However, more general investigations are also necessary after a detailed history and careful clinical examination.

Abnormal physical findings are unusual in patients with urothelial tumours, although a large bladder tumour may be palpable as a suprapubic mass and an enlarged, obstructed kidney may be palpable in the loin. General features, however, such as anaemia, bone tenderness, hepatomegaly and pyrexia may be obvious in patients with more advanced disease.

A full blood picture and ESR are essential, as is measurement of plasma urea, electrolytes and creatinine. A chest X-ray should be performed and an ECG if indicated by the patient's general health. Urine must be cultured for bacteria and microscoped to confirm the presence of red blood cells in the urine. Urine may also be spun down and the sediment stained and examined cytologically for malignant cells. A negative cytological examination does not exclude the presence of a urothelial tumour but a positive result is very useful. Cytology is of particular use in patients with carcinoma in situ where malignant cells are often shed in the urine; in such patients, random biopsy of the bladder mucosa may not show any definite malignancy although biopsy of abnormal areas usually does.

The presence of sterile pyuria (pus cells in the urine without urinary infection) should also raise the possibility of a urothelial tumour. Sterile pyuria may also be caused by calculi, tuberculosis and partially-treated urinary infections.

Intravenous urography is the mainstay of radiological investigations in suspected urothelial cancer. If there is a history of allergy to contrast media, a plain abdominal film and ultrasound may be used as an initial alternative. Although a cystogram tends to show bladder tumours more reliably, the post-voiding film during an IVU often demonstrates tumours in the bladder.

Tumours in the upper urinary tracts usually appear as filling defects in the ureter or renal pelvis. In the kidney, tumours cause loss or distortion of calyces or, very rarely, distortion of the renal outline. If a bladder tumour is seen on the IVU causing obstruction of the ureter, this indicates that the tumour is already invading the bladder muscle. Bladder tumours obstruct the ureteric orifice as a result of muscle invasion; even the largest superficial bladder tumours never obstruct the ureter simply due to their bulk.

If the IVU shows ureteric obstruction above the ureteric orifice, the suspicion is that there is a ureteric tumour. In contrast to lesions in the bladder, a superficial ureteric tumour, if sufficiently bulky, may obstruct the ureter. This situation may be clarified by antegrade or retrograde ureterography, and this can be combined with sampling of urine from the ureter (or kidney) for cytological examination.

Abdominal CT scanning may be useful in certain situations, especially when radical surgery is planned for bladder tumours and when the status of regional lymph nodes needs to be determined.

The crucial investigation, however, is cystoscopy and examination under anaesthesia. This allows bladder tumours to be biopsied for histological assessment and permits clinical staging which is vital in determining subsequent treatment.

## CLINICAL AND PATHOLOGICAL ASSESSMENT OF TUMOUR STAGE

Cystoscopic assessment involves a careful examination of the entire transitional cell lining of the bladder, prostate and urethra. Any visible tumours should be resected and sent for histological assessment. Resection is performed in two stages: first, the exophytic portion of the tumour is resected flush with the bladder wall; second, a deeper biopsy, including bladder muscle, is taken and sent separately for histology (Fig. 16.3).

The bladder should then be washed out and emptied and, with the patient anaesthetised, relaxed and in the lithotomy position, a bimanual examination performed (Fig. 16.4). This determines the clinical stage of the tumour and, when combined with histological analysis, determines subsequent treatment.

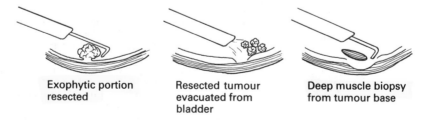

Exophytic portion resected

Resected tumour evacuated from bladder

Deep muscle biopsy from tumour base

**Fig. 16.3** Endoscopic resection of bladder tumour

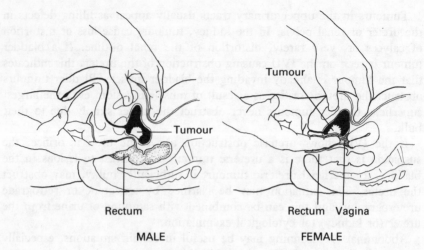

**Fig. 16.4** Bimanual assessment of bladder

Staging of tumours is performed according to the TNM classification (Fig.16.5). Local clinical staging has an accuracy of 80% and this figure is increased by pathological confirmation of stage and grade. Nodal and metastatic spread are difficult to determine for bladder tumours and are usually only assessed if radiotherapy or radical surgery is contemplated (Table 16.4).

Tumours in the upper urinary tract cannot, of course, be staged in this way. Staging for these tumours can usually only be performed pathologically on surgically excised specimens. Pathological stages $pT_3$ and $pT_4$ cannot be determined on bladder biopsy specimens (which contain a partial thickness of bladder wall) but only after total or partial cystectomy.

| Clinical stage | Bladder findings on bimanual assessment after resection | | Histopathological classification | |
|---|---|---|---|---|
| $T_1$ | | No palpable mass | $pT_a$ <br> $pT_1$ | Tumour confined to epithelium <br> Invasion of subepithelial connective tissue |
| $T_2$ | | No mass or thickening | $pT_2$ | Invasion of superficial bladder muscle |
| $T_3$ | | Hard mobile mass | $pT_{3a}$ <br><br> $pT_{3b}$ | Invasion of deep muscle not beyond bladder wall <br> Invasion beyond bladder wall |
| $T_4$ | | Hard fixed mass | $pT_{4a}$ <br><br> $pT_{4b}$ | Deep invasion with involvement of prostate, uterus or vagina <br> Deep invasion with fixation to bony pelvis |

**Fig. 16.5** Staging of bladder tumours

**Table 16.4** Staging of lymph nodes and metastases in bladder cancer

| | | | |
|------|------------------------------------------------------|-----|------------------------------|
| N0 | No nodal involvement | | |
| N1 | Single ipsilateral regional node involved | | |
| N2 | Contralateral/bilateral or multiple regional nodes involved | M0 | No evidence of metastases |
| N3 | Fixed regional nodes involved | M1 | Metastases present |
| N4 | Juxtaregional nodes involved | Mx | Metastatic state unknown |
| Nx | Nodal status unknown | | |

# TREATMENT OF BLADDER TUMOURS

## Ta and T1 tumours

Superficial bladder tumours can, in most cases, be dealt with endoscopically by cystodiathermy under anaesthesia. This may require repeated cystoscopy in some patients. There is, nowadays, an increasing use of flexible cystoscopes and laser treatment for destroying superficial bladder tumours under local anaesthetic. In 30% of affected patients, there are no further tumour recurrences. In all patients, regular endoscopic follow-up is necessary. In some, however, recurrent tumours occur very rapidly and endoscopic measures fail to control the situation. Alternative measures are listed in Table 16.5.

**Table 16.5** Alternative measures for multiple, recurrent superficial tumours

*Systemic chemotherapy*
  cyclophosphamide
  methotrexate
  vitamin A derivatives

*Intravesical chemotherapy* (30–50% response rates)
  mitomycin C
  adriamycin
  epodyl (ethoglucid)
  thiotepa
  cisplatinum
  bleomycin

*Immunotherapy*
  BCG (intravesical or systemic)

*Helmstein balloon distension of the bladder*
  (produces tumour necrosis by compression)

*Bladder hyperthermia*

*Cryosurgery/laser surgery*

*Mucosal stripping of the bladder*

*Total cystectomy and urinary diversion*

The place of radiotherapy in superficial tumours remains to be defined although external irradiation may be useful for G3 tumours. If all other measures fail, then it may be necessary to resort to total cystoprostato-urethrectomy and urinary diversion for superficial tumours.

Partial cystectomy for single large superficial lesions is very rarely indicated. Removal of a tumour-containing segment of the bladder is an illogical operation when tumour recurrence is likely elsewhere in the bladder and there is a real risk of seeding tumour into the wound. Partial cystectomy, however, is still occasionally indicated for adenocarcinomas arising in a urachal remnant or for tumour arising in a bladder diverticulum.

## T2 tumours

Only 15% of bladder tumours fall into this clinical staging category. This is a reflection of the difficulty in detecting induration in the bladder wall after resection. The diagnosis of a T2 tumour is more reliably made histologically.

In patients in whom there is no residual mass palpable in the bladder wall after tumour resection, it is reasonable to assume that the muscle biopsy has removed all the viable tumour. In this situation a well-differentiated tumour can be followed up as if it were a superficial one. If there is thickening palpable after resection or if the tumour is poorly-differentiated, then radical treatment either by external beam radiotherapy alone or by combined irradiation and cystectomy is indicated.

In this country, external radiotherapy alone is generally preferred although the results of cystectomy for T2 tumours are good, especially for women and for patients less than 65.

After radiotherapy, regular endoscopic follow-up for life remains essential. If viable tumour is still present in the bladder 6 months after radiotherapy or if invasive tumour subsequently recurs, total cystectomy and urinary diversion is the treatment of choice. If, however, tumour recurrences after radiotherapy are superficial, they can be managed by repeated cystodiathermy without resort to radical surgery.

## T3 tumours

The mainstay of treatment in the UK for deeply invasive bladder cancer is external beam radiotherapy (40–60 Gy). This should be followed up regularly with cystoscopies. If there is tumour recurrence after radiotherapy or if severe side-effects (bleeding, contracted bladder, incontinence, fistulae) occur, total cystectomy with urinary diversion may be performed (*salvage cystectomy*).

In the USA and in some centres in Britain, there is a trend towards aggressive surgical treatment for T3 bladder cancer. Total cystectomy is performed with urinary diversion after pre-operative radiotherapy. The

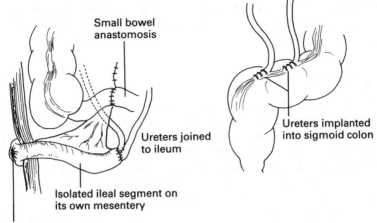

Small bowel anastomosis

Ureters joined to ileum

Ureters implanted into sigmoid colon

Isolated ileal segment on its own mesentery

Conduit opening onto skin

### COMPLICATIONS

**ILEAL CONDUIT**
**(occ. COLONIC CONDUIT)**
Stomal stenosis, prolapse,
excoriation, recession
Ureteroileal obstruction
Reflux and infections
Stone formation
Renal failure

**URETEROSIGMOIDOSTOMY**
Reflux and infection
Ureteric stenosis
Rectal incontinence of urine
Metabolic problems
(hyperchloraemic acidosis)
Tumours at ureterocolic
anastomosis

**Fig. 16.6** Methods of urinary diversion after total cystectomy

results from this are little different from those for radical radiotherapy, except in younger patients and in patients in whom the local or nodal disease downstages after radiotherapy.

Total cystectomy involves removing the lower ureters, bladder, prostate and urethra in men, and the lower ureters, bladder, urethra and gynaecological organs in women. There is a 10–15% risk of tumour developing in an isolated urethra left in situ after total cystectomy and urinary diversion (Fig. 16.6).

CT scanning is useful in planning the management of invasive bladder cancer. Radical pelvic node dissection may be added to cystectomy if there is CT evidence of regional node involvement (seen in 30% of T3 bladder tumours at presentation).

### Advanced (T4) tumours

The prognosis of T4 bladder cancer is extremely poor. Palliative radiotherapy is generally employed to relieve local symptoms such as haematuria. If this cannot be controlled, measures such as intravesical instillation of formalin or alum, internal iliac artery embolisation, supravesical urinary diversion and systemic chemotherapy may produce improvement in the patient's quality of life. The terminal event is often renal failure due to ureteric obstruction.

### Carcinoma in situ

In broad terms, patients with carcinoma in situ fall into two groups. The majority of patients have in situ change alone or changes in association with tumours of other stages in the bladder but few symptoms. These patients can be managed by the means outlined for superficial bladder cancer and this form of carcinoma in situ responds relatively well to intravesical chemotherapy. However, a proportion of these patients develop invasive tumours over a 5-year period and need radical treatment.

A minority of patients with carcinoma in situ have symptoms rather like those of cystitis (*malignant cystitis*). These patients often have tumour in their prostatic ducts and 70% progress to invasive disease within 3 years. In these patients, systemic chemotherapy (cyclophosphamide) may produce good results but many require total cystectomy and urinary diversion.

### Metastatic bladder cancer

Response to chemotherapeutic agents in metastatic bladder cancer is very disappointing. Many drug regimes have been used, characterised more by their toxicity than their efficacy. As single agents, cisplatinum and methotrexate seem to be the most effective in patients with invasive bladder cancer and metastases. Reasonable palliation can be obtained, with a 30% response rate in terms of a measurable decrease in the size of tumour deposits. Chemotherapy seems to be most effective at treating nodal and pulmonary metastases and relatively ineffective against hepatic or osseous secondaries.

## PROSPECTS FOR THE FUTURE IN BLADDER CANCER (Table 16.6)

A non-invasive test of tumour recurrence and some measure of invasive potential are needed. Whilst cytological screening of urine is practised by industries using known carcinogens, a negative cytology does not mean the patient does not have a bladder tumour. Some tumour antigens have been defined in peripheral blood but their presence does not correlate well with tumour recurrence in the urinary tract.

Loss of epithelial surface blood group antigens can be used as an indicator of invasive potential but the results are difficult to assess and the tests are not wholly reliable.

New imaging techniques (e.g magnetic resonance imaging, MRI) and adjuvant chemotherapy may eventually prove useful but their place has yet

**Table 16.6**   Prognosis of bladder tumours

| Tumour stage | 5-year survival |
|---|---|
| Carcinoma in situ | 30–40% |
| pTa | 90–95% |
| pT1 | 40–75% |
| pT2 | 55% |
| pT3 | 25% |
| pT4 | 5–10% |

| | |
|---|---|
| Low risk — | small G1 tumours |
| | pTa tumours |
| | single bladder tumours |
| | normal random bladder biopsies |
| High risk — | large G2/G3 tumours |
| | random biopsies showing dysplasia |
| | multiple tumours |
| | carcinoma in situ |

to be defined. Early results of cisplatinum treatment for invasive bladder cancer are encouraging but further trials are needed to determine whether such treatment is justified.

## UROTHELIAL TUMOURS IN THE KIDNEY AND URETER

Traditionally, the time-honoured treatment for upper tract urothelial tumours has been nephroureterectomy with removal of the kidney, ureter and a cuff of bladder. This requires two incisions, one in the loin to remove the kidney with its upper ureter and one suprapubically to remove the lower ureter and its cuff of bladder. Alternative methods in which the lower ureter is resected endoscopically with the remaining ureter and the kidney being removed through a loin incision are used by some surgeons.

Now that the multifocal nature of urothelial cancer is better recognised, conservative treatment for upper tract tumours is becoming more widespread. Upper tract tumours, however, tend to present late and, as a result, conservative surgery is not always possible.

### Tumours of the calyces and renal pelvis

Local resection by partial nephrectomy may be possible for tumours within the collecting system, although nephroureterectomy is usually necessary. Tumours of the renal pelvis may be dealt with by local resection and reconstruction using either a pyeloplasty-type technique or direct anastomosis of the ureter to the lower pole calyces (*ureterocalycostomy*).

### Tumours of the ureter

Rigid ureteroscopes can now be equipped for ureteric tumour resection so

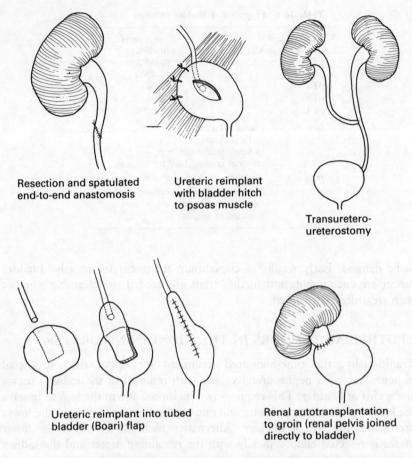

Resection and spatulated
end-to-end anastomosis

Ureteric reimplant
with bladder hitch
to psoas muscle

Transuretero-
ureterostomy

Ureteric reimplant into tubed
bladder (Boari) flap

Renal autotransplantation
to groin (renal pelvis joined
directly to bladder)

**Fig. 16.7** Reconstruction after ureteric resection

that superficial ureteric tumours may be resected endoscopically in much the same way as are bladder tumours. In most cases, however, localised ureteric resection is more appropriate. The method of restoring continuity between ureter and bladder depends on the level of the ureter resected (Fig. 16.7). If direct reconstruction is not possible, nephroureterectomy is the treatment of choice.

The development of percutaneous and ureteroscopic instruments may mean that tumours in the kidney or ureter can be diathermised directly. There is, however, a risk of seeding of tumour into percutaneous tracts and this technique has yet to gain widespread popularity.

# 17

# Bladder outflow obstruction and retention of urine

Obstruction to the flow of urine from the bladder may occur anywhere along the length of the urethra, from the bladder neck to the external meatus, and is much commoner in men. The cause of the obstruction may be structural (e.g. prostatic enlargement) or functional (Table 17.1). Functional obstruction is usually neuropathic in origin and is discussed in Chapter 18.

As a result of outflow obstruction, characteristic changes are seen in the bladder and the upper tracts.

**Table 17.1** Causes of bladder outflow obstruction

*CONGENITAL*
   Urethral valves
   Urethral polyps
   Urethral stricture

*ACQUIRED*

*Structural causes*
   benign prostatic hyperplasia
   carcinoma of prostate
   bladder neck stenosis
   urethral stricture
   urethral carcinoma
   urethral calculi
   external compression
      — faecal impaction
      — pelvic tumour

*Functional causes*
   bladder neck dyssynergia
   detrusor-sphincter dyssynergia

THE EFFECTS OF OBSTRUCTION (Fig. 17.1)

## Changes in the bladder

In addition to the structural changes, the obstructed bladder may show an increased irritability during filling. This leads to involuntary or 'unstable' contractions (*destrusor instability*) which cause frequency and urgency of micturition. If the outflow obstruction goes unrecognised or untreated, the detrusor muscle becomes unable to overcome the obstruction so that residual urine remains in the bladder after voiding and predisposes to chronic infection. This can progress to chronic retention of urine, with a very large capacity bladder from which only a small quantity is voided at a time.

### Changes in the upper tracts

Persistently raised pressure within an obstructed bladder may impair ureteric emptying and lead to dilatation of the ureters and collecting systems (*hydroureter* and *hydronephrosis*). The ureters may also be partially obstructed as they pass through the thickened bladder wall, and vesico-ureteric reflux occurs in some patients due to loss of the valvular mechanism at the ureterovesical junction.

The resulting upper tract dilatation is known as *obstructive uropathy*. If high bladder pressures are constantly transmitted to the kidney via a dilated ureter, there may be a gradual deterioration in renal function; the patient becomes salt-depleted and dehydrated as a result of impaired tubular reabsorption of sodium and inability to concentrate the urine (*obstructive nephropathy*).

## CLINICAL FEATURES (Fig. 17.2)

### History

#### Symptoms

The increased resistance to urine flow through the obstructed urethra results in hesitancy of micturition, a poor or variable urinary stream and terminal dribbling.

In addition, there may be frequency, nocturia, urgency and urge incontinence. These 'irritative' symptoms are often due to associated bladder instability which is present in 60% of patients with outflow obstruction due to benign prostatic enlargement. Frequency, however, may be the result of a reduction in functional bladder capacity due to the development of residual urine and nocturia may be exacerbated in the elderly by changes in the diurnal production of antidiuretic hormone (ADH).

If there is progression to chronic retention of urine, the patient may notice an increase in abdominal girth and complain of incontinence, either as a continuous dribble (*overflow incontinence*) or on coughing and straining (*stress incontinence*). Some of these patients have associated renal impairment and symptoms from uraemia.

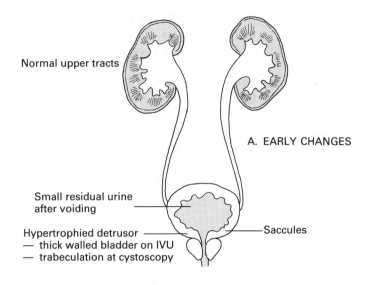

A. EARLY CHANGES

Normal upper tracts

Small residual urine after voiding

Hypertrophied detrusor
— thick walled bladder on IVU
— trabeculation at cystoscopy

Saccules

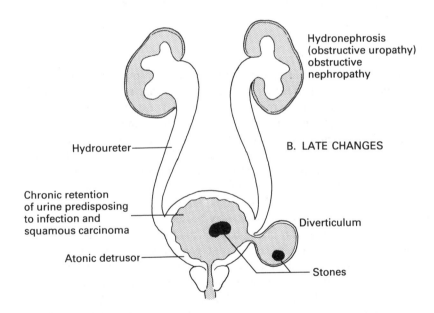

B. LATE CHANGES

Hydronephrosis (obstructive uropathy) obstructive nephropathy

Hydroureter

Chronic retention of urine predisposing to infection and squamous carcinoma

Atonic detrusor

Diverticulum

Stones

**Fig. 17.1** Effects of bladder outflow obstruction on the bladder and upper tracts

Acute retention of urine may occur at any stage in the disease process and may even occur in patients with no preceding obstructive symptoms. Acute retention usually produces severe suprapubic pain from the distended bladder; pain may, however, be minimal in patients with pre-existing chronic retention of urine and a lax bladder (*acute-on-chronic retention*). Factors that are known to precipitate acute retention include drug therapy (e.g. anticholinergics), urethral instrumentation, coincidental surgery (e.g hernia repair) and excessive alcohol intake.

Patients may also present with symptoms caused by the complications of obstruction (e.g. bladder calculi, urinary infection). Urinary infection usually starts as cystitis but may spread to involve the upper tracts (pyelo-nephritis) or the genital tract (prostatitis, epididymitis); septicaemia may also occur, especially after urethral instrumentation in the presence of infection. Haematuria is unusual in bladder outflow obstruction but may occur from veins overlying an enlarged prostate.

*Other features*

Enquiries should be made about previous pelvic fractures, perineal trauma, urethral infection and urethral instrumentation, all of which may cause a urethral stricture. Any neurological symptoms that might indicate a neuro-pathic cause for the patient's symptoms should also be noted.

**Investigations**

A full blood count should be performed and the plasma urea, creatinine and electrolytes measured. The serum acid phosphatase is useful as a baseline measurement if prostatic carcinoma is suspected. An MSU should be exam-ined by microscopy and culture to exclude urinary infection.

A plain abdominal X-ray may show bladder calculi or other stones in the urinary tract and sometimes reveals sclerotic secondary deposits from pros-tatic carcinoma, usually in the lumbar spine, pelvis or upper femora.

The effects of obstruction on the urinary tract are best assessed using ultrasound to look for a thickened bladder wall, residual urine and upper tract dilatation. The prostate itself may be seen by ultrasound but the size of the prostatic impression in the base of the bladder is an unreliable guide to real prostatic size. A coincidental but asymptomatic lesion of the urinary tract such as a renal cyst or tumour may also be detected by ultrasound. An IVU should, however, be performed if there is haematuria.

The patient's voiding pattern and flow rate should be determined using a flow meter, both to help in diagnosis and to give a baseline for comparison during follow-up (Fig. 17.3). Fuller urodynamic assessment (including voiding cystometry) is indicated if the diagnosis of obstruction remains in doubt or if neuropathy is suspected.

Other investigations that may prove useful include an ascending ureth-rogram in patients with a suspected urethral stricture and a micturating cystogram in boys with suspected urethral valves.

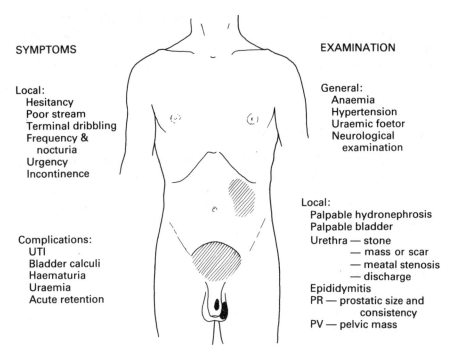

SYMPTOMS

Local:
  Hesitancy
  Poor stream
  Terminal dribbling
  Frequency &
    nocturia
  Urgency
  Incontinence

Complications:
  UTI
  Bladder calculi
  Haematuria
  Uraemia
  Acute retention

EXAMINATION

General:
  Anaemia
  Hypertension
  Uraemic foetor
  Neurological
    examination

Local:
  Palpable hydronephrosis
  Palpable bladder
  Urethra — stone
         — mass or scar
         — meatal stenosis
         — discharge
  Epididymitis
  PR — prostatic size and
              consistency
  PV — pelvic mass

**Fig. 17.2** Clinical assessment of bladder outflow obstruction

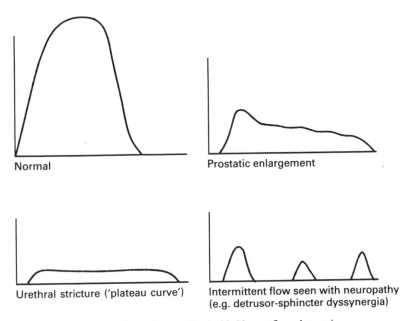

Normal

Prostatic enlargement

Urethral stricture ('plateau curve')

Intermittent flow seen with neuropathy
(e.g. detrusor-sphincter dyssynergia)

**Fig. 17.3** Urinary flow studies in bladder outflow obstruction

The final assessment of the cause of obstruction is made at cystoureth-roscopy when the entire length of the urethra, the prostate and the bladder neck can be inspected. The bladder must also be examined for trabeculation, sacculation or diverticula and for evidence of bladder calculi or tumours.

## PRINCIPLES OF MANAGEMENT

Treatment is aimed at removing the obstruction and correcting or preventing urinary retention, thereby preventing damage to the kidneys. In the majority of patients this involves surgery, the nature of which depends on the cause of the obstruction. Preliminary treatment may be necessary prior to surgery in certain circumstances.

### Urinary infection

Any proven infection should be treated before surgery with antibiotics and antibiotic cover should be given during the peri-operative period to reduce the risk of septicaemia.

### Chronic retention of urine

If renal function is normal and the urine sterile, patients with chronic retention do not require catheterisation before surgery but, if there is evidence of impaired renal function with upper tract dilatation, a period of pre-operative catheter drainage of the bladder is indicated to allow renal function to recover. A urethral catheter is generally preferred although a suprapubic catheter may be needed in some patients.

Catheterisation of patients in chronic retention may precipitate bleeding and result in a post-obstructive diuresis with the production of large volumes of urine and loss of electrolytes. Intravenous fluids may be necessary if the patient is unable to keep pace with his fluid requirements by oral intake alone, but great care should be taken not to precipitate cardiac failure.

A few patients will require pre-operative blood transfusion. Bleeding after catheterisation of patients in chronic retention cannot be prevented by periodic clamping and release of the urethral catheter, so this technique has now been abandoned in favour of continuous drainage without clamping.

Surgery should be delayed until blood urea and creatinine levels have stabilised; persistent elevation after a period of catheterisation may indicate irreversible renal damage, but in some patients levels only return to normal after prostatectomy has been performed.

## Acute retention of urine (Fig. 17.4)

In acute retention, prompt catheterisation should be performed with a small urethral catheter (e.g. 14 French gauge Foley) using full aseptic precautions. If there is any resistance to the passage of the catheter, a suprapubic catheter should be inserted under local anaesthetic.

The practice of placing a patient with retention of urine in a warm bath to encourage spontaneous voiding is occasionally effective but usually accomplishes little.

Subsequent management depends on the cause of the acute retention. If a general cause is suspected (e.g. postoperative, drug-induced), if there are few preceding symptoms or if less than 500 ml of urine is drained from the bladder after catheterisation, a trial of voiding without the catheter is worthwhile. In the majority of patients, however, surgery to relieve the bladder outflow obstruction is necessary. This should not be performed as an emergency (since this is associated with a high morbidity and mortality) but as a semi-elective procedure after correction of any underlying problems.

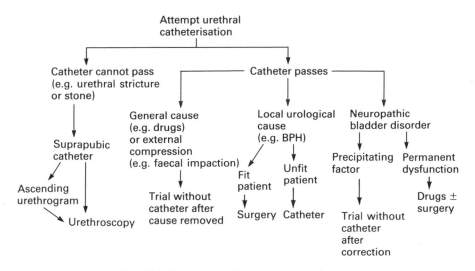

**Fig. 17.4** Management of acute retention of urine

## BENIGN CAUSES OF OUTFLOW OBSTRUCTION IN MEN

### Benign prostatic hyperplasia

The prostate enlarges in most men after the age of 40 but the degree of obstruction produced is highly variable. In the UK, 75% of men have benign nodular hyperplasia of the prostate by the age of 70 but only 10–15% require prostatectomy for relief of obstructive symptoms.

*Pathology* (Fig. 17.5)

The prostate is composed of glandular tissue within a fibromuscular stroma and its activity is regulated both by androgens and oestrogens. From the age of 40 onwards, areas of glandular and fibromuscular proliferation develop in the inner prostatic glands. These areas coalesce to form an adenoma and, as this enlarges, the outer zone of glands is compressed to form a false 'surgical' capsule.

The exact cause of these changes is not known but may be related to an imbalance between oestrogenic and androgenic activity.

Typically, the adenoma enlarges on each side of the midline to form enlarged lateral lobes separated by a median sulcus. A middle lobe of variable size forms between the prostatic utricle and the bladder base. As the prostate enlarges, it may compress the urethral lumen and cause obstruction to the flow of urine. There is, however, a poor correlation between prostatic size and the severity of the obstruction.

Other factors that determine whether an enlarged prostate produces significant obstruction include contraction of muscle fibres in the bladder neck and prostatic capsule (innervated by alpha-adrenergic fibres), vascular engorgement and oedema following prostatic infarcts or infection.

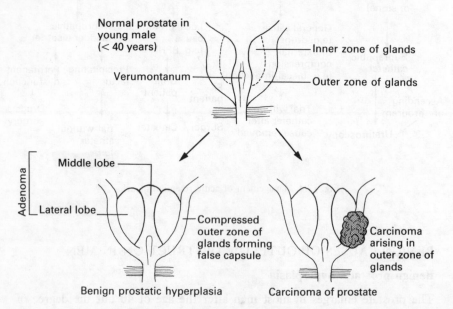

**Fig. 17.5** Pathology of prostatic enlargement

*Clinical assessment*

The patient is usually over 50 and presents with the typical symptoms of outflow obstruction, retention of urine or with complications such as urinary infection and stone formation. Rectal examination provides an approximate assessment of the size of the prostate and helps differentiate benign enlargement from carcinoma of the prostate.

After investigation, a decision must be made on whether treatment is required. The main indications for treatment are retention of urine (acute or chronic), evidence of deterioration in urinary tract function (e.g. residual urine, impairment of renal function), secondary complications (e.g. stones, urinary infection) and severe symptoms which interfere with the patient's normal lifestyle. No treatment is required for the patient with an enlarged prostate who has few symptoms, good bladder emptying and normal renal function.

*Treatment*

Medical treatment is generally ineffective, although it may produce temporary improvement in some patients. Various androgens and progestogens have been used but have proved ineffective. Treatment with alpha-adrenergic blocking drugs (e.g. phenoxybenzamine, prazosin) to inhibit contraction of muscle in the bladder neck and prostatic capsule does help some

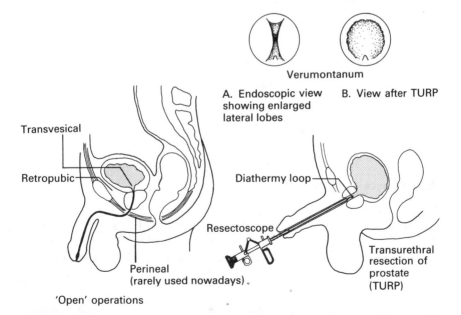

Verumontanum

A. Endoscopic view showing enlarged lateral lobes    B. View after TURP

Transvesical

Retropubic

Diathermy loop

Resectoscope

Perineal (rarely used nowadays)

Transurethral resection of prostate (TURP)

'Open' operations

**Fig. 17.6** Types of prostatectomy

patients. Such drugs improve the urine flow rate and decrease urinary frequency but these benefits are not always maintained.

Prostatectomy remains the most effective long-term treatment (Fig. 17.6). This involves removal of the obstructing adenoma from within the 'surgical' capsule of the prostate, leaving the compressed outer portion of the gland behind. Transurethral resection (TURP) is the procedure of choice for the majority of benign prostates because it has a low morbidity and mortality but open prostatectomy still has a place if the prostate is very large or if open operation is indicated to deal with associated abnormalities in the bladder (e.g. diverticula, stones).

If a patient presenting in retention of urine is deemed unfit for surgery or refuses to have a prostatectomy, a permanent indwelling catheter may be needed.

Complications of prostatectomy are given in Table 17.2.

**Table 17.2**   Complications of prostatectomy

---

*Immediate* (within 48 h)
    primary haemorrhage
    septicaemia
    cardiovascular disturbance (from blood loss and transfusion)
    'TUR syndrome' (from excessive absorption of irrigant)

*Intermediate* (within 14 days)
    secondary haemorrhage
    urinary tract infection
    pulmonary infection
    pulmonary embolism

*Late*
    incontinence (from sphincter damage)
    urethral stricture — meatus
                      — penoscrotal junction
                      — membranous urethra
    bladder neck contracture
    retrograde ejaculation
    recurrent adenoma

---

## Bladder neck stenosis

Fibrous stenosis of the bladder neck may occur after previous surgery on the prostate or bladder neck and causes typical obstructive symptoms. Treatment is by bladder neck incision using a diathermy knife. Resection of the stenosis should be avoided, since this is often followed by recurrent stenosis.

## Bladder neck dyssynergia

In bladder neck dyssynergia, the bladder neck either fails to relax or actively contracts during voiding, causing a functional obstruction. The cause is unknown and there is usually no evidence of a neurological abnormality. This condition usually presents between 20 and 45 years of age. There is often a lifelong history of frequency and a poor stream but many patients come to regard their slow urinary stream as normal. Complications such as urinary infection are sometimes the main presenting feature. The important findings are the lack of neurological signs and the absence of prostatic enlargement. Videocystourethrography is the most accurate method of confirming the diagnosis.

Surgical bladder neck incision is the treatment of choice but may result in retrograde ejaculation and impaired fertility in 20% of patients. Since this disease tends to affect young men who may still wish to father children, surgery should be reserved for severe symptoms or evidence of deteriorating renal function.

Blockade of the alpha-adrenergic receptors in the bladder neck with phenoxybenzamine or prazosin may relieve the obstruction but side-effects (postural hypotension, nasal stuffiness) can make drug treatment intolerable in the long term.

## Urethral stricture (Table 17.3)

### Clinical assessment

The usual presenting complaint is of a slow urinary stream, although any of the typical symptoms of outflow obstruction may be present. Although a stricture may occur at any age, it should be suspected in a patient under the age of 50 who develops obstructive symptoms, especially if there is a

**Table 17.3**  Aetiology of urethral stricture

*Congenital*
  meatal stenosis (e.g. with coronal hypospadias)
  bulbar stricture

*Acquired*
  traumatic
    — perineal trauma
    — ruptured urethra from pelvic injuries
    — urethral instrumentation
  infective
    — gonococcal
    — non-specific urethritis
    — tuberculosis
  inflammatory
    — balanitis xerotica obliterans (meatal stricture)
    — chemical urethritis (e.g. from certain catheter materials)
  neoplastic
    — squamous carcinoma (in areas of squamous metaplasia)
    — transitional cell carcinoma
    — adenocarcinoma

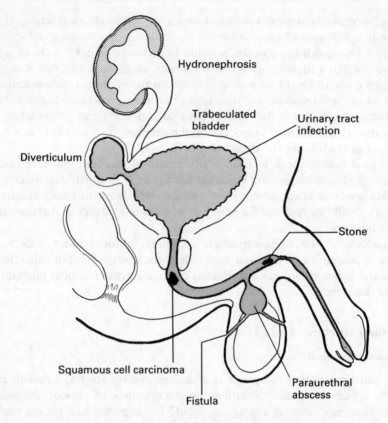

Fig. 17.7 Complications of urethral stricture

history of perineal trauma, previous urethritis or urethral instrumentation. In many patients, however, no precipitating cause can be identified.

Possible complications of urethral stricture are shown in Figure 17.7.

*Investigation*

The urine flow rate is helpful in patients with urethral strictures, the flow curve having a characteristic prolonged plateau appearance.

If a urethral stricture is suspected from the history, an ascending urethrogram should be performed to demonstrate its length, site and calibre. Many strictures, however, are detected only during diagnostic cystourethroscopy.

*Treatment* (Fig. 17.8)

The traditional treatment for a urethral stricture is periodic dilatation under

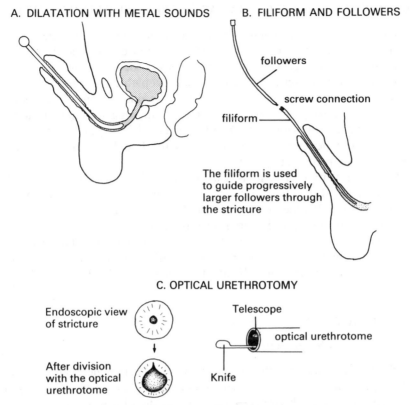

A. DILATATION WITH METAL SOUNDS

B. FILIFORM AND FOLLOWERS

followers

screw connection

filiform

The filiform is used
to guide progressively
larger followers through
the stricture

C. OPTICAL URETHROTOMY

Endoscopic view
of stricture

After division
with the optical
urethrotome

Telescope

optical urethrotome

Knife

**Fig. 17.8** Treatment of urethral stricture

local anaesthetic using metal sounds or plastic bougies. If it proves difficult
to negotiate the stricture with dilators, a fine probe (*filiform bougie*) can be
passed through the stricture first and then larger dilators (followers)
attached to this to ensure that they also pass through the stricture. Although
repeated dilatation may be suitable for an elderly unfit man, a more
permanent solution should be sought in younger patients.

This may be achieved by cutting the stricture with an endoscopic knife
under direct vision (*optical urethrotomy*). The procedure can be repeated if
necessary and cure rates of 50–80% can be expected.

For dense fibrotic strictures or recurrent strictures after urethrotomy,
open operation on the urethra (*urethroplasty*) is indicated. If the stricture
is short, it can be excised and an end-to-end anastomosis performed. For
longer strictures, the narrowed area of urethra is opened longitudinally and
penile or scrotal skin on a vascular pedicle is used to cover the defect. Strictures at the external meatus can be treated by ventral incision (*meatotomy*)
or by reconstruction of the meatus (*meatoplasty*).

## BENIGN CAUSES OF OUTFLOW OBSTRUCTION IN WOMEN

Bladder outflow obstruction is uncommon in women. Genuine urethral stenosis is sometimes seen and should be treated by urethral dilatation or Otis urethrotomy. True bladder neck dyssynergia in women is rare and most types of functional obstruction are neuropathic in origin.

Acute retention of urine in women may be due to general causes (e.g. postoperative, drug-induced) or to extrinsic compression from a pelvic mass (e.g. gravid uterus, complete procidentia, faecal impaction). After catheterisation to relieve the retention, treatment should be directed towards removing the precipitating cause.

Chronic retention of urine is usually the result of detrusor failure rather than outflow obstruction and may follow previous episodes of bladder overdistension. Bladder emptying can be improved by lowering outflow resistance with urethral dilatation or Otis urethrotomy. Drugs to improve bladder contraction can be used but, if all these measures fail to produce satisfactory voiding and bladder emptying, the patient should be taught to perform clean intermittent self-catheterisation of the bladder (CISC).

## MALIGNANT CAUSES OF OUTFLOW OBSTRUCTION

### Carcinoma of the prostate

In the UK, carcinoma of the prostate is the third commonest cancer in men, with approximately 6000 new patients presenting each year. The majority of men affected are between 65 and 85 and the disease is rare before the age of 50. There are racial differences in disease incidence; the disease is relatively rare in Japan but common in the USA.

The cause of prostatic cancer is unknown but it has been postulated that a disturbance in the androgen–oestrogen balance with age leads to over-growth of the prostatic epithelium.

### Pathology

Small foci of prostatic carcinoma are common at autopsy in elderly asymptomatic men. The incidence of such tumours increases with age from 37% at 50–60 years to 77% in men over 80. These latent cancers are much commoner than overt clinical disease and their exact relationship to progressive disease is unknown.

Typically, prostatic carcinoma arises in the periphery of the posterior part of the prostate which has a different embryological origin from the more central site of benign hyperplasia. The tumour may form an isolated nodule or there may be diffuse involvement of one or both lateral lobes.

The majority of tumours are adenocarcinomas which vary from well differentiated to anaplastic; many tumours have a mixed appearance that makes histological grading difficult. The Gleason system of histological grading is the most widely used; this involves five different patterns of differentiation, each given a number 1–5. The two predominant patterns found within the tumour are identified and, by adding their 'scores', nine possible tumour grades have been described. This grading system correlates well with the ultimate prognosis of the patient.

*Spread and staging* (Fig. 17.9, Table 17.4)

Prostatic tumour spreads initially by direct local extension. This may involve penetration of the prostatic capsule and involvement of adjacent structures (e.g. seminal vesicles, lower ureters). Although tumour may infiltrate around the rectum, the fascia of Denonvilliers acts as a barrier to ulceration through the rectal wall. Lymphatic spread is to pelvic lymph nodes and is common in advanced tumours. Haematogenous spread occurs

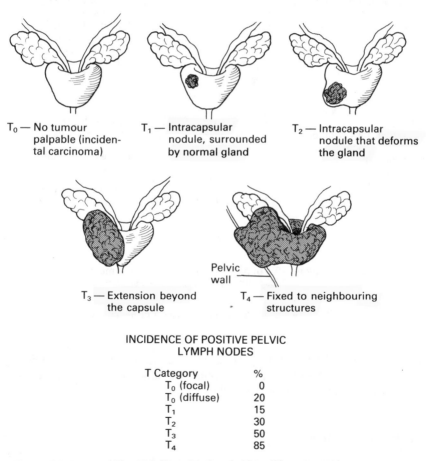

$T_0$ — No tumour palpable (incidental carcinoma)

$T_1$ — Intracapsular nodule, surrounded by normal gland

$T_2$ — Intracapsular nodule that deforms the gland

$T_3$ — Extension beyond the capsule

$T_4$ — Fixed to neighbouring structures

Pelvic wall

INCIDENCE OF POSITIVE PELVIC LYMPH NODES

| T Category | % |
|---|---|
| $T_0$ (focal) | 0 |
| $T_0$ (diffuse) | 20 |
| $T_1$ | 15 |
| $T_2$ | 30 |
| $T_3$ | 50 |
| $T_4$ | 85 |

Fig. 17.9 T staging for carcinoma of prostate

**Table 17.4**   NM staging for prostatic carcinoma

| | |
|---|---|
| Lymph nodes: | N0 regional nodes not involved |
| | N1 single regional node involved |
| | N2 multiple regional nodes involved |
| | N3 fixed regional nodes |
| | N4 distant lymph nodes involved |
| Metastases: | M0 no distant metastases |
| | M1 distant metastases present |

**N.B.** The designation Nx is used if the lymph nodes have not been staged

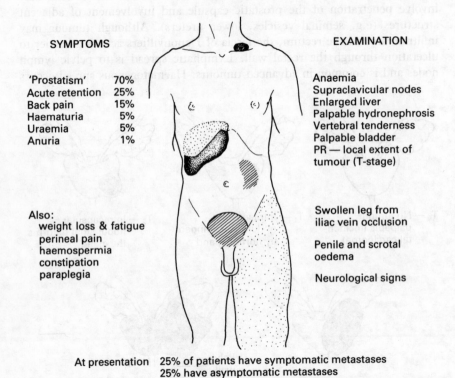

SYMPTOMS

| | |
|---|---|
| 'Prostatism' | 70% |
| Acute retention | 25% |
| Back pain | 15% |
| Haematuria | 5% |
| Uraemia | 5% |
| Anuria | 1% |

Also:
  weight loss & fatigue
  perineal pain
  haemospermia
  constipation
  paraplegia

EXAMINATION

Anaemia
Supraclavicular nodes
Enlarged liver
Palpable hydronephrosis
Vertebral tenderness
Palpable bladder
PR — local extent of
  tumour (T-stage)

Swollen leg from
iliac vein occlusion

Penile and scrotal
oedema

Neurological signs

At presentation   25% of patients have symptomatic metastases
25% have asymptomatic metastases

**Fig. 17.10** Clinical features in carcinoma of the prostate

chiefly to the axial skeleton (particularly the lumbar spine and pelvis) by permeation along Batson's valveless veins. Bloodborne spread to other sites such as lung and liver is occasionally seen.

*Clinical features* (Fig. 17.10)

Typically, a prostatic carcinoma feels hard and irregular on rectal examination. The tumour may initially be palpable as a small nodule, but later the whole gland becomes involved with obliteration of the median sulcus. Tumour may be palpable outside the gland, extending to involve the seminal vesicles or to encircle the rectum.

### Investigations

In addition to the usual investigations performed for bladder outflow obstruction, specific investigations are required for the diagnosis and staging of prostatic carcinoma.

*Diagnosis*. The serum acid phosphatase may be raised, especially in the presence of metastases, although a normal level does not exclude malignancy. Measurement of prostate-specific acid phosphatase increases the sensitivity of this test as a tumour marker and a prostate-specific antigen has now been identified which may help in diagnosis.

Transrectal ultrasound of the prostate is not widely available but is useful to spot small tumours, to assess extracapsular spread and to facilitate needle biopsy of suspicious areas.

Histological confirmation of the diagnosis is essential before commencing treatment, since 50% of palpable prostatic nodules are benign on biopsy. In a clinically suspicious gland, a histological specimen can be obtained either by aspiration of cells for cytology using a Franzen needle or by Trucut needle biopsy (performed transrectally or transperineally). Suspicious prostatic tissue removed during TURP may also be submitted for histology; 15–25% of prostatic carcinomas are discovered incidentally following prostatectomy for a clinically benign gland.

*Staging*. The stage of the primary tumour is normally determined by digital palpation but this tends to be rather inaccurate. Transrectal ultrasound, CT scanning and magnetic resonance imaging (MRI) are now being used to stage prostatic carcinoma more accurately.

Staging of pelvic lymph nodes is difficult and is not routinely performed since treatment depends on the spread of tumour beyond the confines of the pelvis rather than on the presence or absence of nodal metastases. Lymphography is of little help in looking at pelvic lymph nodes. The most accurate method of nodal staging is to remove the pelvic lymph nodes surgically (*pelvic lymphadenectomy*) but this is rarely indicated.

The main site of bloodborne metastases is the skeleton. Bone secondaries may be evident on a radiological skeletal survey as sclerotic lesions but are best detected by bone scintigraphy; a $^{99m}$technetium-labelled isotope is injected into the bloodstream and is taken up selectively by the metastases to produce 'hot spots' in the skeleton when scanned by a gamma camera. Twenty per cent of patients with a normal skeletal survey have a positive bone scan.

A chest X-ray should be performed to exclude pulmonary metastases and liver function tests may detect any derangement due to hepatic secondaries;

ultrasound of the liver may be useful if the liver function tests are abnormal.

*Treatment*

TURP is the treatment of choice in patients with prostatic carcinoma presenting with obstructive symptoms or retention of urine. Open prostatectomy is contraindicated because there is no plane of cleavage between an infiltrating tumour and the prostatic capsule.

Subsequent management of these patients and of those patients with tumour but no obstructive symptoms depends on the grade and stage of tumour. The age and clinical condition of the patient also play an important part in any decision on treatment.

*Incidental carcinoma (T0 Nx M0)*. Treatment depends on the extent and grade of the tumour in the prostatectomy specimen. If the tumour is well differentiated and involves less than 10% of the gland, the prognosis is excellent without treatment. Regular follow-up should be instituted to detect and treat the small proportion of patients who progress to more active disease.

In diffuse or multifocal disease, there is a greater risk of tumour progression and metastases. Further treatment should, therefore, be considered, especially in patients with less differentiated tumours. This usually involves external radiotherapy, although newer techniques such as implantation of radioactive iodine seeds or laser therapy to the prostatic remnant are currently under evaluation.

*Locally confined carcinoma (T1 or T2 Nx M0)*. Patients with well differentiated tumours have a good prognosis and may be kept under surveillance with deferred treatment for those in whom the disease progresses. Radiotherapy is indicated for poorly-differentiated tumours.

Radical prostatectomy is popular in some centres in the USA following preliminary lymphadenectomy, but the procedure carries a significant risk of postoperative impotence and incontinence and has not found favour in this country.

*Locally extensive carcinoma (T3 or T4 Nx M0)*. In locally advanced disease, the pelvic lymph nodes are involved in at least 50% of patients. In this situation, pelvic irradiation may still produce good local control of the tumour. The risk of developing metastases, however, is high and some surgeons favour immediate hormonal manipulation.

*Metastatic carcinoma*. Metastatic disease is treated by hormonal manipulation, although some doubt remains about when this should be commenced. For those patients with symptomatic metastases, immediate hormonal manipulation is best. In patients with asymptomatic metastases, it is not clear whether hormone therapy should be delayed until symptoms appear or given at the outset to try and delay progression of the disease. Clinical trials are currently in progress to try to answer this question.

The main treatment options are orchidectomy or the administration of hormones. Orchidectomy (total or subcapsular) is the simplest form of treatment and produces a response in 70–80% of patients. Similar results can be achieved by the administration of the synthetic oestrogen stilboestrol, 1 mg three times daily. Unfortunately, oestrogenic agents produce unpleasant side-effects, some of which can prove fatal (e.g. stroke, venous thrombosis). Newer hormonal preparations with fewer side-effects include anti-androgens (e.g. cyproterone acetate) and gonadotrophin releasing hormone analogues (e.g. buserelin). The latter group of drugs inhibit the release of the pituitary hormones (chiefly LH) responsible for stimulating testicular production of testosterone. The duration of response to hormonal therapy averages 18 months, although prolonged periods of control are seen in some patients.

For those not responding to hormonal therapy and for those relapsing after an initial response to hormones, the outlook is poor. Adrenalectomy (medical or surgical) to remove extragonadal sources of testosterone production is helpful in some patients but its effect is often short-lived. Hypophysectomy is effective in improving severe bone pain but does not improve survival. Chemotherapy using single agents or combinations of drugs has been tried but has proved disappointing.

The major aim in patients with hormone-resistant disease is palliation of symptoms, usually pain from bony metastases. Opiate analgesia may improve bone pain without over-sedating the patient if the dosage is carefully controlled but the best form of treatment for painful bony metastases is local radiotherapy.

*Other complications.* Ureteric obstruction resulting in renal impairment may require temporary relief by percutaneous nephrostomy or by insertion of a double-J ureteric stent, whilst awaiting a response to hormonal manipulation. Such diversion is not justified in the later stages of the disease when the tumour has escaped from hormonal control.

Surgical intervention may also be needed for bowel obstruction due to a prostatic carcinoma encircling the rectum; this may require a colostomy. Spinal cord compression by an extradural metastasis demands urgent surgical decompression if permanent paraplegia is to be prevented.

*Prognosis*

Well-differentiated tumours confined to the prostate have a good prognosis. Once the prostatic capsule has been breached, the outlook is considerably worse since there is a high incidence of associated pelvic nodal involvement and a considerable risk of developing metastatic disease.

# 18

# Neuropathic bladder disorders

The bladder and urethra act as a single functional unit under complex neurological control for the storage and expulsion of urine. Lesions at any point in the neurological pathway can disturb the continence-voiding mechanism so that bladder dysfunction is a common feature in many neurological disorders (Fig. 18.1).

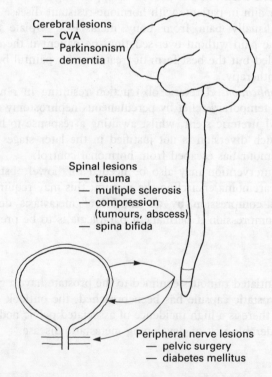

Cerebral lesions
— CVA
— Parkinsonism
— dementia

Spinal lesions
— trauma
— multiple sclerosis
— compression
  (tumours, abscess)
— spina bifida

Peripheral nerve lesions
— pelvic surgery
— diabetes mellitus

**Fig. 18.1** Common causes of neuropathic bladder dysfunction

## CLASSIFICATION OF NEUROVESICAL DYSFUNCTION

The clinical picture in an individual patient can be interpreted on the basis of changes in detrusor and urethral function as measured objectively by urodynamic studies. The detrusor may be either overactive (*detrusor hyper-reflexia*) or underactive (*detrusor areflexia*). Similarly, the urethral closure mechanism may be overactive (causing *detrusor-sphincter dyssynergia*) or underactive (*urethral sphincter incompetence*).

The nature of these changes depends largely on the site of the lesion in the neurological pathway rather than on the underlying cause. Lesions may, however, be incomplete and produce a mixed picture so it is necessary to define the changes in detrusor and urethral function separately (Fig. 18.2).

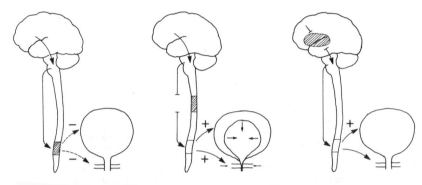

(a) Lesions of sacral cord or peripheral nerves: both detrusor and urethra are underactive

(b) Lesions of supra-sacral cord: loss of inhibitory impulses causes detrusor over-activity: urethra often overactive and uncoordin-ated with detrusor contraction (dyssynergia)

(c) Lesions above pons: loss of cerebral inhibition may produce overactive detrusor. Detrusor and urethral activity remain coordinated

**Fig. 18.2** Effects of lesions at different levels on bladder and urethral function

## FUNCTIONAL CONSEQUENCES

In addition to effects on bladder function (Fig. 18.3), upper tract dilatation may also occur in patients with high intravesical pressures due to detrusor hyper-reflexia and detrusor-sphincter dyssynergia. There may be accompanying vesicoureteric reflux, especially in children with congenital lesions of the spinal cord. The transmission of high pressures to the kidneys may lead to renal damage and chronic renal failure which was, until recent years, the commonest cause of death in patients with spinal injury.

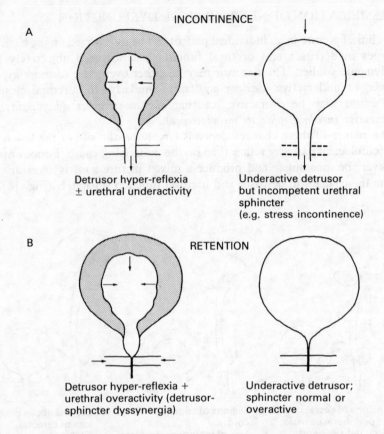

Fig. 18.3 Functional consequences of neuropathic bladder disorders

## ASSESSMENT OF NEUROPATHIC BLADDER DISORDERS

### History

Neurological disorders affecting the bladder produce a wide variety of symptoms. Detrusor hyper-reflexia may cause frequency, urgency and urge incontinence in patients with intact bladder sensation or insensible urine loss if sensation is reduced. Stress incontinence may occur in patients with an incompetent urethral sphincter.

Poor detrusor function or detrusor-sphincter dyssynergia may result in functional outflow obstruction with hesitancy and a reduced urinary stream. Chronic retention may then follow, with overflow incontinence or other associated symptoms (e.g. urinary infection, stone formation, chronic renal failure).

In addition, there may be other symptoms of sacral nerve dysfunction (bowel disturbance, impotence in men) or more generalised neurological symptoms such as weakness, sensory loss and disturbances of co-ordination or cerebral function. Visual disturbances may occur in diabetes mellitus (*retinopathy*) and in multiple sclerosis (*retrobulbar neuritis*).

The onset and duration of symptoms should be determined and any precipitating factors noted (e.g. diabetes mellitus, spinal trauma or disease, pelvic fractures or pelvic surgery). All medications should be recorded, since many drugs, particularly those with anticholinergic or sympathomimetic actions, may interfere with bladder function.

Techniques for examination are described in Figure 18.4.

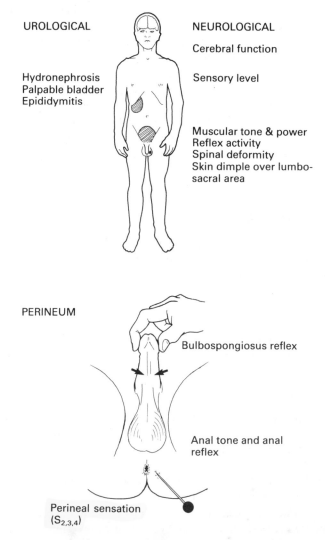

UROLOGICAL

Hydronephrosis
Palpable bladder
Epididymitis

NEUROLOGICAL

Cerebral function

Sensory level

Muscular tone & power
Reflex activity
Spinal deformity
Skin dimple over lumbo-
sacral area

PERINEUM

Bulbospongiosus reflex

Anal tone and anal
reflex

Perineal sensation
$(S_{2,3,4})$

**Fig. 18.4** Examination of patients with neurovesical dysfunction

## Investigations

Initial investigations should include urine culture, blood urea and creatinine estimation and measurement of blood glucose levels.

Intravenous urography (IVU) may reveal calculi on the plain film; following contrast administration, upper tract dilatation may be evident in patients with obstructed voiding and/or vesicoureteric reflux; residual urine after voiding can also be assessed. Other useful investigations include ultrasound for serial measurements of residual urine and micturating cystography to evaluate the bladder neck and urethra and to detect vesicoureteric reflux.

Urodynamic studies are essential for an accurate evaluation of bladder and urethral function. Cystometry allows assessment of residual urine, bladder sensation and bladder capacity; it may also demonstrate normal or uninhibited detrusor contractions. A high detrusor pressure during voiding is suggestive of obstruction, the site of which can be determined by simultaneous radiological screening. Urethral pressure profilometry and pelvic floor EMG are used in some centres to evaluate urethral sphincter activity.

In addition to investigation of the urinary tract, neurological investigations may be required for specific problems. A myelogram is needed if spinal cord compression is suspected (e.g. prolapsed intervertebral disc or spinal tumour) and CT scanning may be useful to exclude cerebral disorders (e.g. frontal lobe tumour).

## PRINCIPLES OF MANAGEMENT

Management depends on accurate diagnosis of the underlying abnormalities in detrusor and urethral function. Treatment is aimed at restoring the normal detrusor-urethral balance.

### Incontinence

This may be due to detrusor hyper-reflexia or to an underactive detrusor in association with urethral sphincter incompetence.

#### Detrusor hyper-reflexia

This may respond to treatment with drugs that have anticholinergic and/or smooth muscle relaxant properties. Agents used include propantheline, oxybutynin and terodiline but side-effects (e.g. dry mouth, blurred vision) are common.

Detrusor hyper-reflexia can be treated surgically by partial denervation of the bladder; this can be achieved by endoscopic injection of phenol into the vesical nerves under the trigone, by injection or division of the anterior sacral nerve roots (*presacral neurectomy*) or by bladder transection. Alternatively, a segment of bowel (usually ileum) can be incorporated into the bladder to increase its functional capacity (*augmentation cystoplasty*) or the bulk of the bladder can be excised and replaced by caecum (*substitution cystoplasty*).

### Incompetent sphincter

Alpha-adrenergic drugs such as phenylpropanolamine and ephedrine may help by increasing bladder outflow resistance.

Surgery to the bladder neck can also be used but is only really applicable in women; the techniques used are similar to those employed for genuine stress incontinence (e.g. colposuspension). Urinary retention can, unfortunately, be precipitated by these procedures but can be treated by clean intermittent self-catheterisation (CISC).

In either sex, implantation of an artificial urinary sphincter may be suitable in carefully selected patients. This involves placing around the urethra a cuff which can be inflated to maintain continence and deflated for voiding.

### Other measures

If incontinence cannot be prevented by the measures described above, a collection device can be used to control urine leakage. In men, a penile sheath or similar appliance can be fitted to the penis, avoiding the need for catheterisation. There is, however, no satisfactory collection device for women and an indwelling catheter may be necessary. If problems arise from leakage around a urethral catheter in patients with detrusor hyper-reflexia, this may be controlled by simultaneous drug therapy.

If incontinence is uncontrollable, urinary diversion may be considered, although the patient's ability to cope with a stoma must be carefully assessed first.

## Retention of urine

This usually results from an underactive detrusor, although it may occur in detrusor overactivity if there is also urethral overactivity resulting in functional bladder outflow obstruction (*detrusor-sphincter dyssynergia*).

### Atonic detrusor

The patients should be taught how to empty the bladder by abdominal straining and suprapubic pressure (Credé manoeuvre). This can be supplemented by drug therapy using agents with either a stimulant action on smooth muscle (e.g. bethanecol) or anticholinesterase activity (e.g. distigmine).

Alternatively, CISC can be used with the patient learning to pass a fine catheter into his/her own bladder 4–6 times per day. This technique requires a certain degree of manual dexterity and the bladder must be of sufficient capacity for the patient to remain dry between catheterisations.

CISC is more socially acceptable to the patient than an indwelling urethral catheter and the incidence of complications (e.g. urinary infection, bladder calculi, urethral fistulae) is low.

### Urethral overactivity

Alpha-adrenergic blocking agents (e.g. phenoxybenzamine, prazosin) or striated muscle relaxants (e.g. baclofen) can be used to lower urethral resistance.

Surgery may be required in some patients; this involves wide urethral dilatation or Otis urethrotomy in women and formal sphincterotomy in men; the latter is accomplished by endoscopic division of the distal urethral sphincter sacrificing continence, if necessary, in order to preserve renal function.

Permanent urethral catheters are poorly tolerated in this group of patients because of accompanying detrusor hyper-reflexia.

### Other measures

Urinary diversion may be needed to protect renal function if the measures described above fail. In young children (e.g. with spina bifida), vesicostomy is a useful temporary form of diversion which can be reversed when the child is old enough to learn CISC. In adults, however, permanent diversion may be necessary (e.g. ileal conduit).

### Upper tract dilatation

In the majority of patients with upper tract dilatation, the cause is high detrusor pressure and chronic retention of urine due to functional bladder outflow obstruction. Dilatation can often be improved by reducing outflow resistance and improving bladder emptying (e.g. by sphincterotomy or CISC). Prophylactic surgery to the bladder outflow is indicated in those patients at risk from high pressure chronic retention (e.g. males with high spinal injuries).

Patients with neuropathic bladders are, of course, prone to many other urological complications, usually related to the presence of residual urine (e.g. urinary infection, stone formation). These are dealt with along the standard lines detailed elsewhere.

## SPECIAL FEATURES OF INDIVIDUAL DISORDERS

### Spinal injuries

Although the eventual activity of the detrusor and urethra depend on the level of the spinal lesion, there is an initial period of *spinal shock* below the lesion which leads to paralysis of the detrusor with retention of urine. Careful attention to the management of the bladder is therefore required from the outset.

### Immediate management

Overdistension of the bladder must be prevented to avoid permanent impairment of detrusor contractility. An indwelling urethral catheter should therefore be inserted before the patient is transferred to a spinal injuries unit. To minimise the risk of complications associated with the catheter (e.g. infection, urethral stricture and fistula), it is best to change either to a regime of intermittent catheterisation (3 or 4 times a day) or to a suprapubic catheter within a few days of the injury.

Intermittent or continuous bladder drainage is continued until the period of spinal shock has passed, as indicated by the return of reflex activity below the level of the lesion.

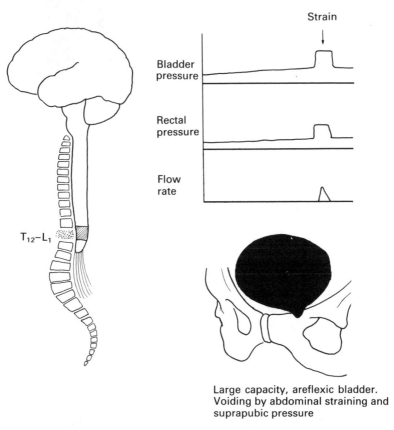

Large capacity, areflexic bladder. Voiding by abdominal straining and suprapubic pressure

**Fig. 18.5** Effects of sacral cord injury on bladder function

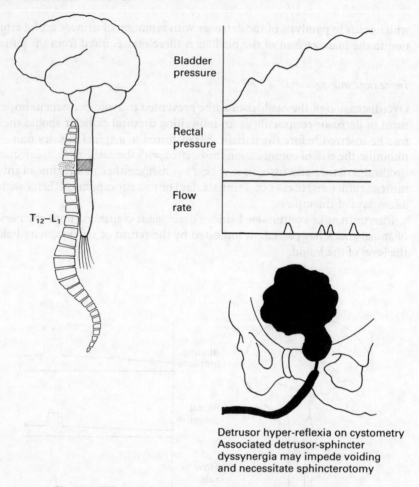

Bladder
pressure

Rectal
pressure

Flow
rate

T₁₂–L₁

Detrusor hyper-reflexia on cystometry
Associated detrusor-sphincter
dyssynergia may impede voiding
and necessitate sphincterotomy

**Fig. 18.6** Effects of suprasacral cord injury on bladder function

*Subsequent management*

The rate of return of detrusor activity after spinal injury is variable but some activity is usually evident 4–5 weeks after injury. Urodynamic studies are helpful at this stage to detect any activity, to evaluate urethral function and to detect detrusor-sphincter dyssynergia.

Eventual bladder function can often be predicted from the level of the spinal lesion (Figs 18.5, 18.6).

In patients with suprasacral cord lesions, a trial of voiding may be attempted using suprapubic tapping to elicit bladder contractions provided detrusor activity can be demonstrated. Voiding efficiency is best demonstrated by serial measurement of residual bladder urine either by catheterisation or by ultrasound.

In patients with sacral cord injuries, spontaneous or induced detrusor contractions do not reappear and effective bladder emptying depends on abdominal straining and suprapubic pressure (Credé manoeuvre).

Specific measures for incontinence or retention are employed as necessary on the basis of the urodynamic findings.

In the longer term, treatment of urological complications (e.g. infection, calculi) may also be needed. Special attention to the skin is essential when using incontinence appliances or catheters in patients with spinal injuries because skin sensation is impaired or absent.

Regular urological follow-up, including periodic evaluation of the urinary tract by IVU or ultrasound, is essential to detect any renal deterioration.

## Spina bifida (Fig. 18.7)

This disorder is due to failure of development of the posterior neural arches; there is a variable degree of neurological deficit.

*Spina bifida occulta* is a common anomaly, with X-ray evidence of a bony lesion (usually L5 or S1) in up to 20% of normal individuals. This may be

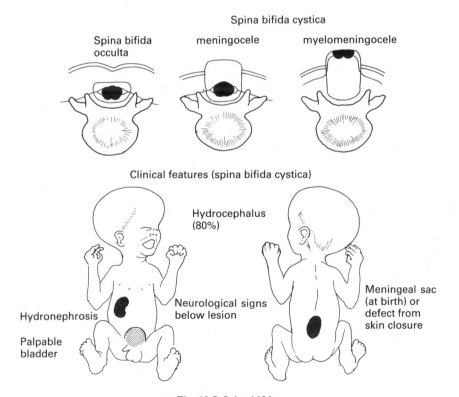

Fig. 18.7 Spina bifida

recognised clinically by the presence of a small pit or tuft of hair on the overlying skin; the defect rarely causes neurological symptoms or bladder dysfunction.

In the more severe form (*spina bifida cystica*), a meningeal sac protrudes
through a defect of the overlying skin. There may be no neural tissue in the
sac (*meningocele*) but, more commonly, neural tissue is present (*myelomen-
ingocele*). Bladder dysfunction is common but forms only a part of the
overall disability.

The number of children born with major neural tube defects has fallen considerably in recent years as a result of effective prenatal screening by measuring maternal alpha-fetoprotein levels.

*Management*

In the newborn child wearing nappies, incontinence is not an immediate
problem and the main priority is to protect the upper tracts from damage by
ensuring adequate bladder emptying. If the bladder is palpable, ultrasound
should be performed to detect upper tract dilatation; if dilatation is present, a
micturating cystogram will exclude vesicoureteric reflux. In the absence of
reflux, bladder emptying can be achieved by regular abdominal compression
by the parents. Alternatively, the parents can be taught to perform clean intermittent catheterisation or a temporary vesicostomy can be fashioned until the
child is older.

In children of school age, achieving continence whilst still preserving renal
function becomes important. Urodynamic assessment at this stage is helpful
to identify the detrusor and urethral abnormalities and allow appropriate treatment as outlined earlier.

Two important forms of treatment have had a significant impact on
improving quality of life for these older children; clean intermittent self-
catheterisation (CISC) for retention and implantation of an artificial urinary
sphincter in selected children with incontinence.

Urinary diversion using an ileal or colonic conduit was formerly used in
many children, especially when there was evidence of hydronephrosis, but
the long-term results are poor due to complications. There is now a trend
towards undiverting some of these children and managing the restored
bladder along the lines already described.

Urinary problems (e.g. recurrent infections, calculi) continue into adult
life, necessitating long-term follow-up.

### Compression of the spinal cord or cauda equina

This usually occurs as a result of a spinal tumour (primary or secondary), spinal
stenosis or a prolapsed intervertebral disc. As before, the nature of the bladder
disturbance is determined by the site and extent of the lesion.

The level of the lesion cannot, however, be accurately determined on the basis of bladder symptoms alone; detailed neurological assessment is necessary to detect the accompanying effects on sensation, muscle power and reflex activity. A myelogram is useful to delineate the site and extent of the lesion, although CT scanning is now preferred in many centres for this purpose.

*Management*

Early recognition of cord compression is essential if permanent damage to bladder function is to be averted. Urgent surgical decompression of the spinal cord is required and this usually involves laminectomy with removal of the cause of the compression. Prompt surgical intervention often results in full recovery of function but any persistent disability should be managed on the basis of urodynamic findings.

## Diabetes mellitus

Neuropathy involving the peripheral nerves is a well-recognised complication of diabetes mellitus and may involve the autonomic nerves to the bladder. Both sensory and motor nerves can be affected.

Typically, loss of sensation causes a delay in the desire to void so that voiding becomes infrequent; on cystometry, the volume at first sensation is high and total bladder capacity is increased. Initially, bladder emptying may be good despite reduced sensation but, eventually, the bladder becomes progressively overstretched, detrusor peformance declines and residual urine develops in the bladder. This may progress to chronic retention of urine with overflow incontinence.

Because of impaired bladder sensation, diabetics often have few symptoms before developing chronic retention. The presence of residual urine predisposes to infection and there may be impaired erections or impotence.

Although a poorly functioning detrusor is the usual cause of bladder disturbance in diabetics, detrusor instability is occasionally found.

*Management*

In the elderly diabetic male it may be difficult to determine whether a large residual urine is due to diabetic neuropathy or prostatic enlargement; prostatectomy is indicated for proven obstruction and to improve emptying of an areflexic bladder. Urethrotomy can be used to lower outflow resistance in women.

Indwelling catheters should be avoided if possible because of the high risk of infective complications in diabetic patients.

## Multiple sclerosis

Bladder symptoms are common in multiple sclerosis and, in some patients, precede other manifestations of the disease.

Involvement of the suprasacral tracts to the bladder results in detrusor hyper-reflexia causing frequency, urgency and urge incontinence. If the pathways to the urethral sphincter are involved, the resulting urethral overactivity may cause voiding difficulty and urinary retention.

Demyelination occasionally affects the sacral segments of the cord directly, resulting in underactivity of the detrusor and retention of urine.

### Management

This involves appropriate treatment for the demonstrated urodynamic abnormalities. Treatment, however, is often difficult because of the fluctuating severity of the disease and the risk of progressive demyelination. A conservative approach to treatment is usually indicated and surgery should, if possible, be avoided since future changes in bladder and urethral function cannot be predicted.

## Pelvic surgery

The pelvic nerves to the bladder may be injured during surgery, especially by operations for pelvic tumours (e.g. abdominoperineal excision of the rectum, Wertheim's hysterectomy).

The resulting injury may be a neuropraxia with recovery after temporary paralysis or the nerves may be divided, resulting in denervation of the bladder. The usual clinical presentation is postoperative urinary retention with inability to void when the catheter is removed a few days after surgery.

Factors other than denervation also contribute to retention of urine after pelvic surgery. There may be mechanical distortion of the bladder and bladder neck due to removal of supporting structures. In men, prostatic enlargement may also be involved; symptomless obstruction of a moderate degree may become significant after partial bladder denervation by pelvic surgery.

### Management

In men with a clear-cut history of prostatic symptoms prior to pelvic surgery, prostatectomy is necessary and should enable those with minor degrees of denervation to void normally. In other patients, drugs to encourage detrusor contraction (e.g. bethanecol) or agents to decrease outflow resistance (e.g. phenoxybenzamine, prazosin) may be tried.

Continued failure to void indicates a marked degree of denervation and may require long-term catheterisation. Functional recovery can take up to 3 months and treatment may be necessary thereafter to achieve bladder emptying.

In women, this may involve abdominal straining and suprapubic compression after lowering outflow resistance by urethral dilatation or Otis urethrotomy. In men, bladder neck and prostatic resection may be necessary. If these measures fail or are contraindicated, catheterisation of the bladder (CISC or indwelling catheter) may be required on a long-term basis.

### Cerebral disorders (Fig. 18.8)

Voluntary control of micturition may be disturbed in many cerebral disorders, the loss of cortical inhibition often leading to detrusor overactivity.

If cerebral awareness of sensation is intact, there may be frequency and urgency with urge incontinence but when sensory perception is impaired, incontinence is unheralded and unnoticed by the patient.

Such disturbances of micturition are common after a stroke and in patients with Parkinson's disease, dementia or cerebral tumours (especially of the frontal lobe).

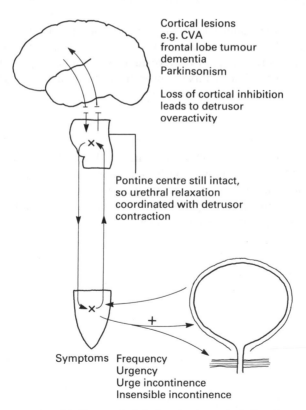

Cortical lesions
e.g. CVA
frontal lobe tumour
dementia
Parkinsonism

Loss of cortical inhibition
leads to detrusor
overactivity

Pontine centre still intact,
so urethral relaxation
coordinated with detrusor
contraction

Symptoms  Frequency
Urgency
Urge incontinence
Insensible incontinence

**Fig. 18.8** Neurovesical dysfunction in cerebral disorders

*Management*

This is often difficult. Meticulous nursing care with regular toileting may help to prevent incontinence in those with limited mobility (e.g. after a stroke). If incontinence is due to uninhibited detrusor contractions, these should be treated with anticholinergic drugs. In many patients, however, lack of cerebral awareness necessitates the use of urine collection devices (penile sheath in men, catheter in women).

For the elderly man with difficulty in voiding and a cerebral disorder (e.g. Parkinson's disease), caution should be exercised in advising prostatectomy since there is a major risk of postoperative incontinence.

## Occult neuropathic bladder

This is a disturbance of micturition which has all the clinical and urodynamic features of a neuropathic disorder but no neurological deficit can be demonstrated. The condition may present in childhood or in adult life. The bladder disturbance is usually one of uninhibited detrusor activity with detrusor-sphincter dyssynergia. This results in either incontinence or retention of urine.

In children, the bladder disturbance is often accompanied by a disordered bowel habit, reflecting a more generalised abnormality of sacral reflex activity. In adults, a proportion of patients have minor spinal defects, particularly spina bifida occulta. This abnormality is, however, so common that a relationship between cause and effect cannot be proved.

*Management*

Uninhibited contractions should be treated with anticholinergic agents. For incomplete bladder emptying in girls or women, urethral dilatation is sometimes helpful but CISC may be necessary. Urinary diversion is rarely necessary. It is important, especially in children, to avoid constipation which can exacerbate the pre-existing bladder problems.

# 19

# Incontinence

Incontinence is the involuntary loss of urine. It is a distressing and socially disabling condition that affects 5% of the population, with women affected more often than men (8% and 3%, respectively). In recent years an increased understanding of the mechanisms responsible for incontinence has resulted in considerable improvement in management.

## CLASSIFICATION OF INCONTINENCE

Loss of urine in the incontinent patient may be via the urethra or from an abnormal extraurethral route (Fig. 19.1).

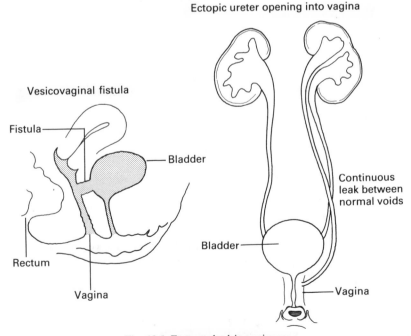

**Fig. 19.1** Extraurethral incontinence

## Urethral incontinence

*Urge incontinence* (Fig. 19.2)

This is the involuntary loss of urine associated with a strong desire to void. It may be due to either motor or sensory dysfunction of the bladder.

Motor urge incontinence due to uninhibited detrusor contractions may be neuropathic (*detrusor hyper-reflexia*) or non-neuropathic (*detrusor instability*); detrusor instability may be secondary to bladder outflow obstruction or idiopathic.

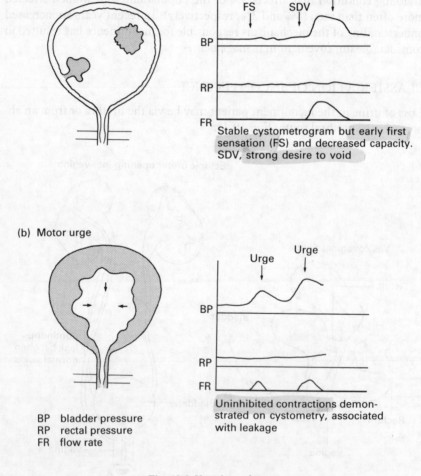

(a) Sensory urge

FS   SDV   Unable to hold and voids

BP

RP

FR

Stable cystometrogram but early first sensation (FS) and decreased capacity. SDV, strong desire to void

(b) Motor urge

Urge   Urge

BP

RP

FR

Uninhibited contractions demonstrated on cystometry, associated with leakage

BP   bladder pressure
RP   rectal pressure
FR   flow rate

Fig. 19.2 Urge incontinence

Sensory urgency may be associated with intravesical pathology (e.g. urinary infection, interstitial cystitis, bladder calculi, bladder tumours), but in some patients there is no demonstrable problem and psychological factors may be involved.

## Stress incontinence

This is the involuntary loss of urine during activities which produce a rise in intra-abdominal pressure (e.g. coughing, straining or lifting). Stress incontinence is a symptom rather than a diagnosis and may occur in a number of different disorders.

In 'genuine' stress incontinence there is weakness of the urethral sphincters so that a rise in intra-abdominal pressure, transmitted to the bladder, exceeds urethral closure pressure in the absence of detrusor activity. Sphincter weakness is commoner in women and is usually the result of obesity, multiparity or childbirth. In men, sphincter weakness may follow pelvic fracture injuries or prostatectomy.

The symptom of stress incontinence also occurs in patients with cough- or strain-induced detrusor instability in whom the leakage is due to the abnormal detrusor activity rather than sphincter weakness; it may also occur in patients with chronic retention of urine.

## Overflow incontinence

This occurs from an overdistended bladder when the intravesical pressure exceeds the urethral closure pressure. It is invariably due to chronic retention of urine secondary either to bladder outflow obstruction or to an unobstructed acontractile bladder.

## Insensible incontinence

This may occur in neurological disorders that interrupt the sensory pathways from the bladder and is often the result of detrusor hyper-reflexia.

Patients with cerebral degeneration may be incontinent without warning because either they have no awareness of a full bladder or they have lost the usual social inhibitions. In these patients, loss of cortical appreciation above the pontine micturition centre results in reflex voiding when the bladder is full.

## Post-micturition dribbling

This is the loss of a small amount of urine after voiding has finished and is not synonymous with terminal dribbling. It occurs predominantly in men. It is occasionally associated with underlying urological disease (Fig. 19.3).

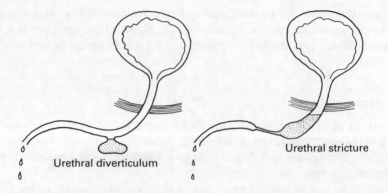

**Fig. 19.3** Causes of post-micturition dribbling

*Nocturnal enuresis*

This refers to bedwetting and the features of this condition are discussed in detail later.

## ASSESSMENT OF THE INCONTINENT PATIENT

### History

It is usually possible to determine the pattern of incontinence from the clinical history. There may be a history of outflow obstruction in patients who have developed chronic retention and overflow incontinence. Dysuria may suggest urinary infection as a cause of urgency and, if there has been haematuria, a tumour of the urinary tract should be suspected. In women with a fistula into the vagina, the patient may recognise that leakage is not from the urethra.

Neurological symptoms should be recorded, including those caused by cerebral degeneration. Bowel function (and sexual function in men) may also be affected in neurological disorders; constipation and faecal impaction may themselves cause incontinence, especially in the elderly.

Previous illnesses and other possible causative factors should also be noted (e.g. urethral surgery, diabetes mellitus, multiple sclerosis). Medications must be recorded and their possible side-effects on bladder and urethral function considered.

### Examination

This should include abdominal palpation to detect an enlarged bladder and inspection of the external genitalia which may be macerated and excoriated by urine leakage.

In women, vaginal examination may reveal atrophic vaginitis due to postmenopausal oestrogen deficiency or a cystourethrocele. Stress incontinence can often be demonstrated by asking the patient to cough with a full bladder, especially if examination is performed with the patient standing; it may be possible to control the leakage of stress incontinence by digital elevation of the bladder neck within the vagina.

Rectal examination may detect faecal impaction but, more importantly, allows anal tone to be determined and the prostate to be assessed.

A detailed neurological examination should be performed to detect any abnormality. Finally, the patient's general level of orientation and motivation should be assessed, since this is important in predicting the success of any subsequent treatment.

### Investigations

The urine should be cultured to detect infection. Haemoglobin and plasma urea levels should be measured, and a blood glucose estimation performed.

Objective assessment of symptoms is often helped by completion of a *frequency-volume chart*; the patient records fluid intake, times and volumes of urine passed throughout a 24-hour period and notes any episodes of incontinence. These charts can also be used to assess the effects of treatment. The severity of incontinence can be determined by quantifying the urine loss; this is estimated by weighing absorbent pads worn over a timed period during regulated activities such as climbing stairs.

An IVU is indicated in most patients. It may be diagnostic in congenital abnormalities (e.g ectopic ureter) or urinary fistulae. Chronic retention of urine may be apparent or the bladder may have the typical 'fir tree' appearance seen in neurological disorders. Other abnormalities such as bladder calculi and tumours may also be seen on urography. An IVU is not strictly necessary in women with uncomplicated stress incontinence.

Specific information about detrusor and sphincter function is best obtained from urodynamic studies. The extent of the test used varies considerably but, for complex problems, full assessment with simultaneous video-cystourethrography is essential. The cystometrogram shows whether the bladder is stable or unstable; in patients with genuine stress incontinence, leakage is often demonstrated on coughing.

The voiding phase of the cystometrogram identifies bladder outflow obstruction or may reveal an atonic detrusor with voiding by abdominal straining. Simultaneous radiological screening helps to demonstrate competence of the bladder neck and allows evaluation of distal sphincter activity in patients with incontinence due to neurological disorders.

Finally, cystoscopy is needed in some patients. This may reveal specific pathology in the bladder (e.g. bladder stone or tumour) and allows assessment of potential bladder capacity. Trabeculation is often present in patients with bladder outflow obstruction and/or detrusor instability. Fistulae from the bladder may be evident and careful examination may reveal the opening of an ectopic ureter. Ascending ureterography can be performed if a ureteric fistula is suspected.

## MANAGEMENT OF INCONTINENCE

Many general factors contribute to incontinence and these should be eliminated if possible. Relative immobility in an elderly patient can convert a moderate degree of urgency into frank incontinence; regular toileting and provision of a bottle or commode may suffice to improve the situation. Faecal impaction must be avoided and careful attention paid to maintaining a regular bowel habit. Drug therapy with diuretics or anticholinergic agents should be modified to see if improvement can be achieved.

Simple treatment of associated disorders such as urinary infection, bladder stones or tumour may successfully restore continence. In many patients, however, simple measures are inappropriate and treatment then depends on the type of incontinence and its underlying cause.

### Urge incontinence

Sensory urge incontinence may resolve after treatment of local intravesical pathology; if this is ineffective or no cause is found, management is along the same lines as for idiopathic detrusor instability.

The treatment of motor urge incontinence in neuropathic bladder disorders is discussed in Chapter 18. If detrusor instability is related to bladder outflow obstruction, the obstruction should be relieved, since instability will disappear after relief of obstruction in 60–70% of patients. Patients with persisting symptoms after surgery and those with idiopathic detrusor instability will, however, require other forms of treatment.

#### Drug therapy and bladder training

Agents with anticholinergic and/or smooth muscle relaxant properties may help. The most useful drugs are propantheline, oxybutynin and terodiline, although side-effects are common.

Functional bladder capacity may also be increased by encouraging the patient to void by the clock, gradually increasing the interval between voids. Drug therapy may be needed at the same time to achieve maximum benefit.

#### Hydrostatic bladder distension

A 5-minute distension can be performed under a general anaesthetic and this undoubtedly helps some patients. More prolonged (*Helmstein*) distension under epidural anaesthesia is useful for severe symptoms. This involves inflation of a balloon within the bladder to a pressure between systolic and diastolic blood pressure for 2–4 hours; although improvement occurs in 60–70%

of patients, recurrence of symptoms is common and there is a risk of bladder rupture during the procedure.

*Surgical treatment* (Fig. 19.4)

Partial denervation of the bladder can be achieved by cystoscopic subtrigonal injection of phenol, surgical division or percutaneous ablation of selected sacral nerves (usually $S_3$) or by division and resuture of the bladder just above the trigone (*bladder transection*). Alternatively the bladder capacity can be increased by cystoplasty.

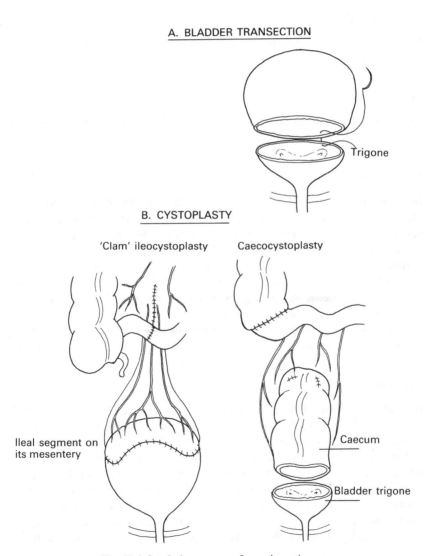

Fig. 19.4 Surgical treatment of urge incontinence

### Appliances

Some patients remain incontinent despite the above measures. In men, a penile sheath may provide control but there is no suitable external collecting device for women. Although incontinence pants may be useful, the volume of urine lost is often considerable during unstable contractions and padding may need to be changed frequently. A permanent indwelling urethral catheter is required in some patients but continued unstable contractions can cause painful bladder spasms with bypassing of the catheter; this can usually be controlled by drug therapy.

### Urinary diversion

A small proportion of patients require urinary diversion as a last resort for intractable incontinence.

## Stress incontinence

Pure sphincter weakness is largely a problem of women and can be treated by surgery or by non-operative measures.

### Non-operative measures

In women with minor degrees of stress incontinence, pelvic floor exercises may improve control; these can be supplemented by electrical stimulation of the pelvic floor muscles using external electrodes (*pelvic faradism*). If the patient is overweight, weight reduction should be encouraged.

Alpha-adrenergic stimulants such as phenylpropanolamine may help by increasing urethral tone. In women with stress incontinence and atrophic vaginitis due to oestrogen deficiency, urine leakage may be reduced by local or systemic oestrogens which cause proliferation of the urethral mucosa.

If there is an associated cystocele, a vaginal pessary that reduces the cystocele may improve continence although, in the long term, surgical repair is preferred.

### Operative measures

If the above measures fail, surgical correction is required. Many operative techniques have been described but the aim is to elevate and support the bladder neck, returning it to its normal position above the pelvic floor muscles.

This can be accomplished by vaginal repair (combined with correction of any associated cystocele) or by suprapubic repair. In the *Marshall–Marchetti–Kranz* procedure, the bladder neck is hitched to the back of the symphysis pubis by sutures placed on either side of the urethra. *Colposuspension* is a modification of this with sutures placed in the lateral vaginal fornices, thus elevating and supporting the bladder neck. A similar effect can be achieved by using slings made from muscle, fascia or synthetic material; the *Stamey* operation uses a long needle passed via a small suprapubic incision to place nylon sutures on either side of the bladder neck.

Other surgical options are occasionally used. Endoscopic injection of Teflon paste on either side of the bladder neck may relieve stress incontinence. Alternatively, an inflatable artificial urinary sphincter can be implanted around the bladder neck, although this is rarely indicated for simple stress incontinence.

### Stress incontinence in men

Non-operative measures such as pelvic floor exercises and alpha-adrenergic drugs do help some patients with minor symptoms but surgery is necessary in men with severe sphincter weakness.

Attempts to reconstruct the bladder neck and proximal urethra by plication or by using slings have been disappointing. As a result, implantable mechanical devices have gained in popularity. A silicone gel (*Kaufman*) prosthesis can be implanted into the perineum to provide constant urethral compression or variable compression can be achieved with an artificial urinary sphincter (*Brantley-Scott*) (Fig. 19.5). These compression devices are prone to complications including urethral erosion, infection and mechanical failure.

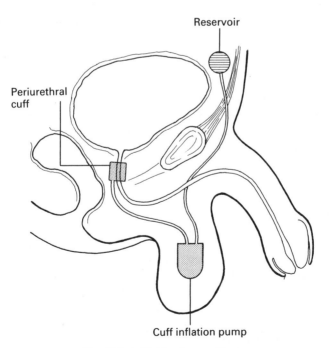

Reservoir

Periurethral
cuff

Cuff inflation pump

**Fig. 19.5** Artificial urinary sphincter

## Combined stress and urge incontinence

The first step should be to correct the underlying detrusor instability using the methods outlined above. If this is successful a weak sphincter may be able to maintain continence once high pressure unstable contractions have been abolished.

If incontinence persists despite treatment of detrusor instability, surgery for sphincter weakness is indicated but the patient should be warned that a cure cannot be guaranteed.

## Overflow incontinence

When overflow incontinence is due to chronic retention, the bladder outflow obstruction should be relieved by prostatectomy (in men) or urethral dilatation/urethrotomy (in women).

If the bladder still fails to empty after relief of outflow obstruction or if an atonic detrusor is the primary problem, bladder emptying can often be improved by cholinergic agents (e.g. bethanecol), by anticholinesterases (e.g. distigmine) or by suprapubic compression (*Credé manoeuvre*) and abdominal straining. Clean intermittent self-catheterisation (CISC) has, however, become more widely used in recent years to achieve adequate bladder emptying.

As a last resort, an indwelling urethral catheter may be needed; this is usually better tolerated and easier to manage in patients with atonic bladders than it is in detrusor instability.

## Insensible incontinence

Patients with insensible loss due to cerebral degeneration are one of the most difficult groups to treat. Regular toileting may be useful but drug therapy is often unhelpful. In most patients, an external drainage device (e.g. penile sheath), absorbent padding or a permanent urethral catheter is needed. Regular supervision is necessary in the long term to deal with the inevitable problems in these patients.

## Post-micturition dribbling

This is usually seen in men. If investigation reveals local urethral pathology such as a stricture or diverticulum, this should be treated appropriately. If no urethral abnormality can be found, the patient should be encouraged to 'milk' the urethra manually after voiding to ensure that it empties completely.

## NOCTURNAL ENURESIS

This can be divided into primary and secondary enuresis; in primary enuresis, the patient has never been dry at night whilst, in secondary enuresis, bedwetting develops in an individual who has previously been dry at night.

### Primary enuresis

In the infant, micturition is a reflex event. As the child grows older, voluntary control is gradually exerted over this reflex and the child becomes aware of the sensation of bladder fullness; daytime continence is normally achieved by 18-24 months. The development of night-time control is more variable, with 67% of children dry at night by the age of 3. In the remaining children, the incidence of bedwetting steadily declines, with nearly 50% becoming dry by 10 years and most of the remainder by 15; about 2% of children remain wet at night after the age of 15.

There is often a family history of bedwetting in parents or siblings. Psychological factors may also contribute to enuresis and information about these can be obtained from the parents or the family doctor. Physical examination is usually normal, although neurological disease must be excluded.

In view of the natural tendency for the condition to improve with age, the extent of investigations should be carefully considered. Urinary infection should be excluded in all patients, but additional investigations are not warranted under the age of 5 unless there are accompanying urinary symptoms. After the age of 5, an IVU or ultrasound is necessary to exclude urinary tract abnormalities.

If no abnormality is found on examination or investigation, reassurance and encouragement about the likelihood of spontaneous improvement is important both for child and parents. Simple measures such as bladder training during the day, fluid restriction before bedtime and 'lifting' the child when the parents go to bed are often effective.

Drug therapy can be employed if no improvement occurs with simpler measures. Anticholinergic agents (e.g. propantheline, oxybutynin) or synthetic ADH analogues (e.g. desmopressin) may help some patients. However, the most widely used drug is *imipramine*. This acts by reducing the depth of sleep (so that bladder fullness is appreciated) and inhibiting the bladder directly.

Another helpful technique is the use of an enuresis alarm. This is a small detector worn in the pants during the night which triggers an audible alarm to wake the child as leakage occurs. Eventually, the child becomes conditioned to appreciate bladder fullness and to wake and pass urine before leakage occurs.

For the 2% of patients whose bedwetting persists beyond adolescence, a formal urodynamic assessment is helpful. Many of these patients have daytime symptoms too and are found to have detrusor instability that requires appropriate treatment.

### Secondary enuresis

This may develop at any age and should always be fully investigated. It is often due to urinary infection, especially in children and in the elderly. It may also occur in patients with chronic retention of urine or be a manifestation of certain neurological disorders (e.g. nocturnal epilepsy). In some children, it is precipitated by a psychologically traumatic event such as the arrival of a new baby in the family.

Treatment is directed at the precipitating cause but, if this is unsuccessful, the measures outlined for primary enuresis should be instituted.

## URINARY FISTULAE

A fistula is an abnormal communication between two epithelial surfaces. Any part of the urinary tract may be affected, communicating either with other internal viscera or with the skin. Acquired fistulae are usually the result of trauma, infection, tumours, surgery or radiotherapy.

### Vaginal urinary fistulae

A fistula into the vagina may follow injury either to the ureter or the bladder. This usually occurs during pelvic surgery, especially hysterectomy. A ureterovaginal fistula develops if the ureter is accidentally cut, ligated or crushed in a clamp; a vesicovaginal fistula occurs after injury to the back of the bladder. In countries with less well-developed obstetric services, vesicovaginal fistula is more often due to prolonged labour with the fetal head causing pressure necrosis of the posterior wall of the bladder. Radiotherapy for carcinoma of the cervix may also be complicated by the development of a vesicovaginal fistula.

The presence of fluid leaking from the vagina is often all too obvious to the patient, although it may not appear until several days after the injury has occurred. The leaking fluid can be confirmed as urine by measuring its urea content which is higher than that of plasma.

The vaginal opening of a large fistula may be visible on speculum examination. If a pack is placed in the vagina and methylene blue instilled into the bladder, blue staining of the vaginal pack indicates that the fistula is from the bladder rather than the ureter.

Investigation should include an IVU which usually shows the side and level of any ureteric injury; a cystogram may be helpful in detecting a small vesical fistula. Cystoscopy will usually confirm a vesicovaginal fistula and can be combined with ureterography to determine the level of the ureteric injury in a ureterovaginal fistula.

There is some debate about the timing of surgery for the repair of vaginal fistulae. Although a delay of 3 months was once recommended, most surgeons now favour early operation providing this can be carried out within the first few days (before the tissues become too oedematous).

For a low ureterovaginal fistula, reimplantation of the ureter into the bladder should be performed; any loss of ureteric length can be made up by hitching the bladder on to the psoas minor tendon (*psoas hitch*) or by using a tubed bladder flap (*Boari flap*). For higher ureteric injuries, the damaged ureter can be swung across the midline and anastomosed to the opposite ureter (*transureteroureterostomy*) although nephrectomy is occasionally necessary.

With a small vesicovaginal fistula, closure may be possible via a vaginal approach. For larger or recurrent fistulae, a suprapubic approach should be used. The bladder is opened down to the fistula posteriorly, the fistula excised and the vagina and bladder closed; the greater omentum is mobilised and brought down between bladder and vagina. For very large fistulae after obstructed labour or radiotherapy, closure may be impossible and urinary diversion (e.g. ileal conduit) is the only available option.

## Vesicointestinal fistulae

Vesicocolic fistula (between sigmoid colon and bladder) is the commonest fistula between bladder and bowel. It is usually the result of diverticular disease, although it may also occur with colonic carcinoma, Crohn's disease and bladder carcinoma. Acute appendicitis and Crohn's disease occasionally cause a fistula between the bladder and the right colon.

Any communication between bladder and bowel invariably leads to urinary infection which is the commonest presenting symptom. The classical symptom is pneumaturia (gas bubbles in the urine) but incontinence is rare.

A mixed growth of faecal organisms is often seen on urine culture and faecal particles may be seen in the urine. Air may be visible in the bladder on a plain abdominal X-ray, giving rise to an air-fluid level on erect films. An IVU should be performed but a barium enema is the most reliable method of demonstrating the fistula and is essential to identify the nature of the bowel lesion. Cystoscopy often shows the opening of the fistula surrounded by oedematous mucosa. Biopsy of this rarely produces histological evidence of the underlying problem; sigmoidoscopy is more reliable in confirming the histological nature of the disease.

Treatment is by resection of the diseased segment of bowel and closure of the bladder defect; partial cystectomy may be necessary in some patients.

## Urethral fistulae

Rectoprostatic fistula is occasionally seen as a complication of prostatectomy, especially after open operation for invasive carcinoma of the prostate. It may also occur after severe pelvic fracture injuries with rupture of the membranous urethra and laceration of the rectal wall.

Some rectoprostatic fistulae will heal after a period of suprapubic catheter drainage of the bladder and diversion of the faecal stream by colostomy. For those fistulae which do not heal, *Park's pull-through operation*, in which a segment of sigmoid colon is pulled down and sutured to the lower rectum, is the simplest form of repair. For complex injuries involving urethral rupture, reconstructive surgery to the urethra may also be necessary.

# 20

# Urethral and sexually transmitted disorders

## URETHRAL DISORDERS

### Urethral caruncle

Urethral caruncles are found exclusively in women. They may cause pain, bleeding after voiding and blood spotting on underwear. The caruncle is composed of vascular connective tissue and appears as a fleshy, red polyp at the urethral orifice. If a caruncle is causing symptoms, it can be excised locally or treated by electrocautery.

### Urethral prolapse

Urethral prolapse occurs in two age groups: first, in young girls where it is related to chronic constipation and second, in elderly women where it is probably due to lack of oestrogenic support after the menopause.

Because the prolapse involves the full thickness of the urethra, it is particularly prone to undergo strangulation when it becomes swollen, blue and painful. Treatment is excision of the entire prolapse (after urethral dilatation) with careful mucosal reapposition, followed by catheterisation for 48 hours. If the prolapse is recurrent, it is best to perform retropubic surgery to support the urethra from above using one of the standard urethropexy procedures.

### Foreign bodies in the urethra

The variety of foreign bodies which have been introduced into the urethra is matched only by the ingenuity of urologists in devising methods of retrieving them. In the male, foreign bodies tend to lodge in the distal urethra resulting in pain, bleeding, urethral discharge and, eventually, urethral stricture. Most foreign bodies can be extracted endoscopically, if necessary after pushing them back into the bladder. Occasionally, direct incision into the urethra is necessary to remove an impacted foreign body. In women, inserted foreign bodies are usually found in the bladder from where they are easily retrieved endoscopically.

## Urethral tumours

Most urethral tumours in men and women are transitional cell tumours and are associated with urothelial cancer in the bladder. Four per cent of patients with bladder cancer have tumours in the urethra, although this figure is higher for patients with multifocal tumours. Primary tumours (usually squamous carcinomas) are unusual and often arise in chronically inflamed urethras as a result of urethral strictures, diverticula or gonorrhoea.

Superficial tumours in the urethra may be diathermised endoscopically although the recurrence rate is high. If they occur in the defunctioned urethra left in situ after total cystectomy, it is best to remove the entire urethra. Squamous tumours spread early to inguinal lymph nodes and the results of radical excision are poor with little long-term survival and high local recurrence rates.

## The urethral syndrome

This is the term often given to a disease pattern characterised by frequency, dysuria and abacteriuria. It may, of course, be secondary to cystitis but, in many cases, is not. Bacteria are found in the urethras of affected patients in 67% but cytological evidence of inflammation is seen in only 33%.

A similar syndrome can be caused by local irritation of the urethral orifice during sexual intercourse (*honeymoon cystitis*). This may be relieved by simple measures such as avoiding the use of condoms, using lubricating (KY) jelly, changing the coital position or emptying the bladder and washing before and after intercourse. Some patients find their symptoms completely relieved by taking a single antibiotic tablet after intercourse.

Chemical irritants such as deodorants, bubble baths and bath salts may produce similar symptoms and, if implicated, should be avoided. The best advice for a woman in this situation is to shower rather than bath and to keep the perineum clean with a separate flannel. Wiping of the vaginal area after voiding should be performed from 'front to back' to avoid contaminating the introitus with bacteria from the anal canal.

In elderly women, such symptoms are often caused by lack of oestrogenic support after the menopause. Typically, the introitus is pale, often with haemorrhagic areas and the urethra often appears stenotic. The situation can be relieved by local application of oestrogen creams or short-term oral oestrogens. Urethral dilatation may be necessary if there is evidence of urethral stenosis.

In many women with the urethral syndrome, no obvious cause is found for their symptoms. Treatment with long-term antibiotics or anti-inflammatory agents helps some patients. Others, however, are helped by wide dilatation of the urethra for reasons which are not clear. Patients with transient symptoms usually respond to urethral dilatation or irrigation of the peri-urethral glands, but persistent symptoms should be fully investigated by X-ray assessment of the urinary tract and cystoscopy.

Sensory denervation of the urethra has been used as a last resort in women with persistent symptoms refractory to any other form of treatment. This is performed by freeing the urethra from its supporting tissues but has little to commend it as a logical procedure.

## SEXUALLY TRANSMITTED DISEASES

There has been a gradual increase in the incidence of all sexually trans-mitted diseases over the last 10 years (Fig. 20.1). This increase is particu-larly marked in non-gonococcal urethritis which has become the commonest sexually transmitted disease.

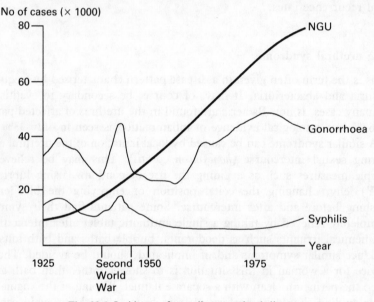

Fig. 20.1 Incidence of sexually-transmitted diseases

### Diseases causing urethral discharge

Urethral discharge is most commonly noticed in men and should be assumed to be a sign of sexually transmitted infection until proved other-wise (Fig. 20.2). Discharge due to urethritis is usually associated with a 'pricking' sensation in the urethra, dysuria and, occasionally, inflammation of the urethral mucosa visible at the meatus.

The first step is to confirm that the discharge comes from the urethra. This is performed using the *two-glass test*. The patient is asked not to void for at least 2 hours, and then passes approximately 20 ml of urine into each

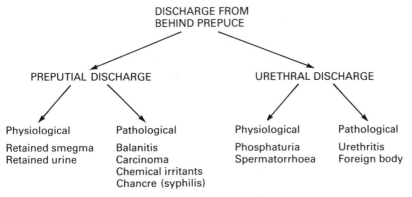

**Fig. 20.2** Urethral discharge in men

of two glasses. If the first glass alone contains a generalised haze or threads and debris, then urethritis is likely. If both glasses are affected, it is more likely that the problem has originated in the bladder or upper urinary tracts. Phosphate deposits will cause a uniform haze in both glasses which clears when the urine is acidified (Fig. 20.3).

The presence of urethritis can be confirmed by the finding of pus cells in a Gram stain of the discharge swabbed from the urethra using a cotton-tipped culture swab. *Neisseria gonorrhoeae* appears as a Gram-negative intracellular diplococcus and may be cultured from the swab. Special culture medium is required for urethral swabs if *Chlamydia* or *Mycoplasma* infections are suspected. A wet slide preparation in saline is the best way of demonstrating *Trichomonas* in urethral smears.

The presence of general symptoms such as pyrexia, rigors, diarrhoea, joint pains and conjunctivitis may help in the diagnosis of patients with urethral discharge. Locally, one should look for meatal inflammation, urethral tenderness and abnormalities in other pelvic organs and in the scrotum.

Haematuria and spontaneous bleeding from the urethra usually suggest a prostatic source for the inflammation, although they may be caused by posterior urethritis. One special problem is the condition known as *juvenile urethritis*, which affects a short segment of the bulbar urethra in children. The disease presents as frequency, dysuria and blood-spotting of the underpants. It is a self-limiting condition which is said not to progress and stricture the urethra, provided the urethra is not instrumented. It is possible the disease may not be as benign as previously thought, since some boys do seem to develop strictures in early adult life.

*Gonorrhoea*

This disease is invariably transmitted by sexual contact and is usually seen

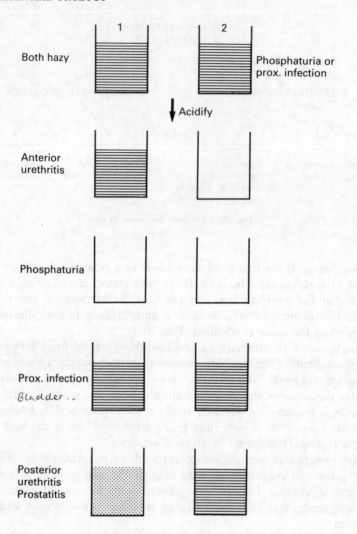

**Fig. 20.3** The two-glass test

in young adults. In men, the anterior urethra is usually affected whilst in women there is infection of the urethra and cervix, which may progress to pelvic inflammation. Homosexuals may have primary rectal involvement or infection of the pharynx.

The incubation period is only a few days. Men usually present with frequency, dysuria and a urethral discharge (in 90%): the discharge is normally thick and purulent. The disease in women is asymptomatic in 70% but may present as vaginal discharge, dysuria or pelvic pain.

The diagnosis is made by Gram stain and culture of a swab from the urethra or cervix. Microscopy shows Gram-negative intracellular diplococci.

Treatment is simple and can be accomplished very rapidly. The standard therapy is oral ampicillin 2 g or intramuscular penicillin combined with probenecid 1 g to maintain high blood levels. This treatment need only be given once but culture of a urethral swab should be repeated at 2 days and 1–2 weeks to determine eradication of the bacteria.

Some strains of *N. gonorrhoeae* are penicillinase producers and do not respond to penicillin. Most laboratories nowadays culture routinely to test for penicillin sensitivity. Resistant strains usually respond to treatment with cephalosporins (e.g cefotaxime).

If there is a history of allergy to penicillin, treatment is instituted with co-trimoxazole or spectinomycin. In the event of systemic complications, treatment should be continued for a period of 2 weeks.

Other organisms such as *Chlamydia* may be acquired concurrently with gonorrhoea and cause persisting urethral discharge after the gonococcus has been eliminated (*post-gonococcal urethritis*).

## Non-gonococcal urethritis (NGU)

This is a general term used to describe urethritis which is not caused by gonococci. It encompasses chlamydial infection, other specific infections and non-specific urethritis (Table 20.1). More than 125 000 cases of NGU were recorded in 1980 in England and Wales and the incidence is rising at the rate of approximately 10% per year.

**Table 20.1**   Possible causative organisms in NGU

| |
| --- |
| *Chlamydia trachomatis* (50–60%) |
| *Trichomonas vaginalis*<br>*Ureaplasma urealyticum*<br>*Gardnerella vaginalis*       } 5–10%<br>*Candida albicans*<br>Herpes simplex<br>Viral warts |
| Unknown in 30–45% (non-specific urethritis, NSU) |

Incubation periods vary considerable for NGU but are usually in the region of 2–3 weeks. Symptoms are seen exclusively in men and there is usually a mucoid urethral discharge with mild dysuria. Pus cells are seen on a urethral smear, but gonococci, yeasts and *Trichomonas* are not seen. When the discharge is scanty, it may be best to examine an early morning urethral smear before the first void of the day. Culture of *Chlamydia* requires a cell line and is not available in all centres but monoclonal antibody tests for *Chlamydia* are now coming into widespread use.

The organisms implicated often respond poorly to antibiotics. The first choice lies between tetracycline or erythromycin, with sulphonamides as a second line. Although 80% of men are said to be cured at 2 weeks, cure is difficult to assess, relapse is common and re-infection from the sexual partner is difficult to exclude.

The sexual partner must be investigated and treated. NGU does not occur as a clinical entity in women but is presumed on the basis of sexual contact with a male sufferer and the culture of *Chlamydia* from cervical swabs. Women should be treated for 2 weeks with tetracycline. Erythromycin should be used to treat NGU in pregnant women.

Complications of NGU are unusual, but can be very distressing for the patient. In men, the commonest are low-grade prostatitis and epididymitis. These respond very poorly to antibiotics and treatment may need to be continued for at least 2 months to produce symptomatic relief. In women, pelvic inflammatory disease may occur, especially after untreated chlamydial infection.

## Reiter's disease

This is an unusual syndrome which is often associated with, although not necessarily caused by, chlamydial infection. There is also an individual susceptibility to the disease, since 67% of affected patients are found to have HLA-B27 antigen; this antigen is also associated with a high risk of developing sero-negative spondarthrosis.

The typical syndrome is of mild urethritis progressing to conjunctivitis and then polyarthritis, affecting particularly the lower limbs. Circinate balanitis and oral erosions are seen in up to 30% of patients and thickening of the plantar skin (*keratoderma blenorrhagica*) is seen in 10%.

Treatment is with tetracycline or erythromycin and anti-inflammatory agents. Involvement of the eyes and joints may require specialist advice. Topical steroids may help the balanitis or oral lesions.

## Diseases causing genital ulceration

### Syphilis

Syphilis is caused by *Treponema pallidum* and is usually spread by sexual contact, although it may be transmitted from mother to foetus and by blood transfusion. Almost 60% of cases of syphilis now seen occur in homosexuals.

The incubation period of the disease is usually 20–25 days, although the range is from 9 to 90 days. The initial lesion is a small pink macule on the genitalia. Typically, this occurs on the coronal sulcus in men, progresses to become papular and eventually ulcerates (*primary chancre*) (Fig. 20.4), often becoming secondarily infected. At this stage, the lesion is highly infectious and is usually associated with rubbery, non-tender, enlarged inguinal lymph nodes. In women, the primary chancre is usually on the

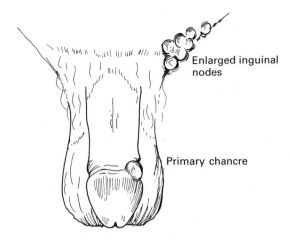

Enlarged inguinal nodes

Primary chancre

**Fig. 20.4** Primary chancre of syphilis

vulva. In homosexuals, chancres may occur in the anus, rectum or mouth: anal lesions are easily mistaken for simple anal fissures.

Secondary bacterial infection can make diagnosis difficult, especially if antibiotic creams have been applied to the genitalia. Diagnosis is confirmed, however, by dark-ground illumination of a smear from the lesion which usually shows the organisms.

Serological tests for syphilis are not always positive in the early stages, although they usually become so over 1–3 months. The VDRL test is the most widely used non-specific test and it can be titrated to assess the activity of the disease; it may, however, be positive in other acute infections. Of the specific tests, the TPHA is the most widely used, being positive in most patients before treatment but often remaining positive despite adequate treatment.

Treatment is with intramuscular penicillin for a total of 10 days. This occasionally precipitates an acute toxic (*Herxheimer*) reaction within a few hours of treatment characterised by fever, pyrexia and oedema or infiltration of the primary chancre. This toxic reaction settles rapidly, although the symptoms may require treatment with anti-inflammatory analgesics.

In patients who are allergic to penicillin, tetracycline or doxycycline are the best alternatives.

Untreated, the primary chancre usually heals within 3–6 weeks. However, the patient may then go on to develop secondary and tertiary syphilis with their well-known systemic manifestations.

Follow-up of patients with syphilis is important. All patients should be subjected to repeated clinical examination and serological testing over the first year. Assessment should be performed monthly for the first 3 months and then 3-monthly for the next year. Thereafter, most genitomedical units recommend follow-up for a further 2 years, although some clinicians would suggest surveillance for life.

*Genital herpes simplex*

This is caused by *herpes simplex virus*, usually type 2 (HSV-2), which has an incubation period of 4–5 days.

There are often prodromal symptoms of malaise, irritability, local skin itching and nerve root pains (usually down the legs). Vesicles then appear on or near the genitalia and these burst to produce erosions which are associated with inguinal lymphadenopathy. Vesicles arise on the prepuce, glans and shaft of the penis or on the vulva. Anorectal lesions are often seen in homosexuals.

Pain and local neuropathy may cause retention of urine and the disease may progress to become systemic, resulting in meningitis or encephalitis.

The diagnosis is made on the typical appearance of the lesions and the virus can be found in scrapings taken from erosions or vesicle fluid. The virus can be grown in tissue culture and identified by its cytopathic effect. It can also be identified on electron microscopy or by enzyme-linked immunosorbent assay (ELISA). Using these methods, a definitive diagnosis can normally be reached within 4–72 hours.

Treatment of primary herpes simplex is with oral acyclovir but this needs to be started within 2–3 days of the appearance of the lesions. Oral analgesics and bathing with warm saline are helpful and any associated infection should be treated with appropriate antibiotics.

Subsequently, the virus lies dormant in the dorsal root ganglia of the spinal cord until re-activated by factors unknown. Recurrences are usually mild but occur in at least 60%. There is, unfortunately, no effective treatment for recurrent disease.

The continuing presence of HSV-2 in the cervix uteri is possibly a risk factor in the development of carcinoma of the cervix and is an indication for regular cytological evaluation of the cervix for pre-malignant change.

## Other ulcerating infections

A number of other sexually transmitted infections produce genital ulceration but are rare in the UK, occurring more commonly in tropical countries.

*Chancroid*

This causes multiple, painful ulcers from which *Haemophilus ducreyi* can be cultured. It usually responds to treatment with co-trimoxazole or ampicillin.

*Lymphogranuloma venereum*

This starts as a small ulcer but is followed by painful inguinal lymphadenopathy and systemic disturbance. Diagnosis is by serology for the appropriate serotype of *Chlamydia trachomatis*. It responds to treatment with tetracycline.

### Granuloma inguinale

This causes painless, destructive genital ulcers with granulation. Tissue smears or biopsy show *Calymatobacterium granulomatis* and treatment is with tetracycline.

### Miscellaneous

Ulceration of the genital mucosa can also occur in systemic conditions such as erythema multiforme or Behçet's syndrome and in drug eruptions. Diagnosis, therefore, requires a careful assessment of the whole clinical picture.

## Other virally-induced sexually transmitted diseases

### Genital warts (Fig. 20.5)

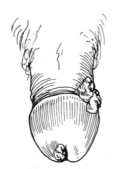

Fig. 20.5 Penile and meatal warts

Genital warts (condylomata acuminata) are caused by *human papilloma virus* (HPV) types 6,11,16 and 18. The incubation period may be as long as 3 months and the warts appear as small flat lesions on the genital skin. In moist areas, the warts may be more hypertrophic and giant warts occasionally develop, especially on the foreskin (Buschke–Loewenstein tumours).

The diagnosis is usually made clinically on the typical appearance of the lesions. HPV antigen may be detected by immunocytochemistry and cervical smears from women with genital warts show typical cells with irregular hyperchromatic nuclei and a perinuclear halo.

Treatment is to keep the affected areas cool and dry. Applications of 10–25% podophyllin for a period of 2–4 weeks is usually sufficient to resolve the problem. Podophyllin is irritant and should be kept off the surrounding skin. If podophyllin fails to resolve warts effectively, applications of 50–100% trichloroacetic acid may be effective. More refractory warts or lesions within the urethral meatus which are not amenable to topical treatment may require treatment by electrocautery, cryotherapy or laser cautery.

The natural history of such warts is that they will disappear spontaneously, in much the same way as palmar warts, when the patient develops immunity. Before they do so, however, some patients are subject to recurrent crops of warts. This has led to a search for specific treatment and interferon has been used to try and stimulate immunity to the causative virus.

There is increasing evidence that the wart virus (especially HPV-16) is involved in the pathogenesis of carcinoma of the cervix uteri.

### Acquired immune deficiency syndrome (AIDS)

AIDS is a viral disease which has probably existed for many years but which only really came to light in 1981. In that year, American health monitoring bodies noticed an epidemic of pneumocystis pneumonia, Kaposi's sarcoma and other opportunistic infections in Los Angeles and New York. Ninety-two per cent of these cases involved homosexual or bisexual men and the current AIDS epidemic was born.

The causative organism has now been identified as an RNA-containing retrovirus, *human immunodeficiency virus* (HIV). The source of this virus is unknown but there is some evidence that it was carried to the developed world from Africa.

Infection by HIV produces a spectrum of disease patterns. The number of symptomless carriers of HIV is unknown but may account for 60% of all patients infected with HIV. Thirty-three per cent of infected patients develop the AIDS-related complex (ARC) or persistent generalised lymphadenopathy (PGL). The clinical features of ARC include pyrexia of unknown origin, loss of body weight, general lethargy, generalised lymphadenopathy, hepatosplenomegaly, hairy leukoplakia and minor oral infections. Laboratory findings include HIV antigen or antibody in the blood, lymphopenia, anaemia, thrombocytopenia and raised levels of cholesterol or immunoglobulins. The diagnosis of ARC is made on the presence of two or more of these clinical features and two or more abnormal laboratory findings persisting over a period of 3 months. PGL may be suspected if enlarged lymph nodes are found in at least two extra-inguinal sites persisting for more than 3 months.

The full-blown AIDS syndrome occurs in 7% of patients infected by HIV and is a disease of cellular immune deficiency not associated with inherited disease and with no known underlying cause or predisposition.

The interrelation between these disease complexes has not been accurately established and, in particular, it is not yet known how many healthy carriers of HIV exist or whether these carriers inevitably progress to one of the disease entities described above. At present, over 25 000 cases of AIDS have been reported, mostly among homosexuals. Over 1200 cases have been reported in the UK, although it is estimated that there may be as many as 30 000 carriers of the virus in this country.

In the UK, 85% of AIDS cases are seen in homosexual or bisexual men with 5.5% occurring in haemophiliacs (from infected blood products) and 1% in intravenous drug users. Heterosexual contact is responsible for AIDS in 5% of patients whilst, in the remaining 3.5%, there is no clear predisposing factor.

Although some patients with mild symptoms do seem to retrogress, the development of full-blown AIDS is universally fatal. The main causes of death are malignancy and opportunistic infection, particularly *Pneumocystis carinii* pneumonia, cryptosporidiosis, cytomegalovirus, toxoplasmosis, cryptococcosis and atypical mycobacterial infection. The mean survival after treatment for patients with pneumocystis pneumonia is 35 weeks, whilst patients developing Kaposi's sarcoma survive, on average, 2 years from the onset of the disease. Other malignancies, in particular non-Hodgkin lymphomas, are more aggressive and may be fatal within a few months.

At present, there is no known cure for AIDS and no effective vaccine against HIV. Prevention of the spread of disease involves the encouragement of 'safe sex', including the use of condoms, screening of all blood for HIV and heat treatment of all blood products to kill the virus. Intravenous drug users who continue to inject themselves should be encouraged not to share equipment and to use clean, disposable needles.

Treatment is, as yet, ineffective. Much research is going into methods of exploiting the specific feature of the virus, which is to produce a reverse transcriptase allowing its genetic material to be incorporated permanently into the genetic structure of the host cell. Azidodeoxythymidine (AZT) is currently under clinical scrutiny in the treatment of a limited number of AIDS patients. Early results suggest that, although it cannot treat the full-blown AIDS complex, it may modify the disease and slow progression.

*Hepatitis B*

There is an increasing fund of evidence showing that the hepatitis B virus may also be sexually transmitted in a proportion of cases. The reader should seek further information on this from specialised texts.

**Contact tracing in sexually transmitted disease**

Counselling and contact tracing for patients found to have sexually transmitted disease is just as important as treating the disease itself. The first step is to ensure that the patient understands the disease enough to co-operate in its treatment and to identify possible sexual contacts.

Primary contacts (the person from whom the disease was caught) are often difficult to trace, whilst it may be easier for the patient to recall secondary contacts (people to whom the patient may have transmitted the disease). Motivation is very important in persuading contacts to attend for testing and to return for follow-up. The tracing of defaulters may be a difficult problem requiring considerable tact and patience; many genitomedical units now have staff trained specifically in contact tracing.

Confidentiality in all matters is vital and firm reassurance is essential, since many patients and contacts feel angry or distressed at having been implicated in a disease chain. Health education, inevitably, plays an important role in counselling patients or contacts with sexually transmitted disease.

The presence of any sexually transmitted disease in children is likely to indicate sexual abuse. Such a problem requires delicate handling and is best left to specialists in this field.

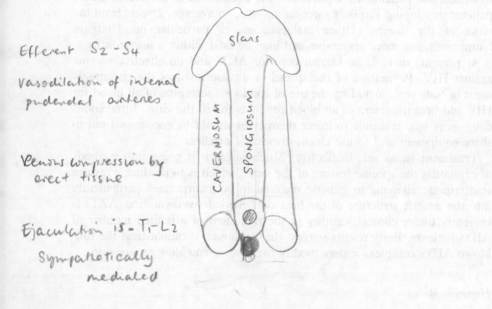

# 21

# Disorders of the penis

## BALANITIS

Balanitis is inflammation of the foreskin; such inflammation usually affects the glans penis and the tissues behind the foreskin (*balanoposthitis*).

All men with balanitis should have their urine tested for glucose. Treatment involves systemic antibiotics if there is evidence of swelling and redness of the foreskin. The mainstay of treatment is careful washing behind the foreskin and, if indicated, installation of chloramphenicol ointment. After successful treatment, all patients should be re-examined carefully and, if they have phimosis, offered circumcision to prevent a recurrence of their balanitis.

## PHIMOSIS

Phimosis is the term given to tightness of the foreskin which prevents it from being retracted fully over the glans penis. An infant's foreskin is normally adherent to the glans penis until the age of 3 years; thereafter, it separates progressively from the glans and is non-adherent by the age of 6 years (Fig. 21.1). No attempt should be made to retract forcibly the foreskin of any boy less than 6 years old.

Children with tight foreskins usually present with balanitis or 'ballooning' of the foreskin during voiding. Ballooning in itself can occur behind a normal foreskin and is not necessarily a sign of phimosis. If the foreskin cannot be retracted by the age of 7 years and this is causing symptoms, then it is justified to recommend circumcision (Fig. 21.2). On occasions, the foreskin may be so tight and adherent that it results in acute retention of urine; this can be relieved by circumcision performed as an emergency. Boys with hypospadias should never be circumcised, since the foreskin may be a vital source of skin for subsequent surgical repair of this anomaly.

Many patients with tight foreskins do not present in childhood. In these patients, phimosis may only become obvious once they start to have intercourse. Circumcision in this situation cures the problem. The tight foreskin, however, often appears thickened and pale or even white at its

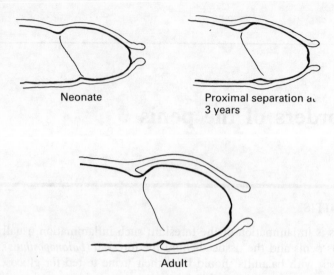

Neonate

Proximal separation at 3 years

Adult

**Fig. 21.1** Separation of foreskin with age

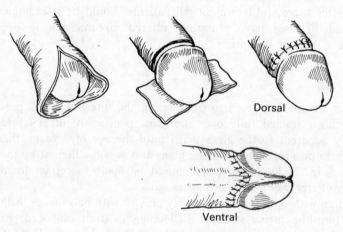

Dorsal

Ventral

**Fig. 21.2** Formal circumcision

tip; this pallor sometimes extends onto the glans penis. This condition is known as *balanitis xerotica obliterans* and is analogous with the atrophic changes (*lichen sclerosus et atrophicus*) occasionally seen on the female vulva. Steroid creams may help but circumcision is eventually curative.

The fibrosis and loss of elastic tissue in balanitis xerotica obliterans may result in narrowing of the urethral meatus for which meatal dilatation or meatoplasty may be required.

Circumcision in the absence of phimosis is occasionally requested in the neonatal period for religious or ritual reasons. This can most easily be accomplished under regional penile block using a *Plastibell* device.

The practice of carrying out a dorsal slit of the foreskin as an alternative to formal circumcision results in a cosmetically unacceptable penis. It may be permitted as an emergency measure, for example, to insert a urethral catheter into an elderly man with a severe phimosis completely covering the urethral meatus.

## PARAPHIMOSIS

This condition is caused by pulling a tight foreskin back over the glans penis. Typically this occurs when the penis is erect during intercourse or masturbation but it may occur after instrumentation of the urethra. Subsequently, the foreskin cannot be pulled forwards again and, as a result, the glans penis swells considerably, making reduction of the foreskin even more difficult.

Treatment can be accomplished under a regional local anaesthetic block. The glans penis and tissue distal to the constricting ring of foreskin are gently squeezed for a few minutes to reduce the oedema. The glans penis is then pulled firmly forwards to elongate it as much as possible and the foreskin 'eased' forwards over the glans. It is wrong simply to try and push the swollen glans backwards through the constriction ring; this will inevitably result in failure.

Reduction of the paraphimosis can be accomplished in most cases but, when it cannot, emergency circumcision may be necessary. All patients who have had a paraphimosis successfully reduced should have elective circumcision performed within 6–8 weeks.

## PRIAPISM

Priapism is defined as a persistent, painful erection which is not associated with an appropriate sexual desire. Although the aetiology in many cases is uncertain, there are some well-recognised causes of priapism (Table 21.1).

**Table 21.1**  Causes of priapsim

*Haematological disease*
  sickle cell anaemia
  leukaemia

*Malignant infiltration of the penis*

*Spinal cord injuries*

*Drugs (often in overdose)*
  anticoagulants
  phenothiazines
  marijuana
  antihypertensives

*Idiopathic*

Typically, the corpora cavernosa are congested but the corpus spongiosum and glans penis remain flaccid. Stasis of blood in the corpora cavernosa results in local hypercapnia, sludging and hyperviscosity. This, in turn, causes oedema of the muscle in the corpora resulting in ischaemia and fibrosis. The final result of this, if priapism is left untreated, is *impotence*.

Priapism should be regarded as a genuine urological emergency and treated as soon as possible. Although a delay in treatment increases the risk of subsequent impotence, late treatment is better than none at all. Clearly, specific treatment of the underlying condition is important where possible, but the crucial step is to relieve the erection and, if possible, preserve potency.

Numerous drugs have been used either systemically or by injection into the penis, but none has proved entirely satisfactory. Only metaraminol and arfonad seem to be effective in reducing priapism but the effects are often only temporary. The most reliable way of treating the problem is to insert large-bore cannulae into the corpora cavernosa under anaesthetic and to wash out the contents with saline. If this fails to reduce the erection, then a *shunt procedure* should be performed (Fig. 21.3).

It is important before any shunt procedure to warn the patient of the possibility of impotence despite adequate treatment. Carefully-performed shunting, however, means that potency rates of 60% can be achieved postoperatively.

In some centres, radiologically-controlled embolisation of one internal pudendal artery is used to treat priapism with good results.

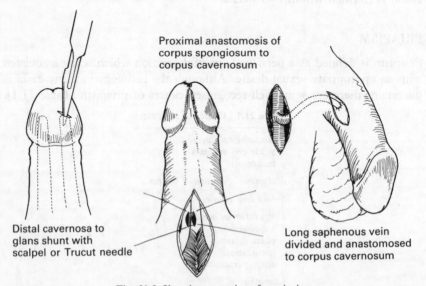

Proximal anastomosis of
corpus spongiosum to
corpus cavernosum

Distal cavernosa to
glans shunt with
scalpel or Trucut needle

Long saphenous vein
divided and anastomosed
to corpus cavernosum

**Fig. 21.3** Shunting operations for priapism

## PEYRONIE'S DISEASE

Peyronie's disease is a fibrotic process of unknown aetiology which affects the tunica albuginea and corpora cavernosa of the penis. It is considered analogous to Dupuytren's contracture in the hands (with which it is often associated) and to idiopathic retroperitoneal fibrosis. The plaque prevents the tunica albuginea from expanding during erection, resulting in erectile deformity (Fig. 21.4).

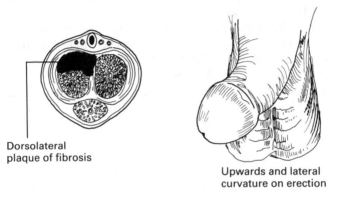

Dorsolateral
plaque of fibrosis

Upwards and lateral
curvature on erection

**Fig. 21.4** Cross-section of Peyronie's plaque and its effect on erection

Some patients give a definite history of coital trauma which has resulted in the development of a plaque of scar tissue in the corpus cavernosum and, in others, drugs such as beta-blockers have been implicated in the development of Peyronie's disease. In the majority of patients, however, there is no identifiable aetiological factor.

Typically, the patient notices pain on erection followed a few weeks or months later by bending of the erect penis. The usual site for the plaque of fibrosis is on the dorsum of the penis, so that curvature on erection is up towards the body. However, the plaques may be found at any site and, indeed, may be multiple. The site and direction of the bend usually tell the clinician where to look for the fibrotic plaque, which is palpable in the penis as an area of induration. If there is any doubt about the siting of the plaque or the direction of bending, a cavernosogram helps to clarify the situation.

Extensive plaques of fibrosis may prevent blood flow to the tip of the corpora cavernosa during erection, resulting either in inability to achieve an erection at all or loss of distal penile tumescence. Cavernosography confirms partial or complete occlusion of the corpora at the level of the plaque.

### Treatment

Mild cases require no treatment at all apart from firm reassurance that the disease often regresses or remains static and that it is not a malignant condition. Provided the patient is able to have intercourse comfortably despite the erectile deformity, no treatment is necessary.

Numerous forms of medical treatment have been tried and all have been shown to be ineffective. Intralesional steroid injections, ultrasound and superficial radiotherapy have gained some popularity in that they relieve the discomfort, but they rarely influence the deformity and their effect is often short-lived. Some therapeutic effect has been claimed by users of vitamin E (200 mg three times daily).

Treatment with potassium p-aminobenzoate is probably effective in reducing pain and improving deformity. However, to be effective, the drug must be given in high doses and the therapeutic effect is only maintained as long as the patient takes the drug.

The most effective treatment is surgery. This is only indicated if the patient's erection is so deformed that he is unable to have sexual intercourse, or if the patient is impotent.

### Surgery for pain and erectile deformity

Excision of the plaque of fibrosis is the obvious solution to the problem, although this usually requires grafting of the defect in the tunica after excision using skin, fascia lata or dura. There is, however, a high incidence of impotence after these procedures and the grafted tissue used does not have the rigidity of the natural tunica albuginea. The best surgical approach, therefore, is *Nesbitt's operation* (Fig. 21.5) which aims to straighten the penis by shortening the corpora cavernosa slightly at a point diametrically opposite to the bend; the plaque of fibrosis is left untouched.

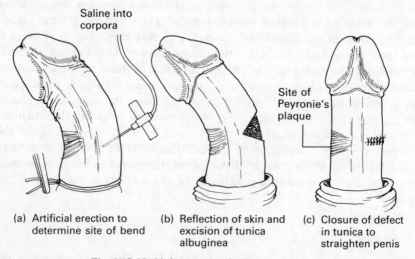

(a) Artificial erection to determine site of bend

(b) Reflection of skin and excision of tunica albuginea

(c) Closure of defect in tunica to straighten penis

**Fig. 21.5** Nesbitt's operation for Peyronie's disease

This procedure inevitably causes up to 1 cm of shortening of the penis and this should be explained to the patient before surgery. The technique has also been used successfully to straighten and restore erections in patients with severe disease and impotence.

### Surgery for impotence in Peyronie's disease

Whilst Nesbitt's operation gives good results, it may fail to restore potency in patients with fibrotic plaques which obstruct blood flow through the corpora cavernosa. In these patients, it is better to incise the plaque to release the curvature and then insert penile prostheses which will give sufficient stiffness to permit intercourse.

## CARCINOMA OF THE PENIS

Malignant tumours of the penis are uncommon, occurring at a rate of 1 per 100 000 of the male population. They are rare under the age of 45 years but, thereafter, the incidence increases with age. Carcinoma of the penis is rare in Jews and other religious groups who are circumcised at birth. Phimosis is present in 25% of patients with carcinoma of the penis.

The implication, therefore, is that the presence of an intact foreskin increases the likelihood of carcinoma developing. This is borne out by experimental observations that smegma may be carcinogenic not only to the male penis but also to the female cervix.

The tumour arises as a warty growth or ulcer on the glans penis or in the coronal sulcus. This is usually hidden by the foreskin and the first presenting symptom may be pain, bleeding or a foul-smelling discharge. Presentation is frequently late in the disease process, partly because the tumour is hidden and partly because the patient often delays seeking medical attention. A few patients delay for so long that the entire penis is eroded at the time of presentation.

Histologically, the tumour is usually a squamous carcinoma, although there may be glandular elements within the lesion. Early spread occurs via

**Table 21.2**  TNM staging of carcinoma of the penis

| | | | |
|---|---|---|---|
| T0 | No tumour present | N0 | No nodes palpable |
| T1 | Lesion < 2 cm diam. & superficial | N1 | Mobile ipsilateral inguinal nodes |
| T2 | Lesion 2–5 cm diam. with minimal infiltration | N2 | Mobile bilateral inguinal nodes |
| T3 | Lesion > 5 cm diam. with deep infiltration | N3 | Fixed inguinal nodes |
| T4 | Large lesions invading adjacent structures | | |
| | M0 | No metastases | |
| | M1 | Metastases present | |

lymphatics to the inguinal nodes, which are enlarged in 50% of patients at presentation. Nodal enlargement, however, may be due to secondary infection rather than tumour involvement.

The initial management consists of a biopsy of the tumour to obtain histological confirmation of the diagnosis, and circumcision is usually required to accomplish this. Staging is performed on purely clinical criteria at the time of biopsy (Table 21.2).

## Treatment

For T1 and most T2 tumours, the alternatives lie between radiotherapy and partial amputation of the penis. Radiotherapy is given directly to the tumour using a protective mould. After treatment, careful follow-up is necessary but a 5-year survival rate of almost 100% can be expected. For this reason, most surgeons now opt for radiotherapy as first choice, reserving partial amputation for tumour recurrence or failure to respond to radiotherapy. If partial amputation is required, the penis is considerably shortened but penetration for sexual intercourse is still possible in 45% of men.

When there is localised involvement of the shaft of the penis, radiotherapy is the best form of treatment, giving a 5-year survival of 80%. Partial amputation can be performed provided a 2 cm proximal clearance of the tumour can be effected and amputation may be required for recurrent disease.

More advanced tumours, involving the shaft of the penis and the scrotal skin, require radical amputation. This involves removal of the penis and scrotal contents, with reconstruction of the urethra as a perineal urethrostomy. Wide involvement of scrotal or perineal skin by local infiltration may require extensive skin grafting. If surgery is not possible in advanced disease, palliative local radiotherapy should be offered.

## Inguinal node enlargement in carcinoma of the penis

Fifty per cent of patients have enlarged inguinal nodes at the time of presentation, but only one third of these are found to contain tumour. However, 20% of impalpable inguinal nodes have been shown to contain tumour deposits. If the inguinal nodes are involved on the affected side, there is a 50% chance that the nodes in the contralateral groin will also be involved. If both groins contain involved nodes, then 30% of such patients will also have involvement of iliac nodes.

The best policy with inguinal nodes is 'wait-and-see'. After treatment of the primary tumour the nodes should be re-assessed at 2 months. If they are still palpable, it is best to perform aspiration biopsy or to excise a single saphenous node for histology. If there is tumour in the node, block dissection of the inguinal nodes should be performed.

Lymph node involvement worsens the prognosis of carcinoma of the penis considerably. Five-year survivals are reduced to 20–50%, depending on the number of nodes involved. There is some evidence that adjuvant systemic chemotherapy with bleomycin, methotrexate or cis-platinum may improve survival in patients with nodal involvement.

## IMPOTENCE

The precise vascular and neurological mechanisms which control erection (Fig. 21.6) are poorly understood. During erection, there is an increased arterial inflow into the erectile spaces of the penis. It is probable that there is also obstruction to venous outflow from the penis to maintain the erection. The means by which these changes are mediated is unknown. It is known, however, that alpha-adrenoceptors and vasoactive intestinal poly-

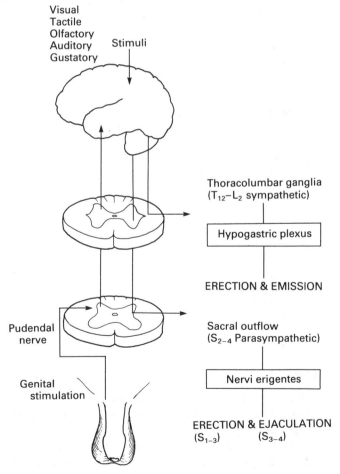

Fig. 21.6 The neurology of erection and ejaculation

peptide (VIP) play a part in the vascular changes because injection of VIP or α-blockers directly into the corpora cavernosa produces erection.

Anatomically, there are helicine arterial branches to the corpora which also have branches piercing the tunica albuginea and supplying the corpus spongiosum. Some of these branches go to the glans penis and act as 'shunts'. It is possible that these 'shunt' arteries close during erection to prevent leakage of blood away from the penis.

The ischiocavernosus and bulbospongiosus muscles can also raise pressure within the penis to maintain erection by contracting under stimulation from the pudendal nerve. This effect, however, is probably short-lasting.

Impotence is the inability to initiate or sustain a penile erection sufficiently to permit penetration for sexual intercourse. It can arise as a result of defects in the complex pathways involved in producing erection or, simply, as a result of mechanical problems with the penis (e.g. phimosis, short frenulum, chordee, Peyronie's disease).

Most mechanical problems are immediately obvious and can be dealt with specifically in the expectation that erections will be restored. The remainder of patients have impaired erections due to other causes (Table 21.3).

**Table 21.3**   Common causes of erectile impotence

| | |
|---|---|
| Diabetes mellitus | 20% |
| Post-operative (pelvic surgery e.g. AP resection, cystectomy, shunting for priapism) | 15% |
| Vascular occlusion (usually atherosclerotic) | 13% |
| Spinal cord lesions | 9% |
| Drugs (incl. alcohol) | 9% |
| Peyronie's disease | 9% |
| Other organic causes (severe debilitating disease, endocrine defects, post-priapism) | 20% |
| Psychogenic | 5% |

## Clinical assessment

Organic impotence is usually insidious in onset, whereas psychogenic impotence often arises quite suddenly. As a general rule, patients with psychogenic impotence have preserved night-time and early morning erections but are unable to achieve erection during sexual stimulation. Similarly, the sudden disappearance of erection prior to intercourse is very suggestive of a psychogenic cause. Incomplete erections may suggest a vascular cause for the problem.

The history, therefore, may give important clues about the origin of impotence. The existence of systemic disease such as diabetes should be determined and it is important to ask what drugs the patient is taking; hypotensive, narcotic and oestrogenic agents are particularly likely to cause impotence.

A full clinical examination should be performed, with special emphasis on peripheral pulses, sacral reflexes and rectal examination. The association of impotence with aorto-iliac occlusive disease (*Leriche syndrome*) is well known, so an absence of peripheral pulses may suggest vascular occlusion as the cause of impotence. The bulbospongiosus reflex should be tested in addition to the anal and lower limb reflexes.

## Investigation

Measurements of testosterone, thyroxine, prolactin and pituitary FSH/LH are useful to exclude hormonal problems.

### Studies of penile blood flow

Penile blood flow can be estimated accurately using either a radionuclide washout method or a Doppler technique. A penile/brachial blood pressure ratio of less than 0.6 is highly suggestive of vasculogenic impotence.

### Nocturnal penile tumescence studies (NPT)

A normal man has three to four erections during the night, each lasting for 20–30 minutes and associated with rapid eye movement sleep. A simple cuff apparatus can be used to monitor night-time erections, although this usually necessitates the patient's admission to hospital for 2–3 nights.

### Cavernosography

This is useful for patients with incomplete erections (who may have abnormal venous leaks), for patients with erections which fade rapidly and for patients with erectile deformity.

## Treatment

All patients with suspected psychogenic impotence should be referred for psychosexual counselling. Once the problem is identified by the impotent man, techniques such as those described by Masters and Johnson can prove very effective in dealing with psychogenic impotence.

Many agents are said to have aphrodisiac properties. Whilst little convincing evidence exists for most of these agents, vitamin E and yohimbine have been shown to increase the frequency and duration of erections. Patients with androgen deficiency can be treated with androgen preparations, whilst patients with hypopituitarism or hyperprolactinaemia are best referred for specialist endocrinological advice.

For the remaining patients with organic impotence and, indeed, for some with psychogenic impotence, the options open are surgery, self-injection of the corpora cavernosa or vacuum condoms.

## Surgery

Patients with small vessel arterial occlusion can be treated by penile revascularisation. This involves using the inferior epigastric artery to take blood either to the dorsal penile arteries or to the deep dorsal vein. If large vessel occlusion is present, balloon angioplasty should be considered to try and restore penile blood flow. Patients with demonstrable venous leaks can have these veins ligated surgically to improve erections.

Mechanical causes of impotence such as phimosis, tight frenulum or Peyronie's disease should be treated appropriately, with good results to be expected in terms of restoring potency.

In patients with neuropathic impotence or in whom no vascular cause can be found, penile prostheses may be inserted to allow intercourse. These are inserted into the corpora cavernosa on each side at operation. Semi-rigid prostheses are made of silicone and produce a permanent erection whilst allowing some flexibility of the permanently erect penis. More expensive inflatable prostheses are available which allow an erection to be created by inflating the prostheses using a reservoir and pump sited in the scrotum.

## Self-administered intracorporal injections

Many patients find the prospect of injecting their own penis with drugs a more satisfactory way of producing an erection than having penile prostheses. Phentolamine, papaverine, phenoxybenzamine or thymoxamine are all effective in producing tumescence when injected directly into the corpus cavernosum. The safety of repeated injections into the penis has not been assessed in the long term and there is a risk of priapism.

## Vacuum condoms

For those patients who cannot or will not agree to any other procedure, the use of a vacuum condom allows erection and penetration for intercourse. This condom is slightly stiff and application of a vacuum inside the condom produces a negative pressure which, in turn, generates an erection. The erection is maintained for as long as the vacuum is kept intact.

## EJACULATORY PROBLEMS

Emission of semen into the urethra is accomplished by contraction of the epididymes, vasa, seminal vesicles and prostate together with closure of the bladder neck. This takes place under control from the sympathetic thoraco-lumbar outflow ($T_{12}$–$L_2$). Ejaculation proper is the result of rhythmic contraction of the striated muscle of the perineum, mediated via the parasympathetic fibres from $S_3$–$S_4$ which form a meshwork in the region of the membranous urethra. The ejaculation centre in the spinal cord is probably functionally separate from the erection centres, since it is possible to ejaculate without erection (*pollutio flaccida*).

Many ejaculatory problems (premature or retarded ejaculation, primary ejaculatory failure) are psychogenic. These usually respond to psychosexual counselling, often supplemented with sexual aids such as vibrators.

Retrograde ejaculation may occur in patients after bladder neck surgery or abdominoperineal excision of the rectum and is almost universal after prostatectomy. Whilst orgasm occurs in these patients, no semen is emitted from the penis. In young men, this causes infertility but sperm can be recovered from the bladder, washed and used to inseminate the female partner artificially. Surgical reconstruction of the bladder neck may also be successful in restoring ejaculation.

# 22

# Benign scrotal disorders

In most benign scrotal disorders, there is swelling of the testis or its adnexae and this may be associated with pain. In some conditions, pain may precede the development of an obvious mass in the scrotum. To make an accurate diagnosis, careful examination of the scrotum and its individual contents is required.

DIAGNOSIS OF A SCROTAL SWELLING (Fig. 22.1)

The cardinal sign of a true scrotal mass is that it is possible to *get above it*; if it is not possible to get above the swelling, it is inguinal in origin and probably an indirect inguinal hernia. A cystic mass can usually be transilluminated and is likely to be either a hydrocele or an epididymal cyst. Solid scrotal masses do not transilluminate.

The scrotum should be examined initially with the patient supine. A varicocele, however, may only be palpable when the patient stands up. Typically, this is felt as a 'bag of worms' due to tortuous engorged veins above the testis, usually on the left. The swelling often has a cough impulse and may disappear when the patient lies down.

If the scrotal skin is inflamed, the inguinal lymph nodes may be enlarged. However, lymphatic drainage of the testis itself is to para-aortic nodes and these may be palpable, when enlarged, in the epigastrium. Rectal examination should be performed to assess the prostate and seminal vesicles, which may also be involved in infective lesions of the epididymis.

CONDITIONS THAT PRESENT WITH ACUTE SCROTAL PAIN

The sudden onset of pain in the scrotum should be regarded as due to torsion of the testis until proved otherwise. Acute scrotal pain should, therefore, be treated as a urological emergency with urgent referral of the patient to hospital if torsion cannot be excluded. Prompt action is paramount in torsion, since the longer a torsion is neglected, the more likely the testis is to be infarcted. The main differential diagnosis is from acute epididymitis; other causes of acute scrotal pain include torsion of a testicular appendage, orchitis and trauma to the testis. It is usually possible to distinguish between these conditions by means of a careful history and examination.

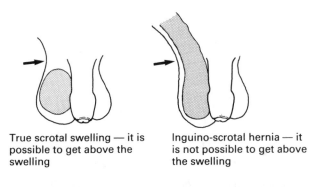

True scrotal swelling — it is possible to get above the swelling

Inguino-scrotal hernia — it is not possible to get above the swelling

True scrotal swellings

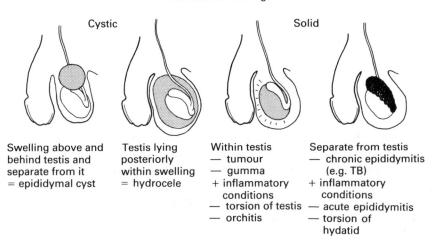

| Cystic | | Solid | |
|---|---|---|---|

Swelling above and behind testis and separate from it = epididymal cyst

Testis lying posteriorly within swelling = hydrocele

Within testis
— tumour
— gumma
+ inflammatory conditions
— torsion of testis
— orchitis

Separate from testis
— chronic epididymitis (e.g. TB)
+ inflammatory conditions
— acute epididymitis
— torsion of hydatid

**Fig. 22.1** Diagnosis of scrotal swelling

## Torsion of the testis (Fig. 22.2)

Torsion of the testis occurs at any age, from the newborn to the elderly, but is commonest between 13 and 16. The underlying mechanism in most cases is an abnormal investment of the testis and epididymis by the tunica vaginalis which extends up onto the spermatic cord. This arrangement allows the testis to rotate within the tunica vaginalis like a 'clapper in a bell' (*intravaginal torsion*). Undescended testes are particularly prone to torsion because of lack of attachment of the cord within the co-existing hernial sac.

Occasionally the testis lies on a long mesentery separate from the epididymis and twists on this mesentery (*congenitally long mesorchium*). In neonates, torsion of the testis occurs together with its covering layers including the tunica vaginalis (*extravaginal torsion*).

When torsion occurs, oedema of the spermatic cord results in obstruction of venous return from the testis and epididymis; this further exacerbates the

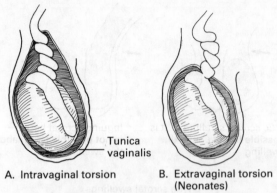

A. Intravaginal torsion     B. Extravaginal torsion
                              (Neonates)

**Fig. 22.2** Torsion of the testis

oedema, causes haemorrhage within the testis and, eventually, arterial occlusion follows leading to infarction of the testis.

### Clinical features

Typically, a young boy complains of sudden severe pain in the scrotum; the pain may radiate to the groin or lower abdomen and is often accompanied by nausea. Fifty per cent of patients affected give a history of previous short-lived attacks of testicular pain that have resolved spontaneously. Urinary symptoms are usually absent.

The patient is usually afebrile. The affected testis typically lies higher than the opposite testis and the overlying scrotal skin is usually reddened. The whole of the testis is tender to touch and the spermatic cord feels thickened and tender.

The opposite testis may also lie abnormally because the predisposing anatomical abnormality is usually bilateral. A torsion which has been neglected may present after several days of pain as a hard craggy mass within the scrotum. This is usually the situation in neonates in whom the torsion occurs in utero; neonatal torsion always results in an infarcted testis.

The diagnosis should be suspected in any patient with acute scrotal pain and swelling of the testis, especially if the vas deferens cannot be felt in the scrotum above the testis. Since epididymitis and mumps orchitis are rare before puberty, torsion must be assumed in this age group until proved otherwise. Radionuclide scintigraphy and Doppler sonography have been used to demonstrate reduced blood flow in the twisted spermatic cord but are rarely applicable in the acute situation.

### Treatment

In some patients it may be possible to untwist the testis manually, the direction of rotation being dictated by the patient's reaction to the manoeuvre. In most patients, however, manual detorsion is not possible and scrotal exploration should be performed as soon as possible. The testis is exposed through a scrotal incision, the torsion untwisted and the viability of the testis assessed. If the testis is viable, its colour improves rapidly and bright red bleeding occurs if the tunica albuginea is incised; a black testis is infarcted and should be removed. A viable testis should be fixed with more than one non-absorbable suture to the wall of the scrotum and the tunica vaginalis should be everted or plicated to prevent recurrent torsion. In all patients the opposite testis should be explored and fixed in the same way.

The viability of the twisted testis is directly related to the time between exploration and the onset of symptoms. If operated on within 5 hours of the onset of symptoms, 80% of testes are viable, but after 10 hours only 20% are viable and, after 24 hours, all twisted testes are infarcted.

In patients with recurrent episodes of testicular pain suggestive of intermittent torsion and patients in whom a torsion has been reduced manually, elective fixation of both testes should be performed at the earliest possible opportunity.

### Torsion of a testicular appendage

This usually affects the hydatid of Morgagni, a pedunculated remnant of the Mullerian duct which lies on the upper pole of the testis, near the head of the epididymis. It causes similar less severe symptoms to torsion of the testis, with pain and swelling on the affected side.

In the early stages, it may be possible to see a small blue pea-like structure through the scrotal skin (*blue-dot sign*) and tenderness may be localised to this nodule. Later, more generalised inflammation of the scrotum obscures this sign and makes it impossible to differentiate from torsion of the testis.

It is usually necessary to explore the scrotum and excise the twisted appendage, both to relieve pain and to exclude torsion of the testis. Since these appendages are not constant findings, there is no need to explore the opposite testis. If the diagnosis can be made confidently and symptoms are minimal, there may be no need for surgical excision since the pain and oedema often subside rapidly.

### Acute epididymitis

Acute infection of the epididymis is rare before puberty but is seen in all other age groups. The infection may reach the epididymis via the bloodstream or by retrograde spread from the prostatic urethra and seminal vesicles. Predisposing factors include urinary tract infection, sexually-transmitted infection and instrumentation of the urethra. In over 50% of affected patients, however, no underlying cause can be identified.

*Clinical features*

The onset is often sudden, with pain and rapidly progressive swelling of the scrotum. There may be systemic symptoms with fever and rigors in severe cases. There is often a history of dysuria, suggesting urinary infection, particularly in older men who often have associated bladder outflow obstruction; some younger patients have an obvious urethral discharge. Recent instrumentation of the urethra, whether performed medically or self-inflicted, should also be noted.

Initially, the epididymis may be palpable separate from the testis; it is usually tender and swollen. There is often a secondary hydrocele present. Later, the inflammation spreads to affect the testis (*epididymo-orchitis*) so that it becomes impossible clinically to exclude torsion of the testis.

Investigation should include microscopy and culture of the urine and culture of any urethral discharge. A full blood count often shows a leucocytosis and blood cultures may be helpful in patients who are systemically unwell. A plain abdominal X-ray is useful to exclude urinary tract calculi as a possible source of infection.

Full investigation of the urinary tract with an IVU or ultrasound is only indicated in children before puberty (associated anomalies of the urinary tract are often present), in young adults with other urinary symptoms and in elderly men (who usually have bladder outflow obstruction). Such investigations can usually be deferred until after the acute illness has settled.

*Treatment*

If the diagnosis can be made confidently, the patient should be treated with bed rest, scrotal support, analgesia and antibiotics. If there is any doubt about the diagnosis, the scrotum should be explored surgically to exclude torsion.

The commonest organisms cultured are *E. coli* in patients with urinary infection and *Chlamydia* in those with a history of urethral discharge. Epididymitis is due to gonorrhoea in only 4% of patients. In many patients, however, no causative organism can be identified.

Trimethoprim, ciprofloxacin or cephalosporins are the first-choice antibiotics for proven bacterial infection or for patients in whom no organism can be identified; doxycycline is effective for chlamydial infection. It is important to stress to the patient that prolonged antibiotic treatment for up to 6 weeks is necessary to guarantee full resolution.

Complications include suppuration and abscess formation which may destroy the testis. A localised abscess may be drained, although orchidectomy is necessary in some patients. In the long term, atrophy of the testis occurs in 20% of patients and fertility may be impaired in men who have had bilateral disease due to fibrosis and obstruction of epididymal tubules.

**Viral orchitis**

Acute inflammation of the testis may complicate a number of viral illnesses including mumps, infectious mononucleosis, rubella and Coxsackie virus infections.

Only the commonest viral infection, mumps orchitis, is discussed here. It occurs in 15–20% of adult males contracting mumps but is very rare in boys before puberty.

*Clinical features*

Pain and swelling of the testis typically starts 3–7 days after the development of parotid enlargement, although orchitis may occasionally be the only manifestation of the disease. There is often an accompanying fever. In most men one testis only is involved but, in 15%, the orchitis is bilateral.

Examination in the early stages reveals a swollen testis and a normal epididymis. As the disease progresses, the whole scrotum becomes inflamed and oedematous, with formation of a secondary hydrocele.

The diagnosis is essentially a clinical one made on the history of parotitis; it can be confirmed by finding a rising titre of antimumps antibodies in the plasma. The urine is usually sterile on culture. As with all acute swellings of the testis, exploration of the scrotum may be needed if torsion of the testis cannot be excluded.

*Treatment*

Conservative treatment with bed rest, scrotal support and analgesia usually results in resolution within a few days. Fifty per cent of men subsequently develop atrophy of the affected testis and, if the disease is bilateral, this may result in sterility.

To prevent late atrophy, some surgeons advocate incision of the tunica albuginea in the acute phase to relieve pressure within the testis; steroids have also been used to suppress the inflammatory response. There is no convincing evidence that these techniques prevent subsequent testicular atrophy.

**Trauma to the testis**

Testicular trauma must always be considered in the differential diagnosis of acute scrotal pain. Its management is discussed in Chapter 7.

## CONDITIONS THAT PRESENT AS A SCROTAL MASS

As has already been seen, some inflammatory conditions can produce a scrotal mass but other disorders present with a mass as the predominant feature. Clinical examination will usually distinguish those swellings that are cystic (hydrocele, epididymal cyst) from those that are solid (tumour, gumma, chronic epididymitis), will determine the relationship of the swelling to the testis and will detect a varicocele.

## Hydrocele

A hydrocele is a collection of fluid in the tunica vaginalis. It may be congenital or acquired; congenital hydrocele is discussed separately in Chapter 6.

An acquired hydrocele may be primary (idiopathic) or secondary and, unlike a congenital hydrocele, does not communicate with the peritoneal cavity. In idiopathic hydrocele, the fluid is thought to accumulate because of an imbalance between the normal secretion and reabsorption by the layers of the tunica vaginalis. A secondary hydrocele may develop in response to intrascrotal disease (e.g. trauma, torsion, infection or tumour).

### Clinical features

A hydrocele may be symptomless or may cause dragging discomfort in the scrotum and groin; large hydroceles can cause considerable cosmetic embarrassment. With a secondary hydrocele, the presenting symptoms are usually those of the primary testicular disorder. Clinically, the cystic swelling lies anterior to the testis, although the testis may be impalpable within a tense hydrocele.

### Treatment

Treatment of a primary hydrocele in the adult is only indicated if it causes symptoms. However, it may be necessary to exclude underlying testicular pathology; simple aspiration of the hydrocele with a trochar and cannula allows palpation of the underlying testis. The aspirated fluid is normally clear yellow; the presence of blood-stained fluid suggests underlying testicular pathology unless the bleeding is fresh and has been caused by a 'bloody' puncture. Ultrasound of the scrotum is very useful in demonstrating a normal testis within the hydrocele sac.

A primary hydrocele can be treated by simple aspiration, although the fluid usually reaccumulates and there is a risk of bleeding or infection with repeated punctures. To prevent fluid reaccumulation, sclerosant agents (e.g. STD, sodium morrhuate, phenol, tetracycline) can be injected after aspiration to obliterate the intravaginal space; sclerotherapy may be complicated by pain and severe inflammatory reactions to the sclerosant.

Surgery is the most effective long-term treatment and involves excision, eversion or plication of the hydrocele sac. The treatment of a secondary hydrocele is usually directed towards the underlying cause.

## Epididymal cysts

Epididymal cysts develop as diverticula of the vasa efferentia as they leave the testis and enter the epididymis. The cysts are typically thin walled and enlarge slowly; they may be multilocular or multiple, replacing much of the epididymis. If communication with the vasa efferentia persists, a whitish fluid containing spermatozoa may be found within the cyst (*spermatocele*). The majority of epididymal cysts, however, contain a clear colourless fluid devoid of spermatozoa.

Epididymal cysts may be asymptomatic or may cause discomfort and cosmetic embarrassment. They are usually non-tender and brilliantly transilluminable; the accompanying testis feels normal.

If symptomatic they should be excised; with extensive involvement of the head of the epididymis, fertility may be impaired in patients undergoing bilateral cyst excision. Aspiration and injection of sclerosant agents can also be used for epididymal cysts.

## Varicocele

This condition is due to varicosities of the veins of the pampiniform plexus. It is seen in 8% of normal males and occurs on the left side in 98% of affected patients. The left-sided dominance is due to the different venous drainage of the two testes; the right testicular vein drains directly into the inferior vena cava whilst the left drains into the left renal vein. Venographic studies have shown that the valve mechanism at the termination of the left testicular vein is either absent or incompetent in patients with a left varicocele.

In a small number of patients, a varicocele develops as the result of venous occlusion by a renal or retroperitoneal tumour; this can occur on the right side as well as the left. A varicocele is often encountered in men attending infertility clinics and there has been much debate about its role in infertility. The scrotal temperature is usually higher in the presence of a varicocele and this may impair spermatogenesis.

### Clinical features

Many varicoceles are incidental findings. When a varicocele does cause symptoms, the patient may notice a dragging discomfort in the scrotum or scrotal swelling. Clinical examination reveals the typical 'bag of worms', best felt when the patient is standing. The affected testis is often smaller than its opposite partner.

### Treatment

In young men a varicocele can be ignored unless it is causing symptoms. The appearance of a varicocele in an older man or the presence of a varicocele on the right are indications for further investigation to exclude venous obstruction by a tumour.

If a varicocele is causing symptoms, it should be treated by venous ligation. This may be carried out in the inguinal canal with the individual veins being ligated as they run in the spermatic cord; retroperitoneal ligation of the testicular vein itself above the inguinal canal is, however, a simpler surgical procedure. Percutaneous embolisation of the testicular vein via a catheter introduced into the femoral vein may also be performed, especially if the varicocele recurs after surgery. The role of varicocele in patients with infertility is discussed in Chapter 24.

## Tumours of the testis

Tumours of the testis and scrotum are discussed separately in Chapter 23.

## Gumma of the testis

Syphilitic infection (*gumma*) of the testis was common in the pre-penicillin era. It is now very rare in the UK, although it is still encountered in underdeveloped countries where the primary disease may go unrecognised and untreated.

## Chronic epididymitis

This usually follows repeated attacks of acute epididymitis but may be an occasional complication of vasectomy. In the tropics, chronic epididymitis may complicate schistosomiasis and filariasis.

Tuberculosis is important as a cause of chronic epididymitis and was quite common before the introduction of modern antituberculous chemotherapy. Tuberculous epididymitis may occur as a primary lesion, although it is usually secondary to infection elsewhere in the genitourinary tract. It is unclear whether infection occurs via the bloodstream or by retrograde spread along the vas deferens, since the disease often involves the vas and seminal vesicle as well.

Typically, there is slowly-progressive swelling of the epididymis with little pain although a more acute onset is occasionally seen. Examination reveals a hard irregular swelling involving the epididymis, often with nodules palpable along the vas deferens. There is commonly evidence of involvement of the seminal vesicles on rectal examination and there may be signs of tuberculosis elsewhere. In advanced cases, the testis becomes involved and cutaneous fistulae develop from the rupture of 'cold' abscesses.

The diagnosis is made by finding tubercle bacilli in the urine or in biopsy material from the epididymis; histological examination of the latter may show the typical appearance of caseation and granuloma formation. An IVU is mandatory to detect any other sites of involvement in the genitourinary tract.

A full course of antituberculous chemotherapy usually effects a cure. Epididymectomy or orchidectomy may be required for a residual painful mass or for a chronic discharging sinus persisting after a full course of chemotherapy.

## DISORDERS OF THE SCROTAL SKIN

### Fournier's gangrene

This is an infection of the scrotal skin caused by the synergistic action of several strains of bacteria (aerobic Gram-negative rods, Gram-positive cocci and anaerobic bacteria, especially *Bacteroides fragilis*). The infection causes gangrene of the scrotal skin, which may slough off to leave the scrotal contents exposed.

The condition is rare but is usually caused by an underlying problem such as diabetes mellitus, perianal sepsis or periurethral abscess. Before the advent of antibiotics, Fournier's gangrene was associated with a very high mortality.

Treatment is by intensive antibiotic therapy (aminoglycosides, penicillin and metronidazole) with careful debridement of devitalised skin. Skin grafting may be required once the infection has been eradicated and can be accomplished by rotation flaps from adjacent areas or by free grafts.

### Idiopathic scrotal oedema

This is an acute oedematous swelling of the scrotal skin that usually occurs in boys under the age of 10. The cause is unknown but the occurrence of localised outbreaks of the disease in small communities suggests an infective aetiology.

The swelling may affect both sides of the scrotum and often extends into the groins and thighs. The onset is rapid but usually painless. The scrotal skin becomes oedematous and takes on a bright pink colour but the scrotal contents are normal to palpation. The diagnosis is made on clinical grounds and the swelling resolves without treatment in a few days.

# 23

# Tumours of the testis and scrotum

## TESTICULAR TUMOURS

Tumours of the testis are relatively uncommon, accounting for only 1–2% of malignant tumours in men. Despite their relative rarity, they are of particular importance because they affect predominantly young men; testicular tumour is the commonest neoplasm in men aged 25–34. In recent years, advances in staging methods and the introduction of effective chemotherapy have resulted in a dramatic improvement in survival rate for testicular tumours.

## Aetiology (Table 23.1)

There is a well-established link between undescended testis and testicular tumour; 10% of men with a tumour have a history of testicular maldescent. From the incidence of the two conditions, it has been estimated that adults with maldescent have a 20–30 times greater risk of developing a testicular tumour than men with normally descended testes. The mechanism for tumour formation, however, is not clear since, in patients with unilateral maldescent, the tumour may develop in the contralateral normally-descended testis.

**Table 23.1** Aetiological factors in testicular tumour

*Undescended testis*

*Infertility*
increased incidence of carcinoma
in situ and invasive cancer

*Carcinoma in situ*
50% risk of developing invasive
cancer after 5 years

*Previous testicular tumour*
5% develop a second primary

*Certain intersex states*
(with Y-chromosome)

310

Controversy exists about the effectiveness of orchidopexy in reducing the risk of malignant change. Orchidopexy after puberty does not alter the risk of tumour development, although it seems likely that early orchidopexy (before the age of 8) does.

Testicular tumours are commoner in Caucasians than in Negroes and there is a higher incidence in patients from high socioeconomic groups.

**Pathology** (Table 23.2)

The two most important types of tumour found are *seminoma* and *teratoma*; occasionally both histological types are found together in a malignant testis to form a *mixed tumour*. *Lymphoma* of the testis is seen in an older age group than either teratoma or seminoma but is relatively rare. Sertoli cell tumours, interstitial (Leydig) cell tumours and mesothelioma of the testis are very rare.

**Table 23.2**  Histological types of testicular tumour

| Type of tumour | % incidence | Peak incidence |
|---|---|---|
| Seminoma | 40% | 30–40 years |
| Teratoma | 32% | 20–30 years |
| Mixed seminoma/teratoma | 14% | 25–35 years |
| Lymphoma | 7% | 60–70 years |
| Other tumours, e.g. | 7% | |
|     interstitial cell (Leydig) tumour | | |
|     sertoli cell mesenchymal tumour | | |
|     gonadoblastoma | | |
|     yolk sac tumour | | |
|     mesothelioma | | |

*Seminoma*

The testis is usually symmetrically enlarged and the tumour itself is well-demarcated with a uniform creamy-white appearance on section. These tumours arise from the seminiferous epithelium and are composed of sheets of large round cells with clear cytoplasm (*classical seminoma*). A histological variant (*spermatocytic seminoma*) is seen in 2% of seminomatous tumours, usually in older patients.

*Teratoma*

The tumour may be cystic or solid and there are often areas of haemorrhage and necrosis. Teratomas arise from primitive totipotential germ cells, so that they may show a wide variety of tissue types; these range from mature tissues (e.g. skin, glandular epithelium, cartilage) to anaplastic sheets of highly malignant cells.

Four histological types have been described according to the degree of differentiation present.

*Teratoma differentiated (TD)*. This is the most benign form of teratoma. Only differentiated tissue is present in this tumour; although no histological evidence of malignancy can be identified, metastases may occur.

*Malignant teratoma intermediate (MTI)*. This is the commonest histological pattern; the tumour contains a mixture of differentiated tissue and areas of undoubted malignancy.

*Malignant teratoma undifferentiated (MTU)*. The tumour is composed entirely of sheets of large pleomorphic cells.

*Malignant teratoma trophoblastic (MTT)*. This is the most malignant variety and contains elements which have the appearance of placental trophoblastic tissue.

### Carcinoma in situ

It is now recognised that carcinoma in situ of the testis often precedes the development of invasive cancer. In situ changes with large bizarre germ cells in the tubules of the testis are often seen adjacent to areas of overt tumour. Carcinoma in situ is seen in the testes of some patients undergoing testicular biopsy for infertility, in the contralateral testis of patients with overt testicular tumours, in patients with pure gonadal dysgenesis and in undescended testes. In the presence of carcinoma in situ there is thought to be a 50% risk of developing invasive testicular cancer over 5 years.

### Spread and staging (Fig. 23.1)

Testicular tumours spread by direct infiltration, via the lymphatics and via the bloodstream.

Direct extension of the tumour is limited by the tunica albuginea. Although 10% of patients with a testicular tumour develop a secondary hydrocele, invasion of the scrotal tissues and spermatic cord is rare.

Lymphatic spread occurs initially to para-aortic nodes; the testicular lymphatics accompany the testicular artery to its origin from the abdominal aorta. Some testicular lymph passes along lymphatics closely associated with the artery to the vas deferens and drains directly into the internal iliac nodes. It is, however, of practical importance to know that the inguinal nodes drain only the superficial scrotal tissues and do not receive lymph from the testes unless there has been previous surgery to the groin or scrotum.

Haematogenous spread occurs late in seminoma but early in teratoma. The commonest sites of distant metastases are the lungs and liver although deposits may also occur in bone, brain or skin.

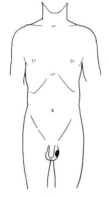

Stage I — Disease confined
to testis

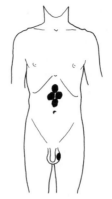

Stage II — Infradiaphragmatic
node involvement
A: <2 cm
B: 2–5 cm
C: >5 cm

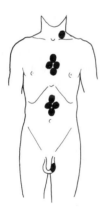

Stage III — Supradiaphragmatic
node involvement

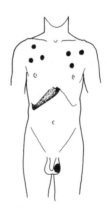

Stage IV — Extralymphatic
disease

**Fig. 23.1** Staging of testicular tumours

## Tumour markers

Alpha-fetoprotein (AFP) and beta-human chorionic gonadotrophin (β-HCG) have both proved useful as tumour markers in teratoma. Seventy-three per cent of patients with teratoma have elevated plasma levels of one or both markers. Tumour markers are less helpful in seminoma, with β-HCG being raised in only a minority of patients.

Tumour markers in the blood are also used in the long term to monitor progress during and after treatment. A patient with persistently raised marker levels after removal of the primary tumour probably has metastatic disease. Fluctuations in marker levels are useful to assess the response to treatment, a fall indicating tumour regression and a rise indicating the need to look for tumour recurrence.

## Clinical features

The majority of patients present with local symptoms, either a discrete lump in the testis or enlargement of the whole testis. In some patients, a painful scrotal swelling due to a testicular tumour is mistaken for epididymitis. There is a history of trauma in 20% of patients and this may obscure the diagnosis initially.

A few patients present with symptoms from metastases (e.g. enlarged nodes in the neck, an abdominal mass, dyspnoea, haemoptysis or jaundice).

An unusual presenting symptom, seen in 2% of patients, is gynaecomastia; this may occur with any type of tumour.

Examination of the scrotum usually confirms the diagnosis by demonstrating a firm testicular swelling or mass. In 10% of patients there is an associated hydrocele, although this is usually lax and rarely obscures the underlying testicular pathology. If there is a tense hydrocele or if the diagnosis is not clear on simple palpation of the testis, scrotal ultrasound is useful to determine whether a palpable mass is, in fact, in the testis and whether the internal architecture of the testis is disrupted by the tumour.

A full clinical examination should always be performed to look for evidence of metastases to abdominal and cervical lymph nodes or to extra-lymphatic sites (e.g. hepatic enlargement, pleural effusion).

## Initial management of a suspected tumour

In most patients, the presumptive diagnosis of a testicular tumour is made from clinical examination; the priority is to confirm this by prompt exploration of the testis.

It is essential that blood be taken pre-operatively for tumour markers since, if elevated, the subsequent behaviour of these markers postoperatively is an extremely useful guide to the presence or absence of metastases. A chest X-ray should also be performed to look for pulmonary metastases.

The testis should not be explored through the scrotum but through the inguinal canal to avoid interference with the superficial lymphatics of the scrotum which drain to the inguinal nodes. The spermatic cord should be temporarily occluded in the inguinal canal to prevent vascular dissemination of tumour whilst the testis is mobilized and delivered into the wound.

If a tumour is confirmed, orchidectomy is performed with division of the spermatic cord at the level of the deep inguinal ring. If no tumour is found, the cord is unclamped and the testis returned to the scrotum.

When there is doubt about the diagnosis at operation, Chevassu's manoeuvre can be employed; after isolating the wound with swabs, the testis is bisected and any suspicious area biopsied for frozen section to confirm the presence of tumour. Should no tumour be found, the testis is reconstituted and returned to the scrotum.

**Staging protocol**

Once the diagnosis of a testicular tumour has been confirmed and the histological type determined, the disease must be accurately staged to determine the appropriate treatment.

This involves serial AFP and β-HCG estimations; in patients with positive markers, a fall in levels slower than the expected biological half-life of the markers indicates the presence of metastases.

Involvement of para-aortic nodes is best assessed by CT scanning of the abdomen and this has now replaced lymphography in most oncology units.

CT scanning of the chest and mediastinum is usually combined with abdominal scanning to look for mediastinal node enlargement and pulmonary involvement; it has proved more accurate than whole lung tomography in detecting small pulmonary metastases.

Since a proportion of patients will subsequently require treatment with potentially toxic chemotherapeutic agents, baseline haematological investigations should be performed together with tests of renal and hepatic function. Sperm banking should be offered before treatment to those patients requiring chemotherapy, since the drugs used produce profound impairment of spermatogenesis which may not recover after treatment.

**Treatment**

*Seminoma*

Seminoma is extremely sensitive to radiotherapy and this remains the treatment of choice in early, small-volume disease (Fig. 23.2). Chemotherapy is used for bulky or advanced metastatic disease.

In stage I disease prophylactic radiotherapy (30 Gy) is usually given to the para-aortic and ipsilateral pelvic lymph nodes. However, a simple policy of surveillance for stage I is now under investigation in clinical trials.

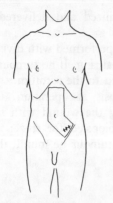 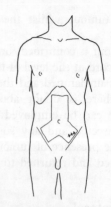

Stage I Irradiation of para-
aortic and ipsilateral pelvic
nodes

Stages II A and II B
Irradiation of para-aortic
and bilateral pelvic nodes

**Fig. 23.2** Radiotherapy for early testicular seminoma

In stages IIA and IIB, radiotherapy (35 Gy) is given as for stage I disease but the fields are extended to include the contralateral pelvic nodes. Prophylactic irradiation of mediastinal and supraclavicular nodes is no longer used because of the risk of damage to bone marrow in the sternum and ribs; this haemopoietic depression can render subsequent chemotherapy hazardous in those who require treatment for relapse after radiotherapy.

In stage IIC disease, primary treatment with radiotherapy is followed by a relapse rate of 40%. These patients with bulky metastases are now treated with chemotherapy using either cis-platinum alone or combination regimes as used in teratoma. Radiotherapy is still used in some patients after initial reduction of the tumour bulk by chemotherapy.

In stage III and stage IV disease, primary treatment with chemotherapy is now preferred with radiotherapy reserved for treatment of individual tumour masses.

## Teratoma earlier blood spread.

Chemotherapy is the treatment of choice for teratoma, since it does not show the same sensitivity to radiotherapy as seminoma.

In stage I disease, all patients were, until recently, given chemotherapy. However, a proportion of patients will be cured by orchidectomy alone so that chemotherapy is unnecessary; 72% of patients not receiving chemotherapy for stage I disease will show no signs of subsequent relapse over the next 5 years.

Those patients with a high risk of relapse after orchidectomy alone can be predicted on the basis of certain histological features in the primary tumour: the presence of venous or lymphatic invasion in the spermatic cord, the presence of undifferentiated tumour are all poor prognostic signs.

Patients who have these histological risk factors have a 2-year relapse rate of 58% if they are not treated and they require chemotherapy; the patients who do not have these features may be treated by surveillance alone.

The surveillance protocol involves monthly measurements of tumour markers and bi-monthly CT scans for the first year. Thereafter, follow-up is at 2–3 monthly intervals for the next 2 years, with chemotherapy being instituted at the first sign of recurrent disease.

In stages II, III and IV teratoma, primary chemotherapy is employed. The first really effective combination of drugs used in teratoma was cis-platinum, vinblastine and bleomycin (PVB). Nowadays, etoposide has replaced vinblastine and carboplatin is beginning to replace cis-platinum because of lower toxicity.

Sixteen-day cycles of bleomycin, etoposide and cis-platinum (BEP) are given at 3-weekly intervals. After four cycles, the patient is reassessed by tumour markers and CT scanning. If complete remission is obtained after four cycles, no further treatment is given; otherwise chemotherapy is continued until complete remission. Thereafter, two further cycles of treatment are given to ensure maintenance of remission.

Complete disease remission is seen in 87% of patients, although further cycles of chemotherapy may be needed at a later date if there is evidence of disease relapse. Tumour markers and CT scanning have an important role to play in follow-up by detecting recurrent disease while the tumour volume is still small.

The response to chemotherapy is dependent on tumour bulk. Patients with low-volume disease fare better than those with bulky metastases, irrespective of clinical stage.

In bulky metastatic disease, a residual mass may remain after chemotherapy (e.g. para-aortic or mediastinal nodes). Excision of residual tumour masses after chemotherapy should be performed to determine whether they are composed of fibrous tissue (34%), mature teratoma (44%) or residual malignancy (22%); if residual malignancy is present, additional chemotherapy should be given.

### Lymphoma

This may be part of a systemic lymphoreticular disorder (usually non-Hodgkin's lymphoma). Systemic treatment is necessary and the favoured chemotherapeutic regime is cyclophosphamide, adriamycin, vincristine and prednisolone.

### Carcinoma in situ

The treatment of carcinoma in situ is difficult. In patients receiving chemotherapy for an invasive testicular tumour, it is reasonable to assume that any in situ change in the contralateral testis will be eliminated by the drugs. If carcinoma in situ is found on testicular biopsy, it may be possible to irradiate the affected testis (20 Gy); this, however, inevitably produces infertility.

## Prognosis

At presentation, haematogenous spread in seminoma is rare. The prognosis, therefore, is good and overall cure rates exceed 90%. In patients with stage I seminoma, death from tumour recurrence is now a very rare event.

Before the advent of effective chemotherapy, high-stage teratoma carried an appalling prognosis. However, intensive chemotherapy now results in cure rates of over 95% in stage I disease; even in disseminated teratoma, 75–85% of patients can be rendered disease free for prolonged periods. The chemotherapy itself, however, has a mortality rate of 3–4%. The worst prognosis in teratoma is seen with liver metastases, which result in a 5-year survival of only 10%.

The prognosis of testicular lymphoma is considerably worse than that of seminoma or teratoma, with only 25–40% of patients surviving 5 years after chemotherapy.

## CARCINOMA OF THE SCROTUM

This disease used to be an occupational hazard in chimney sweeps exposed to the carcinogens in soot, an association described by Percival Pott in 1779. Later, it became prevalent in industries where there was exposure to machine oil (e.g. mule-spinners' cancer). Scrotal cancer is, nowadays, rare.

It presents as a warty or ulcerated growth on the scrotum. This invades the scrotal tissues and the underlying testis, spreading at an early stage to inguinal nodes. Treatment is by wide local excision with orchidectomy if the testis is involved; skin grafting may be required to cover the resulting defect. Block dissection should be performed if the inguinal nodes are involved with tumour.

# 24

# Male infertility

Approximately 1 couple in 10 are infertile during the reproductive period of their lives. Of those couples who are trying to conceive, 80% do so within the first 2 years. Of the 20% who are unable to conceive within 2 years, half will never produce children. The burden upon infertile couples is now all the greater because of the tendency, in Europe at least, to limit family size. As a result, fewer children are being offered for adoption.

Traditionally, investigations for infertility are instituted after 2 years of unproductive intercourse, but most clinicians would probably now accept that this is unreasonable and see any couple who cannot produce children, regardless of the length of time they have been trying.

Male infertility may be associated with a number of abnormalities. Male factors alone are responsible for infertility in one third of couples and contribute to the problem in a further third. Investigation, therefore, should include not only an assessment of the male partner but also a gynaecological assessment of the female partner.

## CLINICAL HISTORY

The initial interview is the single most important part of assessment, since it sets the tone for further discussion and investigation. It is preferable to conduct the initial interview with both partners.

A thorough past history may give important clues. Previous surgery to the genitalia in childhood or adolescence may raise the possibility of testicular or vasal damage. Chronic illnesses such as diabetes, renal failure or hepatic failure and previous acute infections can impair spermatogenesis. Similarly, a past history of genitourinary infection (e.g. mumps, syphilis, gonorrhoea and non-gonococcal urethritis) or epididymitis may be relevant.

One important topic which is often omitted is to inquire about exposure to chemical agents, drugs and irradiation. Many chemical toxins impair sperm production and exposure to these may be accidental. There is a wealth of evidence to suggest that endogenous toxins produced as a result of smoking and drinking alcohol are harmful to sperms, so a full history of social habits is also essential.

Some congenital problems may be associated with subfertility. Epididymal obstruction can occur in patients with recurrent sinusitis and chest infections (*Young's syndrome* and *cystic fibrosis*). Absent sperm motility may also be associated with bronchiectasis, defective cilia in the respiratory tract and situs inversus viscerum (*Kartagener's syndrome*).

It is also vital to determine not only that the couple are having sexual intercourse but that it is timed to occur at the point of maximum female fertility (i.e. ovulation) and that normal ejaculation occurs within the vagina.

## PHYSICAL EXAMINATION

Particular attention should be paid to general body build, hair distribution and the type of underpants worn. The presence of visual field defects suggests the possibility of pituitary problems. The penis, foreskin, external urethral meatus, testes, epididymes and vasa should all be examined with the patient lying down. Rectal examination should be performed to assess the prostate and seminal vesicles. A varicocele may only become obvious when the patient stands and sometimes then only on straining (*Valsalva's manoeuvre*) or by feeling a cough impulse. Ninety-eight per cent of varicoceles are found on the left side.

A full clinical assessment at the first visit will show an abnormality in over 50% of infertile men.

## LABORATORY INVESTIGATIONS

### Seminal analysis

It is helpful to have at least two sperm counts regardless of what previous tests have shown. These should be produced by masturbation after 3 days' sexual abstinence, collected in a plastic (not glass) container and delivered to the laboratory within 4 hours of production, being kept at body temperature in a trouser pocket in the interim period.

All the indicators suggest that a man has a reasonable chance of fertility with a sperm density that exceeds 20 million per ml with more than 30% motility at 4 hours and a semen volume of at least 1.5 ml (Table 24.1). It is possible for a man to be infertile with a normal sperm density due to the

**Table 24.1**  Normal semen parameters

| | |
|---|---|
| Volume | 2–5 ml |
| Sperm density | 20–200 million/ml |
| Motility | > 50% at 4 h |
| Abnormal forms | < 50% |
| Colour | Grey–yellow |

presence of antisperm antibodies. One further condition for fertility, therefore, is that the sperms should produce an adequate post-coital test: this is defined as having at least five sperms present per high-power field in preovulatory cervical mucus.

As a general rule, further investigations should be instituted if the sperm count shows the patient to be oligospermic (density less than 20 million per ml) or azoospermic (no sperms seen).

Laboratory examination of semen may also turn up other significant abnormalities. Cytological evidence of bacteria or white cells in the semen may suggest infection in the seminal tract. Agglutination or immobility of sperms, although not diagnostic, should suggest the presence of antisperm antibodies. Secretory antibodies can be measured in the semen whilst blood-borne antibodies (present in 5–10% of infertile men) can also be assessed by immunological means. Antibodies in 'hostile' cervical mucus (present in 1–2% of the female partners of infertile men) can be assessed by immunological tests.

## Hormonal studies

Traditionally it is believed that the functions of the interstitial cells and seminiferous tubules are controlled separately by luteinising hormone (LH)

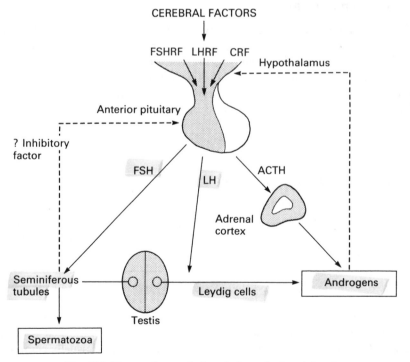

**Fig. 24.1** Hormonal control of testicular and adrenal function

and follicle-stimulating hormone (FSH), respectively. Whilst this is a useful concept in investigative terms, it is probably an oversimplification since the two hormonal pathways do interact to some degree (Fig. 24.1).

Plasma levels of FSH, LH, testosterone and prolactin should be measured in all infertile patients. The combination of small testes, azoospermia and grossly elevated FSH levels suggests *primary testicular failure*, for which there is no effective treatment. Elevated prolactin levels should be interpreted with caution, since they can be raised by stress, drugs and laboratory variations. Persistent elevation, however, suggests a pituitary tumour and, in these patients, full endocrinological assessment is indicated. Similarly, low gonadotrophins should alert the clinician to the possibility of hypopituitarism.

Thyroid and adrenal hormones may be measured if there is any clinical suspicion of abnormality.

## Chromosomal studies

These rarely produce useful information but, in patients with a suspected chromosomal anomaly studies may reveal abnormalities such as Klinefelter's syndrome or translocations.

## Scrotal thermography

This technique can be used to clarify doubts about the presence of a small varicocele. Normal scrotal temperature is approximately 29.5°C, whilst a varicocele may result in a temperature rise up to 32°C. The temperature difference between the two sides of the scrotum should not exceed 1°C. If thermography does not clarify the situation, testicular venography may help by showing abnormalities in scrotal venous drainage. In addition, a skilled vascular radiologist may be able to embolise the abnormal veins during the procedure and occlude the varicocele.

## Vasography and testicular biopsy

Azoospermia with small testes and raised FSH levels is indicative of primary testicular failure. The other major cause of azoospermia is *vasal obstruction*. This is usually associated with normal-sized testes and normal or only marginally raised FSH levels.

If obstruction is suspected, measurement of fructose levels in the semen may be useful. Fructose is produced by the seminal vesicles and is absent in patients with agenesis of the vasa or seminal vesicles and in patients with ejaculatory duct obstruction. In addition, such patients have low semen volumes. Accurate localisation of the obstruction is accomplished by *vasography*. This is performed under general anaesthesia and is usually combined with testicular biopsies to assess the degree of spermatogenesis; this allows an accurate prognosis with regard to the likelihood of conception.

Most patients with obstructive azoospermia have a blockage in the epididymis due to previous infection. If the epididymis is engorged at the time of exploration, epididymo-vasostomy can be performed provided there is microscopic evidence of sperms in an epididymal smear. Such epididymal bypass operations have a success rate of only 40–50%.

## TREATMENT

### Oligospermia

In the first instance, simple non-specific measures should be instituted in oligospermic patients for a period of 3 months after which two more specimens of semen should be examined. This gives the doctor and the patient an idea of what the male partner can do when 'trying his best'. In a proportion of cases this treatment will be all that is necessary if sperm counts rise to adequate levels or a pregnancy results (Table 24.2).

In the remainder of patients, these simple measures fail to produce any improvement in sperm quality. Patients who fall into this category merit further hormonal treatment for a trial period.

**Table 24.2**   Non-specific therapeutic measures

Avoid excessive tiredness
Stop smoking
Reduce alcohol consumption
Treat underlying medical problems
Stop all medications
Wear loose ('boxer') shorts
Twice-daily cold scrotal douches

### *Endocrine therapy*

Gross hormone deficiency is very rare but should not be missed. A reduced sperm count with low gonadotropin levels should raise the possibility of pituitary or hypothalamic failure requiring hormonal replacement therapy.

If there is no gross endocrine abnormality, therapy is somewhat empirical. Anti-oestrogens (clomiphene, tamoxifen) or androgens (mesterolone) are commonly prescribed for a period of 3 months. There is good evidence that some improvement in sperm quality may be expected in 20% of patients on hormonal treatment, but the resulting pregnancy rate remains a disappointing 25% or less. This compares with a pregnancy rate of 20%, over an 8-year period after investigation, in oligospermic men who receive no active treatment.

Further doubts have been cast on the real effect of such endocrine therapy with the discovery that non-steroidal agents such as vitamin C may be equally effective in producing improved sperm quality.

For hyperprolactinaemic men, treatment with bromocriptine occasionally results in a pregnancy. Corticosteroids have little effect on sperm counts in most infertile men but may help when antisperm antibodies are present by reducing IgG and IgA levels.

### Antibiotic therapy

Low-dose antibiotics (trimethoprim, co-trimoxazole, erythromycin, tetra-cycline or ciprofloxacin) and antitrichomonal agents (metronidazole) may be useful in patients with proven chronic prostatitis. Infertile patients with prostatitis-like symptoms do tend to show improvements in semen quality after antibiotics but patients with asymptomatic infection do not.

### Surgical treatment

A varicocele is seen in 20–40% of men attending infertility clinics; this is more frequent than would be expected in the general population. Typically, semen analysis shows oligospermia with poor motility and a high proportion of abnormal forms, but whether a direct relationship exists between vari-cocele and infertility is open to question.

Ligation of a varicocele should be reserved for patients in whom it is causing symptoms (usually aching discomfort), in whom other causes of infertility have been eliminated or who require scrotal exploration for biopsy. The most effective way of ligating a varicocele is to tie off the testicular vein extraperitoneally above the inguinal canal. Improvement in semen quality after surgery is not guaranteed and pregnancy rates of only 50% can be expected. It has been suggested that conception rates are not changed by varicocele ligation and clinical trials are currently in progress to clarify this.

## Azoospermia

With azoospermia due to primary testicular failure, no simple treatment is effective and this should be made clear to the patient and his spouse. In this situation recommendations should be made to adopt or consider arti-ficial insemination with donor sperm (AID). For the benefit of all concerned this advice should be given as soon as possible after diagnosis.

Azoospermia due to vasal obstruction may be helped by reconstructive surgery. Unfortunately the success rate for primary obstruction (agenesis) is poor, whilst that for secondary (post-inflammatory or post-surgical) obstruction is slightly better.

Vasal blockage due to inflammation or previous vasectomy can be

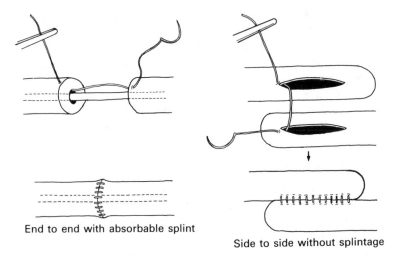

End to end with absorbable splint

Side to side without splintage

**Fig. 24.2** Vasovasostomy

relieved by vasovasostomy (Fig. 24.2). This results in a 40–70% pregnancy rate, the better results coming from accurate microsurgical techniques. Failure is normally due to stenosis at the site of anastomosis, sperm granuloma formation, secondary changes in the epididymis or antisperm antibodies.

Obstruction closer to the epididymis can be relieved by direct anastomosis of the vas to a cluster of epididymal tubules (*epididymovasostomy*) (Fig. 24.3).

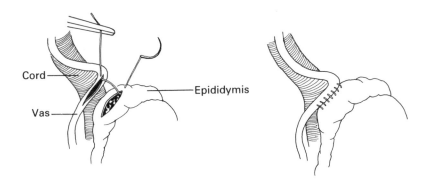

Cord

Epididymis

Vas

**Fig. 24.3** Epididymovasostomy

## Alternative measures

Failure to produce a pregnancy despite successful treatment of a poor sperm count should renew the search for abnormalities in the female partner. In particular, the quality and hostility of the cervical mucus should be tested. A persistently poor post-coital test may be overcome using artificial insemination with semen from the male partner (AIH).

Patients with the unusual problem of retrograde ejaculation due either to drugs which relax the bladder neck or to previous bladder neck surgery can be treated. The urine is first alkalinised by giving oral sodium bicarbonate for 2–3 days, then semen is recovered from the bladder, washed and inseminated artificially.

## Unexplained infertility

In a small proportion of men a male factor for infertility cannot be excluded even when all investigations are normal. In these patients it is useful to assess the ability of sperm to penetrate oocytes. This may be performed using zona-free hamster oocytes in vitro, although human oocytes are also used nowadays. The heterologous oocyte penetration test (HOP) is negative in 40% of infertile men for no obvious reason.

The place of in vitro fertilisation (IVF) still remains to be defined. IVF may prove most useful when both partners have significant problems contributing to their inability to conceive. IVF requires the presence of at least 500 000 motile sperms in the ejaculate and is probably indicated when the post-coital test shows no penetration of cervical mucus by sperms.

The newer technique of gamete intra-fallopian tube transfer (GIFT), involving laparoscopic placement of an ovum into the fallopian tube and fertilisation in situ with semen, is still under assessment but may prove an effective method of producing pregnancy in some couples.

# Suggestions for further reading

---

**Chapter 1**

Geiger S R 1986 Handbook of physiology. American Physiological Society, Bethesda
Guyton A C 1986 Textbook of medical physiology. Saunders, Philadelphia
Keele C A, Neil E, Joels N 1982 Samson Wright's applied physiology. Oxford
  University Press, Oxford
Kiil F 1972 The function of the ureter and renal pelvis. Oslo University Press, Oslo


**Chapter 2**

Ansell I D 1985 Atlas of male reproductive pathology. MTP Press, Lancaster
Mundy A R 1987 Scientific basis of urology. Churchill Livingstone, Edinburgh


**Chapter 4**

Mundy A R, Stephenson T P, Wein A J 1984 Urodynamics: principles, practice
  and application. Churchill Livingstone, Edinburgh
Sherwood T 1980 Uroradiology. Blackwell Scientific, Oxford


**Chapter 5**

Stephens F D 1983 Congenital malformations of the urinary tract. Praeger, New
  York
Whitaker R H, Woodard J R 1985 Pediatric urology. Butterworths, London


**Chapter 8**

Asscher A W 1980 The challenge of urinary tract infections. Academic Press,
  London
Maskell R 1982 Urinary tract infection. Current topics in infection series. Edward
  Arnold, London


**Chapter 9**

Ransley P G, Risdon R A 1980 Reflux and renal scarring. British Journal of
  Radiology, Suppl 14

## Chapter 10

Pyrah L N 1979 Renal calculus. Springer-Verlag, Berlin
Wickham J E A 1979 Urinary calculous disease. Churchill Livingstone, Edinburgh
Wickham J E A, Miller R A 1983 Percutaneous renal surgery. Churchill Living-
stone, Edinburgh

## Chapter 11

O'Reilly P H 1986 Obstructive uropathy. Springer-Verlag, Berlin

## Chapter 12

Black D A K, Jones N F 1980 Renal disease. Blackwell Scientific, Oxford

## Chapter 15

Lohr E 1979 Renal and adrenal tumours. Springer-Verlag, Berlin
Skinner D G 1983 Urological cancer. Grune & Stratton, New York

## Chapter 16

Zingg E J, Wallace D M A 1985 Bladder cancer. Springer-Verlag, Berlin

## Chapter 17

Blandy J P 1978 Transurethral resection. Pitman Medical, London
Blandy J P, Lytton B 1986 The prostate. Butterworths, London
Hinman F 1983 Benign prostatic hypertrophy. Springer-Verlag, Berlin

## Chapter 19

Stanton S L, Tanagho E A 1980 Surgery of female incontinence. Springer-Verlag,
Berlin

## Chapter 20

King A, Nicol C, Rodin P 1980 Venereal diseases. Baïlliere Tindall, London

## Chapter 23

Peckham M J 1981 The management of testicular tumours. Edward Arnold,
London

## Chapter 24

Amelar R D, Dubin L, Walsh P C 1977 Male infertility. Saunders, London
Edwards R G, Purdy J M 1982 Human conception in vitro. Academic Press, London

## General reading

Blandy J P 1976 Urology. Blackwell Scientific, Oxford
Mundy A R 1987 Scientific basis of urology. Churchill Livingstone, Edinburgh
Whitfield H N, Hendry W F 1985 Textbook of genitourinary surgery. Churchill Livingstone, Edinburgh

# Index